AF771548

Infant Feeding Practices

Pranee Liamputtong
Editor

Infant Feeding Practices

A Cross-Cultural Perspective

Springer

Editor
Pranee Liamputtong
School of Public Health
La Trobe University, Bundoora
Victoria 3086, Australia
pranee@latrobe.edu.au

ISBN 978-1-4419-6872-2 e-ISBN 978-1-4419-6873-9
DOI 10.1007/978-1-4419-6873-9
Springer New York Dordrecht Heidelberg London

Library of Congress Control Number: 2010936427

© Springer Science+Business Media, LLC 2011
All rights reserved. This work may not be translated or copied in whole or in part without the written permission of the publisher (Springer Science+Business Media, LLC, 233 Spring Street, New York, NY 10013, USA), except for brief excerpts in connection with reviews or scholarly analysis. Use in connection with any form of information storage and retrieval, electronic adaptation, computer software, or by similar or dissimilar methodology now known or hereafter developed is forbidden.
The use in this publication of trade names, trademarks, service marks, and similar terms, even if they are not identified as such, is not to be taken as an expression of opinion as to whether or not they are subject to proprietary rights.

Printed on acid-free paper

Springer is part of Springer Science+Business Media (www.springer.com)

To all the children in my life:

Kristin, Daniel, Zoe, Wiranut, Emma, Lalita, Nonthapat, Natthapat, Bunnalin, Marlo, Peeyapat, Thanavanit & Max

Preface

This book is born out of my personal life. I breastfed my two children for a long period. My first daughter, Zoe, was breastfed for 2 years, and Emma, my younger one, was breastfed for 4 years. Often, people made comment about my behaviour, saying that it was unusual for a mother to breastfeed her children this long. But then, they also said that since I was born in Thailand, things might be different for Thai people. So, my ethnicity was seen to be my excuse. But others congratulated me for doing so. I even won a prize at a breastfeeding conference in Melbourne for practising prolonged breastfeeding. My curiosity grew as I observed what other women do in regard to infant feeding; and since I commenced my research on reproduction and motherhood, infant feeding issues have always been my great interest.

Breastfeeding is a contentious issue. It is seen as beneficial for both a newborn infant and a mother. It is also profoundly supported by both lay individuals and professionals. However, infant feeding practices occur within the social and cultural context of the society in which women live. And as we have witnessed, not all women and their families necessarily see such benefits. There are many reasons that has prevented or stopped women from breastfeeding their newborn infants. There are other important issues that may impact on infant feeding practices of women and these include social class, ethnicity, socio-economic status and geographical location. These discussions will be included in this book.

In the past few decades, we have also seen a dramatic increase in the rates of women living with HIV/AIDS and many of these women are also mothers with young infants. Due to the infection, women living with HIV/AIDS are advised not to breastfeed their infants. Most of these mothers are from poor backgrounds and their poverty has a great impact on their feeding practices. How do these mothers deal with these issues? What can the government and local authorities do to assist these women? Some of these questions will be discussed in several chapters in this volume.

In this book, I also bring together salient issues regarding cultural beliefs and practices in different societies. I shall show that despite advanced medical knowledge in infant feeding, traditions continue to exert influence on how the women and their families manage to feed their infants in their societies. Women have attempted to preserve valued traditional beliefs and practices although they accept innovations in the management of infant feeding in response to social and cultural changes. Likewise, traditions surrounding infant feeding practices continue to live despite the fact that many societies have been modernised. Some explanations will be discussed through some of the chapters in this volume.

The book provides a comprehensive coverage of infant feeding issues from a cross-cultural perspective. The book comprises chapters written by researchers who carry out their projects in different parts of the world. Each chapter contains empirical information, which is based on real life situations. This can be used as an evidence for health care providers to implement socially and culturally appropriate services, which will assist women who are mothers and their young babies in many societies.

The book will be of interest to health care providers who have their interests in working with women and infant feeding practices from a cross-cultural perspective. They will be useful for students and lecturers in courses like midwifery, anthropology, sociology, social work, nursing, public health and medicine. The book will also attract many lay readers and those in organisations which are interested in infant feeding practices from a cross-cultural perspective.

In bringing this book to life, I owe my gratitude to many people. First, I should like to thank all contributors in this volume, who worked hard in constructing their chapters and getting it to me in the required time. Second, I should like to thank Springer for believing in the value of this book. Last, I am grateful to Rosemary Oakes, my dear friend who helped reading through several chapters for me. I dedicate this book to all the children in my family.

Bundoora, VIC, Australia
February 2010

Pranee Liamputtong

About the Book

This book comprises four parts. It begins with an introduction which aims to set the scene of this book. Pranee Liamputtong introduces issues which are salient to infant feeding beliefs and practices across cultures. These include infant feeding within a socio-cultural context, cultural beliefs and practices regarding infant feeding in diverse cultures, infant feeding practices and mothers' employment outside the home, the impact of HIV and AIDS on infant feeding practices, and authoritative knowledge of health professionals regarding infant feeding practices.

Part I is dedicated to the socio-cultural perspective of infant feeding and policy framework. It is composed of four chapters. In Chapter 2, Orit Avishai writes about how women manage the lactating body by making reference to the 'Breast-Feeding Project in the age of anxiety'. She contends that public health campaigns aimed at increasing breastfeeding rates in the United States rest on the twin premises that the 'breast is best' and that breastfeeding is 'natural'. Her chapter draws on interviews with class-privileged American mothers to demonstrate that far from 'natural', breastfeeding decisions, practices and experiences are shaped by historical, cultural, political and social norms and customs. The chapter examines how this group of women makes decisions about infant feeding and their breastfeeding practices. Orit demonstrates that these women construct the lactating body as a carefully managed site and breastfeeding as a mothering project – a task to be researched, planned, implemented and assessed, supported by expert knowledge, professional advice and consumption. Viewed in this light, 'the breast is best' and 'breastfeeding is natural' are impoverished slogans that do not capture the extent to which both the science and the imagery of breastfeeding are shaped by normative assumptions and middle-class experiences. The chapter also diverges from the emphases on pleasure, embodied subjectivity, relationships and empowerment that characterise much of the recent breastfeeding literature across the humanities, arguing that these normative/political agendas do not reflect empirical realities.

Chapter 3 is written by Jane Scott on attitudes to breastfeeding. Jane suggests that a women's decision to initiate and continue breastfeeding is influenced by her attitude towards breastfeeding as well as the breastfeeding attitudes of significant referent people (e.g. partner, family and friends), and society in general. If she perceives that her breast milk will adequately nourish her infant and that breastfeeding is convenient and better for the health of her infant, then she will have positive attitudes towards breastfeeding. However, her efforts to breastfeed may be undermined by the attitudes of those around her particularly, in Western cultures, the attitude of her partner. Fathers have been shown to participate in and influence the choice of infant feeding method by acting as key supports or deterrents to breastfeeding by the mother. Without the emotional and practical support of their partners most mothers will struggle to successfully establish and maintain breastfeeding. In Western cultures, while most people acknowledge that breastfeeding is the best way to feed infants, there is still a common perception that breastfeeding is a private function and that breastfeeding in public is inappropriate. This perception is formed in part by Western society's inability to dissociate the functional and sexual role of the breasts. Furthermore, the way that breastfeeding is portrayed in the media does much to promulgate this perception. On the whole, breastfeeding is seldom portrayed in the entertainment media and, when it is, it is often presented as being problematic. The positive portrayal of breastfeeding on television and film and in other public arenas will go a long way towards making it 'normal' in our society; positively influencing a woman's perception that breastfeeding is the social norm when it comes to feeding her infant.

In Chapter 4, Athena Sheehan and Virginia Schmied discuss about the imperative to breastfeed from an Australian perspective. They point out that research demonstrates many women choose to breastfeed their baby based on the concept that 'breast is best'. This is not surprising given that the benefits of breastfeeding are broadly promoted and a number of strategies have been deliberately employed globally and nationally to actively support and promote breastfeeding. They argue that in Australia, there is an imperative to breastfeed both socially and professionally. In this chapter, they explore the imperative to breastfeed in Australia from two perspectives. The chapter opens with an overview of International and National breastfeeding strategies and policies to illustrate the Public Health imperative to breastfeed, and examines the professional perspective on breastfeeding and the impact of these policies on their practice. To further examine the imperative to breastfeed, they present findings from a study that explored women's infant feeding experiences and decision-making in the first 6 weeks post-birth. This study demonstrates from the women's perspective the personal, social and professional imperative to breastfeed and the concomitant impact on their experiences and interpretations. For example, women not only believe breastfeeding is presented as the 'best' nutritionally but they also believe it is promoted as 'easy' 'doable' and fixable' with an underlying expectation that a good mother breastfeeds. These beliefs, when unfulfilled, can lead to a loss of confidence and a need to justify their position as a mother. They use women's stories to demonstrate these interpretations as well as others and the impact these understandings have on women's experiences. Finally, they conclude the chapter with a discussion examining the tensions and possible contradictions arising out of the public health, professional, social and personal discourses that influence breastfeeding practices. They argue that far more effort needs to be placed on supporting women to breastfeed using strategies identified by women themselves to achieve their breastfeeding goals in the weeks and months following birth.

Ellie Lee writes about infant feeding and the problem of policy in Chapter 5. She argues that how a mother feeds her baby is a decision for her to make. Yet, infant feeding is surrounded by conventions and precepts about appropriate maternal decisions. British women feed their babies in a policy context where no ambivalence is associated with attaching breastfeeding to only important benefits for individual children, mothers and the wider society. Social scientific research indicates that the presumptions of policy are to some extent widely shared; assessments of mothers' attitudes to infant feeding show they mostly agree 'breast is best'. Yet, practice departs greatly from official advice. One interpretation of this difference is that mothers are more ambivalent about the benefits of breastfeeding in practice than in the abstract. Research utilising social scientific methods has largely not concerned itself with exploring maternal ambiguity and ambivalence, as the paradigm informing most studies is a public health perspective. A small number of studies have, however, utilised social science methods to generate important insights about the tensions between policy and maternal practice and experience. This chapter summarises findings of her work indicating three major themes: breastfeeding promotion and the individualisation of social problems; 'scientisation' and the effacing of maternal choice; and moralisation and the problem of moral jeopardy. It concludes by indicating future possibilities for socio-cultural research about infant feeding.

Part II is about motherhood, work and infant feeding practices. It comprises four chapters. Chapter 6 focuses on social and cultural factors that shape decision-making around sustaining breastfeeding and is written by Joyce Marshall and Mary Godfrey. They suggest that in the United Kingdom, women's beliefs, attitudes and behaviours around breastfeeding are shaped by myriad influences and by changing social and structural factors and cultural mores. Whilst public health discourse equates breastfeeding with 'good mothering' and health professionals emphasise 'breast as best', these normative values compete with other standards or criteria of 'good mothering' held by others within women's social networks that exert influence on them. Moreover, cultural and structural factors affect the pattern of women's labour market participation. Specifically, when public policy that emphasises return to paid work is aligned with policies directed at reconciling work and family, this can act as constraints on sustaining optimal breastfeeding, that is, exclusive breastfeeding for 6 months as advised by the World Health Organisation. For women in their study, initiating and sustaining breastfeeding was subject to a complex process that contributed to multiple-valued outcomes: nurturing thriving and healthy babies, experiencing themselves as 'competent' mothers, successfully managing shifting identities and negotiating competing pressures in the real-life context of their daily lives and relationships with 'significant others'. Even as women struggled to present and see themselves as 'good mothers', they were active agents and not just acted upon. They sought to reconcile the value they placed on breastfeeding with seeing themselves and being seen by others as 'good mothers'. Thus, they sought out situations where breastfeeding was highly valued (such as support groups), and developed strategies to counter or avoid threats to their sense of themselves as nurturing and competent mothers that was related to, but not synonymous with, sustaining breastfeeding. Midwives and health visitors in their study encouraged women to breastfeed, but not in the way that this is generally portrayed in much of the current literature. Analysis of observed interactions between women who had chosen to breastfeed and midwives and health visitors suggests more of a negotiated encounter in which these health professional considered the whole situation of the woman and her struggle to be a 'good mother'.

Following on from Chapter 6, Caroline Jane Gatrell dedicates her discussion on managing the work of breastfeeding and employment in Chapter 7. Caroline's chapter considers how, while breastfeeding is promoted within health policy as the ideal form of infant nutrition, such policy fails to address two major obstacles faced by new mothers who are attempting to breastfeed. The first obstacle concerns the idea that breastfeeding is a 'natural' activity, an assumption which overlooks the problems experienced by women who struggle to breastfeed. The second obstacle relates to the chasm between health expectations that 'good' mothers should breastfeed, and wider social attitudes towards breastfeeding, which are discouraging. Finally, the chapter observes how mothers who 'struggle' to breastfeed are affected by feelings of guilt and anxiety.

Issues relevant to breastfeeding practice among employed women from a Thai cultural perspective is written by Susanha Yimyam in Chapter 8. She suggests that breastfeeding is a natural female function, and is also a customary method of infant feeding. In Thailand, breastfeeding initiation is a nearly universal practice. However, the breastfeeding duration was shortened. Her chapter derives from a combined qualitative and quantitative study, which investigated the relationship between socio-economic, cultural factors and breastfeeding among 300 employed women in Northern, Thailand. Susanha found that Thai women have positive attitudes towards breastfeeding and breast milk in terms of the nutritious, immunological, behavioural and economic benefits. The peak rates of breastfeeding at 1 month also coincide with the period of confinement called '*yu daun*'. Within this period, the women have to rest at home and are relieved of all household chores, only caring for their infants for a month. Generally, these traditional beliefs and practices provide an opportunity for the women to adjust to their new role as a mother. Since both mother and baby always stay together, they can learn from each other. Moreover, strong social endorsement of the value of breastfeeding (and the obligation it places on the next generation) reinforces the benefits of breastfeeding during confinement. However, some cultural beliefs and practices can act as barriers to breastfeeding. These include perceptions that 'breastfeeding can cause infant illness', 'there is no breast milk in the first few days', 'breast milk later in lactation is inadequate in nutritional value', and the practice of giving a bottle of water or formula at an early age. Together with a lack of knowledge about the mechanics of breastfeeding, or how to solve breastfeeding problems, these notions may diminish confidence and lead to early weaning. Therefore, it appears that cultural beliefs and practices, combined with support from family members, may be the most important factors influencing breastfeeding practices in the first month in northern Thailand.

In Chapter 9, Pranee Liamputtong and Somsri Kitisriworapan discuss issues relevant to good mother and infant feeding practices in northern Thailand. They argue that breastfeeding is profoundly supported by both professionals and lay individuals. It is claimed that breastfeeding is beneficial for both a newborn infant and a mother. However, not all women and their families necessarily perceive it as such. Infant feeding practices occur within the social and cultural context of the society in which women live. Although women understand the value of breast milk, many women choose not to breastfeed their infants or may try to combine breastfeeding with bottle-feeding. In the several past decades, rapid social and economic transformations have changed women's lives in many parts of the world. Thai women have also been caught in this change. Since the 1960s when the country's economy has become increasingly dependent on the global market economy, women in Thailand have entered the labour force as a way to increase their family income. Many women in the North work outside the home as well as perform housework. Labour force participation for women in the childbearing years has increased rapidly, particularly in the non-agricultural sector. These changes have profoundly affected women, motherhood and infant feeding practices. In this chapter, Pranee and Somsri discuss discursive practices regarding infant feeding amongst mothers in Northern Thai society. In particular, they focus on how mothers perceive and experience breastfeeding and how they feed their infants.

Part III is dedicated to issues relevant to infant feeding practices and HIV/AIDS. There are four chapters in this part. In Chapter 10, Lucy Thairu writes about the historical account of HIV/AIDS transmission through breast milk in sub-Saharan Africa. She points out that in the 1980s, the finding that HIV can be transmitted through breast milk resulted in heated controversies over the potential benefits of breastfeeding versus bottle-feeding for HIV+ mothers in resource-poor settings such as in Africa. The early part of the 1990s was marked by ambiguity, uncertainty and fear about the rising rates of paediatric HIV/AIDS due to mother-to-child transmission. By the late 1990s, the results of various epidemiological studies had shown that, in the absence of antiretroviral therapy (ART), HIV-free survival was similar for breastfed versus bottle-fed infants. By the turn of the century, it was clear that exclusive breastfeeding before 6 months of ages increased the risk of HIV transmission. At the close of this decade, the results of epidemiological research indicate that, compared to replacement feeding, exclusive breastfeeding and antiretroviral therapy (ART) result in similar HIV-free survival. Breastfeeding, in conjunction with ART, is considered the best intervention in resource-poor settings as it reduces the risk of HIV transmission through breast milk and has the added advantage of improving the health of HIV-positive mothers. Looking ahead, the provision of consistent information about the importance of exclusive breastfeeding, coupled with early ART initiation, will be critical in efforts to improve child health and survival in the context of HIV/AIDS.

In Chapter 11, challenges and opportunities regarding infant feeding in the era of HIV is written by Tanya Doherty. Accordingly, Tanya suggests, child health specialists and health care workers in many resource-limited settings are challenged by the infant feeding dilemma posed by HIV. Whereas previously breastfeeding, especially exclusive breastfeeding, was a key child survival strategy, the finding that HIV is present in breast milk has led to a re-assessment of the benefits of breastfeeding. This has led to reduced efforts globally to promote exclusive breastfeeding, a key child survival intervention. Although the World Health Organisation, UNICEF and Inter-agency Task Team (WHO/UNICEF/IATT) have been at the forefront of developing simple consistent approaches and tools for infant feeding in the context of HIV, challenges of implementation remain. For HIV-positive women, the transmission of HIV through breast milk has created a dilemma; the benefits of breastfeeding, and the risks of not breastfeeding, have to be weighed against the risk of HIV transmission through breastfeeding. Whilst intrauterine and intrapartum transmission can be substantially reduced through improved drug regimens, modifying infant feeding practices in order to reduce postnatal transmission is complex and difficult to achieve. This chapter reviews the evidence with regard to infant feeding and HIV with a particular focus on the experiences of HIV-positive women and challenges of implementing recommended feeding methods. It will also present interventions and strategies for supporting women in their feeding choices and opportunities to strengthen infant nutrition in the general population.

Alice Desclaux and Chiara Alfieri discuss issues facing competing cultures of breastfeeding: the experience of HIV-positive women in Burkina Faso in Chapter 12. They suggest that in low-resource areas of West Africa, where infant feeding patterns are dominated by prolonged breastfeeding, the prevention of mother-to-child HIV transmission requires new feeding practices: formula feeding or exclusive breastfeeding limited to 6 months followed by rapid weaning. Both patterns are innovations for the majority of women in all social categories at the local level. As innovations, these practices are applied only under certain conditions met by mothers. They also have social consequences. Two ethnographic studies conducted in 1998–2000 and in 2003–2007 explored women's perceptions about 'good infant feeding' with implications for 'good mothering', and the social relationships that are involved in infant feeding management in a setting shaped by a patrilinear organisation. These studies also show the contradictions that HIV-positive women face in two local sub-cultures of breastfeeding: the one involving the baby's father, the family and neighbourhood, and the other involving health services and PLHIV support organisations. Women must rely on a range of strategies to face difficulties related to the lack of economic or social autonomy or support from the child's father, the risk of stigma, social norms regarding breastfeeding and contradictory discourses among health workers. HIV-positive mothers' experiences bring to light several key features of local infant feeding cultures, including the changes that occurred over the last 10 years regarding the role of the fathers, the impact of infant feeding conceptualisation in biomedical institutions and the promotion of a model of infant care based on the dual mother-and-child relationship. These dimensions are considered in relation to general social trends in a West-African society regarding the autonomy of women, the role of the couple in the household, and the medicalisation of infant feeding.

In Chapter 13, relevant to infant feeding and HIV, Rachel Bezner Kerr, Laura Sikstrom and Laifolo Dakishoni discuss what they refer to as 'fluid boundaries' and multiple meanings of the illness '*moto*' in northern Malawi. They suggest that, for over two decades, high levels of child malnutrition have been observed in Malawi, and have been linked to infant and complementary feeding practices. Previous research in northern Malawi indicated that early introduction of non-breast milk foods and liquids had negative effects on child growth, and grandmothers were actively involved in early child feeding decisions. The objectives of their study were to examine local child care practices, knowledge of childhood illnesses and the underlying explanatory theories that give meaning to people's practices and observations when children become ill. Sixty-eight qualitative, in-depth interviews, two focus groups, ethnographic observation and participatory workshops were held over a 4 year period as part of an ongoing participatory agriculture and nutrition research project in Mzimba district, Malawi, in the region surrounding the town of Ekwendeni. The purpose of the research was to understand child feeding practices and concepts in order to develop a culturally appropriate strategy for the prevention and treatment of child malnutrition. One child illness, called '*moto*', which means fire or heat in chiTumbuka is considered a syndrome of symptoms including fever, coughing, weight loss and diarrhoea that affects primarily young children and sometimes elderly people. The cause of this illness is conceptualised as '*wajumpikha*' or the idea of 'crossing over' cultural taboos and expectations. In this case, crossing the boundary refers to having sex, either postpartum (considered a 'taboo' period for marital sexual relations) or extra-maritally. These types of sexual practices were considered to have dire effects on the health of young children, and had a direct impact on child feeding practices and care. This chapter discusses these research findings in relation to Malawi's high HIV prevalence and chronic food shortages, and discusses areas of further inquiry and the possible implications for community-based nutrition education programs.

Part IV focuses on infant feeding beliefs and practices within specific sociocultural context. There are eight chapters in this last part. In Chapter 14, Gerd Holmboe-Ottesen and Penjani Kamudoni write about issues from traditional breastfeeding practices to optimal breastfeeding practices, using the cases of the Gambia and Malawi as example. They suggest that the scientific evidence for the health benefits of breastfeeding has increasingly grown and is undisputable. These benefits are maximised when breastfeeding is initiated immediately after birth, without any feeds or liquids before, and is exclusive in the first 6 months, lasting until at least 2 years even after other feeds are introduced. Such practices have therefore been optimal breastfeeding. Policy recommendations have since followed to promote optimal breastfeeding through the public health care system at both global and national government levels. However, traditionally breastfeeding is perceived differently within the context of customs and taboos. This is well illustrated among the Yao people in Malawi; as well as among the Chagga, Wagogo and Haya in Tanzania. For these tribal groups, it is customary to give pre-lacteal feeds to prevent some childhood illnesses. Among the Chagga introducing supplementary foods early is perceived as a way of familiarising the child to other foods. The discrepancy between the strongly scientifically grounded policy recommendation for optimal breastfeeding and the reality of breastfeeding in a traditional setting raises the discussion of what it will take to build a new culture of optimal breastfeeding. Interventional programs at both policy and community levels have to an extent bridged the gap, although limited to the groups exposed to the interventions. A notable policy intervention has been the Baby Friendly Hospital Initiative, whose primary purpose is to support mothers to optimally breastfeed and to protect them against infant formula influences. In health facilities where the initiative has been implemented, longer breastfeeding duration and early breastfeeding has been noticed. Community-based interventions have been shown to influence mothers in prolonging the period of exclusive breastfeeding. The chapter discusses whether interventions on optimal breastfeeding will have a lasting effect. This seems to be dependent on the scope of focus and extent of scaling up of interventions, and will thus depend on availability of resources.

Marewa Glover and Chris Cunningham write about the perceptions of Māori women and their whānau (family) towards barriers in achieving best outcomes in infant breastfeeding in Chapter 15. Accordingly, breastfeeding was the only way babies were fed in pre-European times, which for Māori was only 150 years ago. Today, however, Māori are more likely than other cultural groups in New Zealand to feed their infants artificial baby milk from birth. The perceptions of Māori women and their whānau (family) towards barriers in achieving best outcomes in infant breastfeeding were explored in this chapter. It focuses on factors perceived as barriers and on issues to do with health services. Exploratory interviews with 59 Māori women aged over 16 years who had given birth in the previous 3 years, and 27 whānau members were undertaken. Women who solely artificially fed their babies were under-represented in the research. Although mothers and whānau members felt positively towards breastfeeding, and generally expected to fully breastfeed children, these expectations remained unmet in many cases because of lack of support soon after childbirth when establishing breastfeeding. Other determinant factors include lack of support when life circumstances change, lack of timely, culturally relevant and comprehensible information, confusion about bed-sharing and tobacco smoking while feeding, and self-imposed beliefs of the lack of acceptance of public breastfeeding. The relatively high rates of tobacco use by Māori created a tension for mothers' breastfeeding, and this was identified by women as a reason for breastfeeding ending prematurely.

Chapter 16 focuses on breastfeeding among Indigenous mothers in Australia and is written by Jane Scott and Colin Binns. They suggest that traditionally, the Australian Aboriginal people were hunter-gatherers and breastfeeding was universal and prolonged. European colonisation and the subsequent loss of traditional lands disrupted this hunting and gathering existence and the ensuing years of European settlement saw a gradual drift of Indigenous clans from their nomadic lifestyle to settlement in, or on the fringes of, rural towns and major cities. This increasing urbanisation was accompanied by a decline in traditional feeding practices and today Indigenous mothers are less likely to initiate breastfeeding than non-Indigenous mothers. However, Indigenous mothers in remote communities are more likely to breastfeed than Indigenous mothers living in urban areas and continue to breastfeed for longer than both urban Indigenous and non-Indigenous women. Infections (mainly respiratory, gastrointestinal and otitis media) are far more prevalent in Indigenous children than non-Indigenous children. Breastfeeding is one way to ensure that short- and long-term health benefits are passed on to Indigenous children and should be actively promoted and supported as a means of *closing the gap* between the health outcomes of Indigenous and non-Indigenous children and adults.

In Chapter 17, issues relevant to breastfeeding, vertical disease transmission and the volition of medicines in Malawi are discussed by Robert Pool, Christopher Pell, Blessings Nyasilia Kaunda, Don Mathanga and Marjolein Gysels. Their chapter is based on data collected in central Malawi as part of a large multi-centre acceptability study of intermittent preventive treatment of malaria in infants (IPTi). It describes women's perceptions of breast milk as being 'good' or 'bad', their beliefs about the transmission of malaria and other diseases through breastfeeding, and the effect of malaria medication taken by the mother on the disease of her infant. It discusses the notion that medicines have volition and are only efficacious in the individual for whom they are intended. As a result, even though women may think that malaria medication they have taken can be passed on to their infant through breastfeeding, they think that this medicine will have no effect on their infant because it is only meant for the mother. The implications of using these ideas to improve adherence to medication administered at home are also discussed in this chapter.

Chapter 18 focuses on infant feeding beliefs and practices in Islamic societies, focusing on Turkey as a case in point and is written by Meliksah Ertem. She suggests that culture profoundly influences health knowledge, attitudes and behavior and this is particularly true of infant feeding practices. The benefits of breastfeeding to mother and the health of infants have long been known and breastfeeding is practiced in Turkey. In this chapter, Meliksah describes infant feeding practices of women living in rural areas of Turkey in the context of beliefs, traditions, and cultural values. In Turkey, nearly 1.5 million new births take place each year and 95% of newborns are breastfed. Turkish mothers both in rural and urban have positive opinion on breast milk. They consider breast milk as the best nutrient for infants; and according to their opinion, it should be introduced without interruption. So as not to interrupt breastfeeding, when a mother is away from her infant, another breastfeeding mother may continue. However, there is a wide range of beliefs, perceptions and practices in infant feeding, which negatively affect appropriate breastfeeding. For example, in rural Turkey, colostrum is deemed unsuitable for babies. Some also believe that babies should not be fed anything before 'three calls to prayer (*ezan*)' or that sugar water should be introduced first, before breast milk, to 'clean' the stomach. Exclusive breastfeeding is very rare in Turkey. Mothers supplement breast milk before 6 month by introducing liquids or solid foods. Mothers believed in the contraceptive effect of breastfeeding. Some mothers prolonged breastfeeding to avoid pregnancy, controversially some of them stop to have new baby. In rural Turkey, mothers breastfeed their infants anywhere whenever the baby needs it. This is an accepted norm and men just turn their eyes away with respect and walk from the area. How mothers obtain their health-related information also affects infant feeding practices. Often, the source of the information is older people living in the same family, and health professionals do not have the desired influence on mothers' behavior on infant feeding practices. For example, in rural area of Southeastern region of Turkey, nearly 60% of mothers are illiterate and cannot speak the official language of Turkey. Those mothers have a poor chance to be informed about infant feeding. Certain beliefs centre surround mothers during postpartum periods. The new mothers and their infants are vulnerable to supernatural powers. Both the woman and her baby should not be left alone by themselves at home, and a needle, bread, knife and onion are put under their pillows to protect them against supernatural powers. Insufficient milk appears to be the major reason for early introduction of weaning foods. If baby cries after breastfeeding, or if they feel that their infant is small, mothers interpret that as the result of insufficient breast milk. The reasons shown by mothers for insufficient breast milk included mothers' nutrition, sadness and hereditary features.

Yuko Nakao and Sumihisa Honda, in Chapter 19, write about early initiation of breastfeeding and its beneficial effects in Japan. They point out that in Japan, the proportion of mothers who breastfed exclusively at 1 month was 71% in the 1960s; this figure decreased to 32% in the 1970s and has been low ever since (42% in 2005). In 2005, there were only 40 baby-friendly hospitals in Japan, which represents only 1.3% of the total number of Japanese maternity hospitals. Kangaroo mother care for low birth weight infants was introduced in Japan in 1998. Kangaroo mother care has now expanded to include full-term infants in most Japanese maternity hospitals, since kangaroo mother care has been shown to have some beneficial effects, including promotion of mother's milk secretion. Early skin-to-skin contact is also common in Japanese maternity hospitals. However, the Japanese tradition of bathing a baby immediately after birth continues, as does the use of supplemental feeding with sugar water. The World Health Organization recommends helping mothers initiate breastfeeding within a half-hour of birth in Step 4 of *Evidence for the Ten Steps to Successful Breastfeeding*. However, there is controversy about the importance of breastfeeding within 30 min after delivery. Their previous study showed that early breastfeeding after delivery was significantly associated with continuation of full breastfeeding. Logistic regression analysis indicated that the proportion of mothers who continued full breastfeeding at 4 months was 2.5-fold higher in those who breastfed their baby within 2 hours compared with more than 2 hours. Moreover, maternal satisfaction with first breastfeeding was also associated with early initiation of breastfeeding within 2 hours. Some mothers described their feelings about breastfeeding in a questionnaire as 'I felt motherly love', 'I felt calm' and 'I had greater pleasure with childbirth'. Early breastfeeding not only increased the proportion of mothers maintaining full breastfeeding but also produced positive mental effects in the mothers. They contend that helping mothers initiate early breastfeeding, especially within 2 hours, is strongly recommended for child and maternal health.

Chapter 20 focuses on socio-cultural determinants of infants' feeding patterns within 6 months postpartum in rural Vietnam and is written by Dat Van Duong. The chapter is based on a longitudinal study investigating socio-cultural factors, which influence infant feeding patterns within 6 months postpartum amongst women residing in rural Vietnam. The study was conducted during August 2002–June 2004 in Quang Xuong district, Thanh Hoa Province of Vietnam. In the first phase, 463 women were prospectively examined at weeks 1, 16 and 24 postpartum. During the second phase, sixteen qualitative focus group discussions were conducted to obtain complementary information. It found that exclusive breastfeeding dropped from 83.6% at week 1 to 43.6% at week 16, and by week 24, no infant was exclusively breastfed. Home-cooked solid food was introduced by 4.8, 40.9 and 74.3% of women at weeks 1, 16 and 24, respectively. Mother-related factors such as education level, occupation and comfort to breastfeed in public places significantly influence infants' feeding patterns. In addition, father-related factors such as occupation, feeding preference, satisfaction with the infant's sex were significant determinants of infant feeding practices of mothers. Moreover, the study found influences of close relatives and friends to the mother's decision on infant feeding practices. It also revealed a strong influence of commercial advertisement of formula industries on mother's decision. It suggests that community mobilisation for sharing the workload with women could help them to cope with employment and breastfeeding. Dat concludes that health education on breastfeeding should target at both mother and father taking into account local socio-cultural features.

The last chapter in this volume, Chapter 21, is related to attitudes and practices about infant feeding of women born in Turkey and Vietnam following migration to Australia and is written by Helen McLachlan and Dalla Forster. They contend that cultural variations exist in the proportion of women who initiate and continue breastfeeding, and for some cultural groups, migration to a new country is associated with a reduction in both initiation and duration of breastfeeding. This chapter describes the initial infant feeding attitudes and practices of women born in Vietnam, Turkey and Australia who gave birth in Australia. One hundred Turkish-born, 100 Vietnamese-born and 100 Australian-born women who gave birth in a large, tertiary referral hospital in Melbourne, Australia, were interviewed in hospital prior to discharge. Almost all Turkish women initiated breastfeeding (98%) compared with 84% of Australian women. Vietnamese women had the lowest rate of breastfeeding initiation (75%). They also perceived their partners to be more negative about breastfeeding and did not value the health benefits of colostrum to the same extent as women born in Turkey and Australia. Despite the 'Baby Friendly' status of the hospital where the study was conducted, 40% of Vietnamese women gave their baby formula in hospital. The hospital environment is a key area where care providers can make a difference to breastfeeding initiation. Given the widely known benefits of breastfeeding, further research should explore interventions that may increase the proportion of Vietnamese women who breastfeed following migration.

About the Editor

Pranee Liamputtong holds a Personal Chair in Public Health at the School of Public Health, La Trobe University, Melbourne, Australia. Pranee has previously taught in the School of Sociology and Anthropology and worked as a public health research fellow at the Centre for the Study of Mothers' and Children's Health (now Mothers and Child Health Research), La Trobe University. Pranee's particular interests include issues related to cultural and social influences on childbearing, childrearing, and women's reproductive and sexual health.

Pranee has published several research method books. Her first research method book is titled *Qualitative Research Methods: A Health Focus* (with Douglas Ezzy, Oxford University Press, 1999, reprinted in 2000, 2001, 2003, 2004); the second edition of this book is titled *Qualitative Research Methods* (2005, reprinted in 2006, 2007, 2008); and the third edition is authored solely by herself (*Qualitative Research Methods, 3rd edition*, 2009). Pranee has also published a book on doing qualitative research online: *Health Research in Cyberspace: Methodological, Practical and Personal Issues* (Nova Science Publishers, 2006). Her new books include: *Researching the Vulnerable: A Guide to Sensitive Research Methods* (Sage, London, 2007); *Undertaking Sensitive Research: Managing Boundaries, Emotions and Risk* (with Virginia Dickson-Swift and Erica James, Cambridge University Press, 2008); *Knowing Differently: Arts-Based and Collaborative Research Methods* (with Jean Rumbold, Nova Science Publishers, 2008); *Doing Cross-Cultural Research: Ethical and Methodological Issues* (Springer, 2008); *Research Methods in Health: Foundations for Evidence-Based Practice* (Oxford University Press, 2010): and *Performing Qualitative Cross-Cultural Research* (Cambridge University Press, 2009). She is completing a book on *Focus Group Methodology: Principles and Practices* for Sage, London, which will be published in early 2011.

In her own research, Pranee has published several books and a large number of papers in these areas. These include: *Maternity and Reproductive Health in Asian Societies* (with Lenore Manderson, Harwood Academic Press, 1996); *Asian Mothers, Western Birth* (Ausmed Publications, 1999); *Living in a New Country: Understanding Migrants' Health* (Ausmed Publications, 1999); *Hmong Women and Reproduction* (Bergin & Garvey, 2000); *Coming of Age in South and Southeast Asia: Youth, Courtship and Sexuality* (with Lenore Manderson, Curzon Press, 2002);

Health, Social Change and Communities (with Heather Gardner, Oxford University Press, 2003). Her more recent books include: *Reproduction, Childbearing and Motherhood: A Cross-Cultural Perspective* (Nova Science Publishers, 2007); *Childrearing and Infant Care Issues: A Cross-Cultural Perspective* (Nova Science Publishers, 2007); *The Journey of Becoming a Mother amongst Thai Women in Northern Thailand* (Lexington Books, 2007); and *Population, Community, & Health Promotion* (with Sansnee Jirojwong, Oxford University Press, 2008). She is now completing a book on *Motherhood and Postnatal Depression: Narratives of Women and their Partners*, for Springer (with Carolyn Westall), and will be published in 2011. She is also an editor in the series of books on HIV/AIDS and the Social Sciences. Two books are being edited: *Stigma, Discrimination and Living with HIV/AIDS: A Cross-Cultural Perspective*, and *Motherhood and Living with HIV/AIDS: A Cross-Cultural Perspective*.

About the Contributors

Chiara Alfieri is an ethnologist member of Centre de Recherche Cultures, Santé, Sociétés (Université Paul Cézanne d'Aix-Marseille and Institut de Recherche pour le Développement, France). She has been doing research on infant care practices particularly amongst the Bobo-Madare around Bobo-Dioulasso (Burkina Faso) for more than 15 years.

Orit Avishai is an Assistant Professor of sociology at Fordham University. Her work on breast-feeding has appeared in *Qualitative Sociology* and in the *Journal of the Association for Research on Mothering*. Her entry on breast-feeding is forthcoming in the *Encyclopedia of Gender and Society* (Sage Publications). Her current work focuses on women's experiences with conservative religions.

Rachel Bezner Kerr is an Assistant Professor in the Department of Geography at the University of Western Ontario. She has collaborated in a participatory agriculture and nutrition research project, the Soils, Food and Healthy Communities (SFHC) project, for the past 8 years in northern Malawi. She conducts research on feeding practices, agricultural methods, social dynamics and historical precedents that have implications for improved food security, child nutrition and soil fertility in the region. Rachel and her husband Wayne live in London, Ontario, Canada with their two children, but spend considerable time each year in Ekwendeni, Malawi.

Colin W. Binns was foundation of Head of the School of Public Health at Curtin University, a position he held for 21 years and continues as Professor of Public Health. He was Vice-President of the Asia Pacific Academic Consortium for Public Health and is now Deputy Editor in Chief of the Asia Pacific Journal of Public Health. He holds visiting professorial positions at Kagawa Nutrition University, Tokyo and University of Ryukus, Okinawa in Japan, Tonji Medical College Wuhan and Changsha Children's Hospital, PR China and Inje University, Korea. He has served on 17 committees of the National Health and Medical Research Council, including Chair of the Dietary Guidelines Committees for infants, children, adults and elderly Australians. He has published 330 articles in scientific journals in the areas of breastfeeding, public health nutrition and epidemiology. In 2004, he was given the award of Senior Western Australian of the Year and was awarded an honorary PhD from Inje University, Korea for public health research in Asia.

Chris Cunningham is Professor of Maori Health and Director of the Research Centre for Maori Health & Development at Massey University. His research interests include whanau (family) health, cancer, diabetes, ethics and Maori workforce development. He is currently supervising 18 doctoral students – the majority indigenous – in New Zealand, Australia and the United States.

Laifolo Dakishoni started working with Ekwendeni Hospital's Soils, Food and Healthy Communities project in 2001. He studied at the Malawi College of Accounting, where he earned a diploma in accounting. His passion for improving child nutrition through participatory method drove him to become involved with the SFHC project. Laifolo has been actively involved in the qualitative research on child feeding and is an adept interviewer. He lives in Mzuzu with his wife Brenda and his four children.

Alice Desclaux is MD and Professor in Medical anthropology at Université Paul Cezanne d'Aix-Marseille (UPCAM, France). She has done extensive fieldwork on social transformations related to HIV, mainly in West Africa, regarding women and children in the health system. Presently, she works on the anthropology of long-term treatment amongst HIV-positive persons in Dakar (Sénégal) for Institut de Recherche pour le Développement (IRD, UMR 145).

Tanya Doherty is a specialist scientist at the Medical Research Council in South Africa. She has qualifications in Nursing, Public Health, and a PhD in International health with a focus on HIV and infant feeding. Since 2002, she has undertaken research on the PMTCT (prevention of mother to child transmission of HIV) programme in South Africa. This has included two national evaluations, a prospective cohort study and a community intervention trial.

Dat Van Duong holds the first degree on pharmacy. He also has a Master of Public Health and PhD from Curtin University of Technology, Western Australia. He has strong experiences in maternal and child health related issues in developing countries. He is currently working as a head of reproductive health unit at United Nations Population Fund in Vietnam.

Meliksah Ertem is a Professor at the Department of Public Health Faculty of Medicine, Dicle University Diyarbakir, Turkey. Born in Diyarbakir, Turkey, in 1965, she graduated from Medical School in 1989 and received her degree of 'Public Health Specialist' in 1995. She has held a position as a Professor of Public Health since 1995. Her research topics of interest are reproductive health and maternal and child health, especially breastfeeding, vaccination and malnutrition.

Della A. Forster is a Midwifery Consultant at the Royal Women's Hospital in Melbourne, and a Senior Research Fellow at Mother and Child Health Research, La Trobe University. Her research interests include all aspects of pregnancy, birth and the postnatal period, and her PhD was based on a large randomised controlled trial investigating the effect of antenatal education on breastfeeding initiation and duration.

Caroline Jane Gatrell is a Lecturer in Management Learning and Leadership at Lancaster University Management School. Her research focuses on the maternal body and work, and she is engaged in examining relationships between birth and maternal labour in the context of heteronormativity and professional employment, family practices, and the maternal body. Caroline's new research monograph 'Embodying Women's Work' was published in 2008.

Marewa Glover (Tribe: Ngā Puhi) is Director of Auckland Tobacco Control Research Centre, the University of Auckland. She works on building contemporary Māori knowledge and research capacity to improve indigenous health. Her areas of research include: smoking cessation, smoking in pregnancy, infant feeding and Māori attitudes to Assisted Human Reproduction.

Mary Godfrey is a Senior Research Fellow at the Leeds Institute of Health Sciences, University of Leeds. A sociologist, her substantive research interests are lay conceptions of health and illness and user defined outcomes to inform models of integrated health and social care service systems. She has a particular interest in involving participants in all aspects of the research process and in exploring the impact of professional/lay research partnerships in generating knowledge.

Marjolein Gysels studied African linguistics at the University of Ghent (Belgium), and received a PhD in 1996 in cultural anthropology from the University of Amsterdam. She has carried out ethnographic research in D.R. Congo on Swahili and oral literature. She also worked on HIV/AIDS related projects in Tanzania focusing on female infertility, commercial sex workers and truck drivers. Then, at King's College London, she carried out research on palliative care for 5 years. More recently, she has been involved in the literature scoping on the delivery and organisation of generalist services for adults at the end of life for a project funded by the UK NHS Service Delivery and Organisation (SDO), and she has managed a programme on breathlessness in advanced and progressive disease. In 2006, she joined CRESIB, where she managed a programme investigating the acceptability of intermittent preventive treatment in Infants (IPTi), in five African countries, and is currently managing a component of the PRISMA project aimed at developing understanding of cultural issues in end of life care.

Gerd Holmboe-Ottesen holds a PhD in Nutrition Epidemiology and is a Professor in community nutrition. She has worked with child nutrition with more focus on child feeding practices, child nutrition status and its correlation to caregivers in agricultural occupation in Sri Lanka, Tanzania and Botswana.

Sumihisa Honda is an Associate Professor in the Department of Public Health, Nagasaki University School of Medicine, Japan. He has been actively involved in many epidemiologic studies with his expertise in biostatistics.

Penjani Kamudoni is a PhD fellow at the Institute of Community Health and General Practice. She is a community nutritionist. As part of her PhD work, she will work on an intervention study on promoting optimal breastfeeding through peer support. She has previously worked with therapeutic child feeding in Malawi.

Blessings Nyasilia Kaunda is a Social Scientist based at Malaria Alert Center (MAC), an autonomous institution affiliated with the University of Malawi, College of Medicine. She is a graduate of Chancellor College, a constituent of University of Malawi with a major in Sociology and a Public Administration minor. Her main research interests include anthropological work and sociology in relation to public health. She has presented a paper on the acceptability of intermittent preventive treatment of malaria in infants (IPTi) at national level and is in the process of drafting papers for publication on the same. Currently, she is managing four malaria sentinel sites across the country and plans to pursue a masters degree in medical anthropology.

Somsri Kitisriworapan is an Associate Professor at the Kasetsart University's Demonstration School, Thailand. She teaches social science, history and Thai language at both primary and secondary levels. Her main interests are on the health and psychology of children and her research has involved children's understanding of health and social issues.

Ellie Lee is a Senior Lecturer in social policy at the University of Kent. Her research interests are in the sociology of reproduction, health and the family. Her publications include *Abortion, Motherhood and Mental Health* (Aldine Transaction 2003) and *Real Bodies* (Palgrave 2002). Her most recent research projects are about teenage pregnancy and abortion, and second trimester abortion (with colleagues from the University of Southampton), and about infant feeding (with Professor Frank Furedi, University of Kent). The results of these studies are published, to date, in the journals *International Journal of Law, Policy and the Family, Reproductive Health Matters, Health, Risk and Society,* and *Sociology of Health and Illness*. Ellie is the co-ordinator of Parenting Culture Studies www.parentingculturestudies.com

Joyce L. Marshall is a Lecturer at the University of York in the United Kingdom. She is public health researcher with a clinical background in midwifery. Her research has focused on maternal and child health, the use of knowledge in clinical practice, breastfeeding and knowledge and education.

Don Mathanga is a graduate of the College of Medicine, University of Malawi. He obtained his advanced training in epidemiology from the University of Michigan from which he received a PhD in 2004. His research interests include understanding the determinants of malaria risk and analysing programmatic efforts to link malaria interventions to other health programs. Currently, Don is the Director of Malaria Alert Centre and a senior lecturer at the College of Medicine, University of Malawi.

Helen L. McLachlan is a Senior Lecturer in Midwifery in the Division of Nursing and Midwifery and a Senior Research Fellow at Mother and Child Health Research, La Trobe University. She has a background as a clinical midwife and worked across the pregnancy, birth and postnatal spectrum. Her research interests include culture and childbirth, models of maternity care and breastfeeding. Her PhD thesis explored the views and experiences of women born in Turkey, Vietnam and Australia on giving birth in Australia.

Yuko Nakao is an Associate Professor in the School of Health Sciences, Nagasaki University, Japan. She teaches midwifery and perinatal care in the Department of Nursing. Her substantive interests include breastfeeding practice of mothers, breast care of lactation, feeding behavior of newborn infants and qualitative research methods in mother and child health.

Christopher Pell is currently a Research Fellow in the anthropology research group based in the Barcelona Centre for International Health (CRESIB). He has a MSc in the Anthropology and Ecology of Development and has worked for over 3 years in applied anthropological research, participating in multi-site projects based in several sub-Saharan African countries, such as the Acceptability of IPTi and the Social and Cultural Context of Malaria in Pregnancy. He has also been involved in qualitative health research in South America and Spain.

Robert Pool studied cultural anthropology at the University of Amsterdam, where he received a PhD in 1989. He has carried out ethnographic research on food taboos in India, local explanations of illness in Cameroon, and euthanasia decisions in the Netherlands. After spending 8 years in Tanzania and Uganda doing social scientific research relating to various aspects of HIV/AIDS, he moved to the London School of Hygiene and Tropical Medicine where he coordinated the medical anthropology course for 5 years and, as a member of the Gates Malaria Partnership, carried out research on the socio-cultural aspects of malaria in various African countries. He is currently a research professor at the Barcelona Centre for International Health Research (CRESIB) and professor of global health and inequality at the University of Amsterdam.

Laura Sikstrom is a doctoral student in medical anthropology at the University of Toronto. She worked as a research intern with the Soils, Food and Healthy Communities project from 2004 to 2005, during which time she was actively involved in the qualitative research about child feeding in the region. Laura will be conducting her doctoral research on paediatric HIV in northern Malawi.

Virginia Schmied is an Associate Professor at University of Western Sydney. She is a nurse and midwife with tertiary qualifications in sociology and women's studies. As a researcher, she has built a program of nursing and midwifery research using both quantitative and qualitative methodologies to study the transition to parenthood, childbirth and parenting programs, breastfeeding, supporting parents with infants in neonatal nurseries, models of midwifery care and postnatal care and the role of child and family health nurse.

Jane A. Scott is an Associate Professor. Her research has focused primarily on the epidemiology of breastfeeding, namely the determinants of breastfeeding initiation and duration. She has been principle or co- investigator on number of longitudinal infant feeding studies including the two Perth Infant Feeding studies conducted in 1992 and 2002, as well as the INFABIO study, a large multi-centre study funded by the European Union. She has also conducted a number of qualitative studies investigating the relationship of breastfeeding attitudes and outcome. She has authored more than 50 refereed papers and has published her work in high-ranking international paediatric and nutrition journals including *Pediatrics*, *ActaPediatrica*, *Birth* and the *European Journal of Clinical Nutrition*.

Athena Sheehan is a Senior Lecturer at Avondale College, Australia. She is a nurse and midwife with a considerable research background. Her main research interests focus on infant feeding and support for women both during pregnancy and in the postnatal period. She has a particular interest in how professionals support women learning to breastfeed. Her PhD explored women's infant feeding experiences and decisions in the first 6 weeks post birth.

Lucy Thairu is a Postdoctoral Fellow in the Division of Infectious Diseases at Stanford University Medical School. Born and raised in Kenya, she studied Biochemistry in Nantes University in France, and completed a PhD in International Nutrition at Cornell University in the United States. Her research on breastfeeding and HIV has received several awards including the 2001 Abraham Horwitz award from the UN Committee on Nutrition.

Susanha Yimyam is an Associate Professor and a faculty member in OB-GYN Nursing of the Faculty of Nursing, Chiang Mai University Thailand. She obtained her PhD from the University of Melbourne Australia in 1997. She has conducted more than 20 research projects, mostly using combined (mixed) methods of qualitative and quantitative approaches. She was awarded as an excellent nursing researcher from the Thai Nursing Council in 2003. Her research interests include health care policy and health promotion in working women, breastfeeding, HIV/AIDS and infection control.

Contents

Contributors

Chiara Alfieri Institut de Recherche pour le Développement (UMR 145), Université Paul Cézanne d'Aix-Marseille, CReCSS/MMSH, 5 rue du Château de l'Horloge, 13100 Aix-en-Provence, France, ch.alfieri@gmail.com

Orit Avishai Fordham University, 407 Dealy Hall, Rose Hill Campus, Bronx, New York, NY 10458, USA, avishai@fordham.edu

Rachel Bezner Kerr Department of Geography, University of Western Ontario, SSC 2409, 1151 Richmond Street N., London, Ontario, Canada N6C 2B5, rbeznerkerr@gmail.com

Colin W. Binns School of Public Health, Curtin University of Technology, Perth, Western Australia, Australia 6848, cbinns@health.curtin.edu.au

Chris Cunningham Research Centre for Māori Health & Development, Massey University, PO Box 756, Wellington, New Zealand, cwcunningham@xtra.co.nz

Laifolo Dakishoni Soils, Food and Healthy Communities Project, Ekwendeni CCAP Hospital, PO Box 19, Ekwendeni, Malawi, dakishoni@yahoo.ca

Alice Desclaux Hôpital de Fann, Institut de Recherche pour le Développement (UMR 145), Université Paul Cézanne d'Aix-Marseille, BP 1386, 18524 Dakar, Sénégal, alice.desclaux@ird.fr

Tanya Doherty Health Systems Research Unit, Medical Research Council, Francie van Zyl Drive, Parrow, Cape Town, South Africa, tanya.doherty@mrc.ac.za

Dat Van Duong United Nations Population Fund in Vietnam, UN Apartment Building, 2E Van Phuc Compound, Kim Ma Street, Ba Dinh District, Hanoi, Vietnam, dat@unfpa.org.vn

Meliksah Ertem Department of Public Health, Faculty of Medicine, Dicle University, Diyarbakir, Turkey, mertem@dicle.edu.tr ; mertem85@hotmail.com

Della A. Forster Mother and Child Health Research, La Trobe University, Bundoora, Victoria, Australia 3086, d.forster@latrobe.edu.au

Caroline Jane Gatrell Department of Management Learning and Leadership, Lancaster University Management School, Lancaster University, Lancaster, LA1 4YX, UK, c.gatrell@lancaster.ac.uk

Marewa Glover Social & Community Health, School of Public Health, University of Auckland, Private Bag 92019, Auckland, New Zealand, m.glover@auckland.ac.nz

Mary Godfrey Leeds Institute of Health Sciences, University of Leeds, Charles Thackrah Building, 101 Clarendon Road, Leeds LS2 9LJ, UK, m.godfrey@leeds.ac.uk

Marjolein Gysels CRESIB (Barcelona Centre for International Health Research), Hospital Clinic – University of Barcelona, Rosselló 132, sobreático 1a., 08036 Barcelona, Spain, marjolein.gysels@cresib.cat

Gerd Holmboe-Ottesen Department of General Practice and Community Medicine, Faculty of Medicine, Institute of Health and Society, University of Oslo, P.O. Box 1130, Blindern 0318 Oslo, Norway, gerd.holmboe-ottesen@medisin.uio.no

Sumihisa Honda Department of Public Health, School of Medicine, Nagasaki University, Sakamoto, Nagasaki 852-8523, Japan, honda@nagasaki-u.ac.jp

Penjani Kamudoni Department of General Practice and Community Medicine, Faculty of Medicine, Institute of Health and Society, University of Oslo, P.O. Box 1130, Blindern, 0318 Oslo, Norway, p.r.kamudoni@medisin.uio.no/ penjanius@yahoo.com

Blessings Nyasilia Kaunda Malaria Alert Center (MAC), University of Malawi, Pvt Bag 360, Blantyre, Malawi, bkaunda@mac.medcol.mw

Somsri Kitisriworapan Kasetsart University's Demonstration School, Kasetsart University, Paholyotin Road, Bangkok 10900, Thailand, somsri_kus@hotmail.com

Ellie Lee University of Kent, Canterbury, Kent CT2 7NF, UK, e.j.lee@kent.ac.uk

Pranee Liamputtong School of Public Health, La Trobe University, Bundoora, Victoria, Australia 3086, pranee@latrobe.edu.au

Joyce L. Marshall Maternal and Child Health, University of Huddersfield, Harold Wilson Building, The University of Huddersfield, Queensgate, Huddersfield, HD1 3DH, joyce.marshall@hud.ac.uk

Don Mathanga Malaria Alert Centre (MAC), University of Malawi, Pvt Bag 360, Blantyre, Malawi, dmathang@mac.medcol.mw

Helen L. McLachlan Division of Nursing and Midwifery and Mother and Child Health Research, La Trobe University, Bundoora, Victoria, Australia 3086, h.mclachlan@latrobe.edu.au

Yuko Nakao School of Health Science, Nagasaki University, Sakamoto, Nagasaki 852-8520, Japan, ynakao@nagasaki-u.ac.jp

Christopher Pell CRESIB (Barcelona Centre for International Health Research), Hospital Clinic – University of Barcelona, Rosselló 132, sobreático 1a., 08036 Barcelona, Spain, christopher.pell@cresib.cat

Robert Pool CRESIB (Barcelona Centre for International Health Research), Hospital Clinic – University of Barcelona, Rosselló 132, sobreático 1a., 08036, Barcelona, Spain; Centre for Global Health and Inequality, University of Amsterdam, Spui 21, 1012WX Amsterdam, The Netherlands, robert.pool@cresib.cat

Virginia Schmied School of Nursing and Midwifery, University of Western Sydney, Building ER Parramatta Campus, Penrith South DC 1797, Penrith NSW, Australia 1797, v.schmied@uws.edu.au

Jane A. Scott School of Medicine, Flinders University, Adelaide, South Australia, Australia 5042, jane.scott@flinders.edu.au

Athena Sheehan Faculty of Nursing and Health, Avondale College, 185 Fox Valley Rd, Wahroonga, Australia 2076, athena.sheehan@avondale.edu.au

Laura Sikstrom Department of Anthropology, University of Toronto, 19 Russell St., Toronto, ON, M5S-2S2, Canada, lsikstrom@yahoo.ca

Lucy Thairu Division of Infectious Diseases, Stanford University School of Medicine, Stanford, CA, USA, thairu@stanford.edu

Susanha Yimyam OB-GYN Nursing Department, Faculty of Nursing, Chiang Mai University, Chiang Mai 50200, Thailand, syimyam@mail.nurse.cmu.ac.th

Chapter 1
Infant Feeding Beliefs and Practices Across Cultures: An Introduction

Pranee Liamputtong

Contents

1.1 Introduction

> Breastfeeding practices within a given culture represent the ways in which women negotiate and incorporate dominant ideologies and institutional and cultural norms with the realities of their embodied experiences, personal circumstances and social support systems (Dykes 2005, p. 2283).

Infant feeding practices in every society occur in accordance with the social and cultural norms of the society. In all societies and cultures, infant feeding practices, particularly breastfeeding, have 'a rich symbolic content' (Desclaux & Alfieri 2009, p. 822), are shaped by local understanding of breastfeeding (Liamputtong 2007a; Scavenius, van Hulsel, Meijer, Wendte, & Gurgel 2007), and can be a 'highly emotive debate' issue (Coutsoudis 2005, p. 87). We have witnessed that mothers throughout the world see breastfeeding as the best option for their infants (see other chapters in this volume). However, there are certain circumstances that may prevent or stop mothers from breastfeeding their infants. These include socio-economic status, cultural beliefs, illnesses such as HIV/AIDS, and advice from health professionals. Hence, infant feeding practices entail more than breastfeeding. This may

P. Liamputtong (✉)
School of Public Health, La Trobe University, Bundoora, Victoria, Australia 3086
e-mail: pranee@latrobe.edu.au

P. Liamputtong (ed.), *Infant Feeding Practices*, DOI 10.1007/978-1-4419-6873-9_1,
© Springer Science+Business Media, LLC 2011

involve artificial feeding and other supplementary foods. It is also a contentious issue. Often, the decision on how to feed their infants is not made by the mother alone, but others such as family and society can impact on the choices of infant feeding that women have to make. And at certain times and under certain circumstances, women are made to choose other infant feeding options. However, women are not homogenous in their decisions and often their choices between infant feeding options are made within the socio-cultural contexts in which they live (Scavenius et al. 2007; Desclaux & Alfieri 2009).

This chapter introduces issues relevant to infant feeding beliefs and practices. In particular, I focus on infant feeding within a socio-cultural context, cultural beliefs and practices regarding infant feeding in different cultures, infant feeding practices and mothers' employment outside the home, the impact of HIV and AIDS on infant feeding, and authoritative knowledge of health professionals regarding infant feeding practices.

1.2 Beliefs About Breast Milk

In most societies, the use of breast milk is taken seriously as crucial to infant well-being (Baumslag & Michels 1995; Riordan 2005). However, ideas about breast milk may vary in different cultures. One notable pattern is the beliefs concerning colostrum. According to the medical view, colostrum is seen as beneficial since it contains anti-infective and immunological properties (Morse, Jehle et al. 1990; Baumslag & Michels 1995; see Chapters 8 and 14 in this volume). In many cultures throughout the world, however, colostrum is believed to be of no value or harmful to a newborn infant (Jelliffe & Jelliffe 1978; Morse 1984; Conton 1985; Dettwyler 1987; King & Ashworth 1987; Fernandez & Popkin 1988; Fishman, Evans, & Jenks 1988; Gunnlaugsson & Einarsdottir 1993; Liamputtong 2002a; Riordan 2005; see also Chapters 8, 13, 14, 18, and 21 in this volume). In the world survey of the timing of postpartum breastfeeding, Jane Morse and colleagues (1990) found that the reasons for discarding colostrum are varied in different cultures, but most societies believe that colostrum is dirty, poisonous, and contaminated. Some societies hold that colostrum makes the newborn ill and causes vomiting and diarrhea (see Chapters 8, 13, 14, 18, and 21 in this volume).

Similarly, in the Republic of Guinea-Bissau in Africa, Balanta mothers believe that colostrum is 'dirty, insufficient and capable of causing any disease, in some cases even the death of the infant' (Gunnlaugsson & Einarsdottir 1993, p. 284). Hence they discard the colostrum and delay breastfeeding until the 'real milk' comes between 2 and 5 days following birth. Mothers also believe that under circumstances the mature breast milk may differ in quality from one mother to another. If the child is strong and looks healthy, the milk is good. If the milk is bad, the child will not grow properly and is always sick.

In a study of the beliefs and practices regarding a mother's milk in Mithila, all women were found to believe that colostrum should not be fed to the baby under any circumstances, believing it will cause vomiting (Reissland & Burghart 1988).

Women viewed colostrum as analogous to the birth blood. As it has stagnated in the womb for many months, it is considered a foul substance (Reissland & Burghart 1988).

In discussing why colostrum is so widely disliked, Gunnlaugsson and Einarsdottir (1993) argue that it is mainly due to the color and consistency of colostrum which seem to make mothers feel that it can be infectious and stale. Baumslag and Michels (1995) and Riordan (2005) point out that mothers in many parts of the world distrust colostrum due to its yellow color, which resembles 'pus' or 'poison.' Hmong mothers identify colour and consistency of the colostrum as an indication of 'bad milk' (Liamputtong Rice 2000). They also use its taste as a way to differentiate good milk and bad milk. Hmong women also believe that 'first milk' (colostrum) only occurs with the first birth. Since they continue to breastfeed until they give birth to the next child, they do not believe that they have the colostrum again and hence they do not need to discard their first milk. This means that Hmong infants do in fact receive colostrum (Liamputtong Rice 2000).

However, some studies show that women in some parts of the world, such as Thailand (Family Health Division 1994) and Pakistan (Fikree, Ali, Durocher, & Rahbar 2005), view colostrum as beneficial to their infants. Uzbek women believe that colostrum is much more nutritious than breast milk and that one drop of colostrum equals 100 drops of breast milk, coining the term 'gold milk' (Semenova 2001, p. 192). Similarly, the Fula and Mandinga women of Guinea-Bissau believe that colostrum gives the baby strength and protects her/him against disease (Tsianakas & Liamputtong 2007).

Although the results of Liamputtong Rice and Naksook (2001a, b) show that Thai women in Melbourne believe colostrum is beneficial to the newborn infants, there are also those who believe that it causes ill health in their infants. The differing ideas of women on the value of colostrum may be due to differences in women's social circumstances such as education, region of residence, and the amount of contact with Western health care. However, women in the latter group changed their practices in their new homeland since all offered colostrum to their newborn infants after being told about its value. This has also been evident with immigrant women living in Western societies like Australia (Liamputtong Rice 2002b; see Chapter 21 in this volume).

Additionally and importantly, in most societies, women see breast milk as the most valuable food for newborn infants and young children (Moffat 2007; see also several chapters in this volume). There is also a common belief within some cultures that breast milk is 'human milk,' while infant formula is seen as 'animal milk' (Morse 1985; van Esterik 1988; Vong-Ek 1993; Yimyam 1997; Liamputtong Rice & Naksook 2001a, b; Liamputtong 2006). This 'moral' value of breast milk assists the women to believe their breast milk, i.e., breastfeeding, is the best way to nourish their children. This may explain why the majority of women in many cultures breastfeed their infants.

Women also view breastfeeding as beneficial to women's health (Liamputtong Rice & Naksook 2001a, b). For example, Thai women believe that women who do not or never breastfeed are at risk of developing breast cancer or other abnormalities in their breasts. This understanding of the benefits of breastfeeding coincides with scientific evidence, which indicates that women who have breastfed are less likely to develop cancers of the breasts, ovaries, or cervix, and osteoporosis (WHO 1993; Riordan 1997, 2005).

Many mothers also believe that breast milk is developed from blood within the chest of a mother. This is why breastfed children are believed to have closer ties to their mothers than bottle-fed children. In Thai culture, for instance, this belief reflects the Thai custom of honoring one's mother since it is she who nurtures her child from her own blood. This shows a mother's great sacrifice for her children. Children, when grown up, are therefore expected to take care of their mother when she is no longer capable of looking after herself in old age (Yimyam 1997; Liamputtong Rice & Naksook 2001a, b; Liamputtong, Yimyam, Parisunyakul, Baosoung, & Sansiriphun 2004; Liamputtong 2007b; see also Chapter 9 in this volume).

1.3 Infant Feeding Practices and Social Structures

Infant feeding practices have been found to vary with the mothers' social structures (White, Freeth, & O'Brien 1992; Foster, Lader, & Cheesbroughet 1997; Nadesan & Sotirin 1998; Guttman & Zimmerman 2000; Li & Grummer-Strawn 2002; Cricco-Lizza 2005). Mothers' socio-demographic characteristics, which are positively associated with higher breastfeeding rates, include non-White ethnicity (Robinson, Hunt, Pope, & Garner 1993; Timbo, Altekruse, Headrick, & Klontz 1996; Wiemann, DuBois, & Berenson 1998; Li & Grummer-Strawn 2002; Beal, Kuhlthau, & Perrin 2003; Cricco-Lizza 2005), higher educational status (Spisak & Gross 1991; Quarles, William, Hoyle, Brimeyer, & William 1994; Giugliani, Caiaffa, Vogelhut, Witter, & Perman 1994; Scott & Binns 1999), older maternal age (Giugliani et al. 1994), and being married (Giugliani et al. 1994; Institute of Medicine 1991). Callen and Pinelli (2004, p. 285) reviewed the incidence and duration of breastfeeding for full-term infants in Canada, United States, Europe, and Australia. The review shows that 'women who initiate and continue to breastfeed are older, married, better educated, and have higher family incomes than women who do not breastfeed.'

The rates of breastfeeding among low-income mothers tend to be lower than those of the middle-class, higher income mothers (Eckhardt & Hendershot 1984; Gabriel, Gabriel, Lawrence 1986; Ryan & Martinez 1989; Kistin, Benton, Rao, & Sullivan 1990; Buxton, Gielsen, Faden, & Brown 1991; Ryan, Rush, Krieger, & Lewandowski 1991; Brent, Redd, & Dworetz 1995; Ross Laboratories 1995; Guttman & Zimmerman 2000; Mistry, Freedman, Sweeney, & Hollenbeck 2008). Although breastfeeding has been extensively promoted, breastfeeding rates among socio-economically disadvantaged mothers continue to be about 35% points below the recommended levels (Cunningham, Jelliffe, & Jellife 1991; Jacobson, Jacobson, & Frye 1991; National Center for Health Statistics 1996; Guttman & Zimmerman 2000; Li & Grummer-Strawn 2002).

Guttman and Zimmerman (2000, p. 1468) reveal in their study that breastfeeding, for low-income mothers, has 'the connotation of social class deprivation.' Breastfeeding was regarded 'as a luxury, an inconvenience, and as distasteful' among the working-class mothers in their study of breastfeeding choices among women in different income categories (Guttman & Zimmerman 2000). One working-class woman portrayed a breastfeeding mother as someone who 'has a lot of time on her hands.' The comment of the working-class mothers represented 'a social distinction that allocates the material luxuries of breastfeeding to middle-class mothers.' Many low-income women contended that women who were in more privileged positions than themselves would find it easier to breastfeed. Thus, for the working-class women, the notion that breastfeeding is good for the baby and that good mothers should breastfeed may result in 'tensions' more than pleasure. As Guttman and Zimmerman (2000, p. 1457) contend, feeding young infants today presents women with not only choices and desires but also obligations and constraints. Ironically, the working-class women who wished to breastfeed received little social support from their family and friends. This was due to a shared perception that breastfeeding was inappropriate, or even 'nasty.'

As Nadesan and Sotirin (1998, pp. 223–224) argue, the tensions organised around breast- and bottle-feeding underlines 'the material and social distinctions under patriarchal, capitalist orders.' They suggest that material and class structures influence women's decisions to breast- or bottle-feed. Nadesan and Sotirin (1998, pp. 223–224) point out, the middle-class women have a choice to stay at home with her children or go to work. They are able to take longer maternity leaves or choose to work on flexible schedule. Those who work may have better access to a private space for breast-pumping. Clearly, these women are more likely to breastfeed. On the contrary and all too often, the employments of the working-class women are concentrated in 'gender-stratified fields,' which have 'less worker autonomy, less break time, and less economic flexibility.' These women would then be more likely not to initiate or continue breastfeeding. As such, Nadesan and Sotirin (1998, pp. 223–224) argue, breastfeeding 'performs class as well as gender.'

I contend that breastfeeding not only 'performs class and gender' but also ethnicity (see Timbo et al. 1996; Wiemann et al., 1998; Li & Grummer-Strawn 2002; Beal et al. 2003; Cricco-Lizza 2005; Mistry et al. 2008; see also Chapters 18 and 21 in this volume). Li and Grummer-Strawn (2002), who examined breastfeeding rates among women from different socio-economic and racial backgrounds in the United States, found that 60% of the ever breastfed children were from non-Hispanic white mothers whereas only 26% of black children had been breastfed. Black infants also had a lower rate of exclusive breastfeeding at 4 months than white infants. In their study, they conclude that black mothers had consistent lower breastfeeding rates than white mothers regardless of their socio-demographic levels. In addition, significant differences between high and low socio-economic classes among black women clearly indicate that social class status has a major influence on breastfeeding practices among black mothers. Cricco-Lizza (2004, 2005, p. 526), in her study with black women attending a WIC (BWEW) clinic in New York, found that bottle-feeding was commonly practiced by these women. The infant feeding beliefs of these women were reflections of their lived experiences: 'a preponderance of loss and daily stress in their everyday lives,' and their 'experiences with financial hardship, abuse, discrimination, and fears of safety throughout pregnancy and the postpartum.' These women also received little education and support from health professionals during their pregnancy and postpartum care. It is not surprising then to see low rates of breastfeeding among these women.

In Thailand, this situation is reversed. It has been a consistent pattern in Thailand that rural poor women tend to initiate and prolong breastfeeding in comparison to those from urban and educated Thai women (Knodel, Chayovan, & Wongboonsin 1990; Yimyam, 1997). In Knodel et al.'s work, they found that urban women breastfed their children for a shorter period than rural mothers and only small numbers of rural women did not breastfeed their infants. Knodel et al. (1990) also found different regional differentials in breastfeeding patterns. The shortest durations of breastfeeding was found among children in Bangkok, the capital and most modern city in Thailand. Knodel and colleagues (1990, p. 148) conclude in their study that there are several social and economic influences that have discouraged breastfeeding practices among urban educated women. These include 'the rising level of education of women in the reproductive age groups, urbanisation and increasing labor force activity among women outside of agriculture.'

Knodel et al.'s results (1990) are in line with those of Durongdej (1991), who conducted a large-scale study on infant feeding patterns in Bangkok. Durongdej (1991) found that mothers born in Bangkok and older mothers were less likely to initiate breastfeeding. Bangkok-born mothers tended to stop breastfeeding sooner than mothers from higher income families and mothers of lower parity. The average breastfeeding duration from this group was just over 6 months. Interestingly, Durongdej (1991) also found that women who had a paid employment often had higher educational and income levels. Therefore, they were more able to obtain suitable supplementary foods for their infants.

The situation in Thailand is also similar to that in Indonesia. In Hull, Thapa, and Pratomo's study (1990, p. 625) in Indonesia, they found that past durations of breastfeeding declined with education, and breastfeeding durations were shorter among employed women.

> Breastfeeding is not, however, always in step with the forces of modernization. In many contemporary developing countries, breast-feeding is typically shorter for more educated, affluent and younger women.

The highly educated women believed that breastfeeding might ruin the shape of their breasts. They were also concerned that they might have insufficient breast milk. Hull and colleagues (1990) also found that only a small number of women were not breastfeeding because they had to go back to work. The common reasons tended to concentrate on problems associated with breastfeeding such as nipple soreness, engorged or sore breasts, and a perception of insufficient breast milk. In some cases, women did not initiate breastfeeding because their infants were premature or weak, or because the mother did not feel well. Interestingly, Hull et al. (1990, p. 632) conclude their study that 'the women who were not breast-feeding were predominantly the victims of inadequate knowledge and poor breast-feeding management rather than women who made a voluntary choice based on sound advice.' See also Chapters 8, 9, and 12 in this volume.

1.4 Employment and Breastfeeding Practices

Maternal employment outside the home is an important factor in the decline of breastfeeding in many countries in the past several decades (Wright, Clark, & Bauer 1993; van Esterik & Menon 1996; Blum 1999; Yimyam, Morrow, & Srisuphan 1999; Duncan, Edwards, & Reynolds 2003; Galtry 2003; Yimyam & Morrow 2003; Dykes 2005; see also Chapters 4, and 7 in this volume). Dykes (2005, p. 2291) points out that globally increasing numbers of women will return to paid employment during early motherhood. This common pattern, Dykes (2005, p. 2291) argues, 'creates many dilemmas for women as they juggle the demands upon their time and bodies' (see also Blum 1999, Yimyam et al. 1999; Galtry 2003; Yimyam & Morrow 2003). In many societies, working is seen as being incompatible with breastfeeding among mothers and their families (Durongdej 1991; Yimyam 1997; Yimyam et al. 1999; Guttman & Zimmerman 2000; Yimyam & Morrow 2003). According to Yimyam and colleagues (1999, p. 9571), breastfeeding 'becomes increasingly complex when women are employed, especially outside the home.' It has been found that women who either choose to work, or for the many poor women who must return to work for financial survival, tend to have a shorter period of feeding than those who do not work (Richter & Yoddumnern-Attig 1992; Hills-Bonczyk, Avery, Savik, Potter, & Duckett 1993; Yimyam 1997; Guttman & Zimmerman 2000; Yimyam & Morrow 2003).

Yimyam and Morrow (1999), for example, point out in their work with Thai women in Northern Thailand that returning to paid employment negatively influenced the rate and duration of breastfeeding. They report that 'at 6 months postpartum, women who worked inside the home breastfed more than those working in the formal sector at jobs with inflexible hours (home, 80%; public sector, 37%; private sector, 39%).' Women who had to work outside the home for long periods and those who had shift jobs faced many challenges and problems to continue breastfeeding. Most abandoned it within 1 month of returning to paid work. In his study in Bangkok, Thailand, Durongdej (1991) too found that work outside the home was an important influence on infant feeding practices for the subgroup of women who are so employed. The overall effect was the increased introduction of early bottle-feeding and the decrease of breastfeeding duration.

Romito and Saurel-Cubizolles (1996), in their study in a small town in Italy, have also suggested another interesting pattern of breastfeeding and employment. They identified the effect of the length of maternity leave on breastfeeding duration; the longer the leave, the longer mothers breastfed their infants. One third of mothers continued to breastfeed their infants after the resumption of their employment. This confirms that many working mothers had high motivation to continue breastfeeding.

Of those who stayed at home longer, many suggested that they would be happy to go back to work but still continue to breastfeed their babies in the morning and in the afternoon. Romito and Saurel-Cubizolles (1996) suggest that their findings were positive and this was due to the social context of Italy, particularly a generous maternity leave provided for new mothers. This is also what Philipona (1994) has shown in her study in Norway, where the numbers of employed mothers is high. Many women in her study had important political positions, and the incidence and duration of breastfeeding was the highest in the developed world. This is because, as Philipona (1994) contends, maternity leave is generous in this society.

Literature in Western societies suggests that women who are employed in high-status jobs as professionals tend to combine more working with breastfeeding than women who are not working (Hills-Bonczyk et al. 1993). Women in professional employment had a longer period of breastfeeding than women in non-professionals positions such as those in the sales or technical areas (Yimyam 1997). This is because, Yimyam (1997, p. 32) argues, ‘women working as professionals have greater flexibility and more control over their work environment.’ And this allows them to have ‘a more satisfactory relationship between the demands of employment and infant feeding.’

The woman’s ability to combine employment and breastfeeding, Morse and colleagues (1989) suggest, is depended on the nature of their employment or work. Rural work in, for example, agricultural or marketing industries seems to be compatible with breastfeeding and child care in general. Most mothers can keep their infants while working (Selvaratnam 1988; Podhisita, Havanon, Knodel, & Sittitrai 1990). But, for women working in the formal and urban settings, breastfeeding becomes problematic as their work occurs outside the home and it is more difficult to balance the demands placed on them. This seems to be more marked within the formal sector where child care provision is not available. Yimyam (1997, p. 247, original emphasis) also clearly documents in her thesis on breastfeeding patterns in northern Thailand, that her study ‘present[s] a compelling argument that it is not **employment** per se, but **inflexible hours of work** and **separation from the infant** which make the crucial difference to breastfeeding among employed women.’ This is in line with the argument of van Esterik and Greiner (1981) who suggest that employment may not be an important factor, but the conditions in the work environment that impact on breastfeeding among Thai women.

Despite general evidence suggesting that paid employment had negative impacts on the duration of breastfeeding, some studies have interestingly revealed that maternal employment is associated with a longer period of breastfeeding (Kurinij, Shiono, Ezrine, & Rhoads 1989; O’Gara 1989; Wright et al. 1993; Ross Laboratories 1995). Employed women practiced mixed-feeding for longer periods of time. Wright and associates (1993) found in their study with Navajo women that mothers who started work outside the home after 3 months initiated formula feeding later and breastfed longer than others, including unemployed mothers. They suggest that paid employment may not influence duration if breastfeeding is firmly established before mothers’ return to work. Furthermore, women who work outside the home may have higher motivation to continue breastfeeding for a longer period, as breastfeeding permits the maintenance of intimacy with their infant after separation during the day (Wright et al. 1993). Wright and colleagues (1993) suggest that breastfeeding rates among employed Navajo women equal or exceed those of other women when employment is postponed despite the fact that working is seen as a barrier to breastfeeding. As such, maternal employment may influence breastfeeding only under some circumstances. See also Chapters 7 and 8 in this volume.

1.5 Infant Feeding Practices and HIV/AIDS

Globally, it has been estimated that in 2007 about two million children were living with HIV. In the same year, 370,000 HIV-positive children were infected mainly through mother-to-child transmission (UNAIDS 2008). Overwhelmingly, these children were born in poor nations, particularly in sub-Saharan Africa. It is predicted that the HIV epidemic will continue to grow over the next decade. Increasingly and disturbingly, the majority of infected persons in poor countries will be young women (Del Rio 2005). In Haiti, for example, young women of childbearing age are at highest risk of contracting HIV and the chance of transmitting the disease to their infants is very high. Vertical transmission from infected mother to infant through gestation, childbirth, or postpartum breastfeeding continues to be the main channels of transmission of HIV to infants (Del Rio 2005; Piwoz et al. 2006). Transmission through breastfeeding contributes to about 40% of mother-to-child transmission of HIV worldwide. However, the main factor in this high rate of transmission can be attributed more to the prevalence of mixed feeding methods (Coutsoudis & Rollins 2003; Deschamps et al. 2009; *see also* Chapter 12 *in this volume*).

Breastfeeding, according to Chisenga and colleagues (2005, p. 226), contributes to nearly half of mother-to-child HIV transmissions among breastfeeding populations, particularly those in sub-Saharan Africa. In many poor countries, where prolonged breastfeeding is commonly practiced and antiretroviral treatment (ART) is still not readily available, the risk of postnatal mother-to-child-transmission (MTCT) of HIV remains considerably high. In Africa, it accounts for 42% of HIV infections in infants and young children (Breastfeeding and HIV International Transmission Study Group [BHITS], 2004). However, the risk of death from other infectious diseases, particularly diarrhea, is six times greater in bottle-fed than breastfed children in poor nations (WHO 2000). Fortunately, studies have indicated that infants who are exclusively breastfed have a lower risk of being HIV-infected than those who are partially breastfed or receive mixed feeding (Coutsoudis, Pillay, Spooner et al., 1999; Iliff et al., 2005). Although the mechanisms are not clearly known, it is theorised that exposure to microbes in water or food may cause micro-trauma to infants' bowels, and this in turn provides an entry point for HIV transmission (Buskens, Jaffe, & Mkhatshwa 2007, p. 1101). See also Chapters 10 and 11 in this volume.

However, breastfeeding continues to be the backbone of child health and child survival in poor nations. Exclusive breastfeeding (EBF), that is, breast milk and nothing else except prescribed medicines, is seen as having a lower risk of HIV transmission than mixed feeding of breast milk and other foods. And it has been recommended as a potential solution to the dilemma of infant feeding in HIV-prevalent sub-Saharan Africa (Coutsoudis, Pillay, Kuhn et al. 2001). Currently, international policy recommends that HIV-infected mothers who have no access to a consistent supply of safe and nutritionally complete replacement foods should exclusively breastfeed their infants (United Nations Children's Fund/Joint United Nations Program on HIV/AIDS/World Health Organization 1998).

For HIV-infected mothers who breastfeed their infants, exclusive breastfeeding is recommended since it helps to protect the infants from having diarrhea and other infections (Doherty, Chopra, Nkonki, Jackson, & Persson 2006; Piwoz et al. 2006; Desclaux & Alfieri 2009). In a study in South Africa (Coutsoudis et al. 1999), it showed that in comparison to mixed feeding, exclusive breastfeeding was associated with reduced risk of HIV transmission. Coutsoudis and Rollins (2003) found higher rates of HIV infection in children who were mixed fed with breast milk and other liquid and solid foods than in children exclusively breastfed for at least 3 months, or children who were exclusively formula fed in South Africa. And in a study in Zimbabwe (Iliff et al. 2005), it was found that exclusive breastfeeding increased HIV-free survival. This study also showed that early mixed feeding resulted in a fourfold increased risk of breastfeeding-associated HIV transmission at 6 months. There have been some proposed explanations for this increased risk of HIV transmission, and these include higher viral load in breast milk, increased gut inflammation and permeability to infection, and higher breast health problems among mothers who mixed feed (Kourtis, Butera, Ibegbu, Beled, & Duerr 2003; Piwoz et al. 2006).

However, as we have witnessed, a large number of women still do not exclusively breastfeed for the recommended 6 months (Rollins, Meda, Becquet, Coutsoudis, Humphrey, Jeffrey, Kanshana, Kuhn, Leroy, Mbori-Ngacha, Mcintyre, & Newell 2003; Kiarie, Richardson, Mbori-Ngacha, Nduati, & John-Stewart 2004). In fact, as Omari, Luo, Kankasa, Bhat, and Bunn (2003) and Chisenga et al. (2005) point out, due to poverty and other health issues, HIV-infected mothers may not be able to successfully achieve the recommended infant feeding practices. See Chapter 12 in this volume.

In order to balance the risks in areas of high HIV sero-prevalence and poor access to water, health and sanitation infrastructure, the World Health Organization (2001) recommends the following:

- Avoidance of all breastfeeding by HIV-infected mothers is recommended, but replacement feeding should be done in a way that is acceptable, feasible, affordable, sustainable, and safe for the mothers and infants. If this is not feasible, exclusive breastfeeding is recommended during the first months of life.
- To reduce the risk of HIV transmission, breastfeeding must be stopped as soon as feasible. However, this must be done in accordance to local situations, the individual woman's circumstances, and the risks of replacement feeding (including infections other than HIV and malnutrition).

- When HIV-infected mothers choose not to breastfeed from birth or stop breastfeeding later, they must be provided with specific guidance and support for at least the first 2 years of the child's life in order to ensure sufficient replacement feeding. Programs must be carried out to improve conditions that will make replacement feeding safer for HIV-infected mothers and their infants.

Nevertheless, Buskens and colleagues (2007) contend that exclusive breastfeeding followed by rapid cessation of breastfeeding necessitates careful planning of how best to provide alternative feeding to mothers, comfort options for the infant, and avoid breast health problems such as mastitis in the mothers. It also requires family and community acceptance, participation, and support (see also Dewey, Nommsen-Rivers, Heinig, & Cohen 2003; Doherty et al. 2006). Although the guidelines for HIV and infant feeding have been revised (WHO/UNAIDS/UNICEF/UNFPA 2004a, b), there is still no clarity on how to balance the risks of breastfeeding and not breastfeeding for each HIV-positive mother. There is no clear guidance on how to make a safe transition from exclusive breastfeeding to exclusive replacement food or even how to make a practical stop to breastfeeding (Buskens et al. 2007, p. 1101). For many resource-poor nations, where prolonged breastfeeding is the norm for social, cultural, or economic reasons, making HIV-positive mothers exclusively use replacement feeding with their infants is indeed a challenging task (see Chapter 12 in this volume).

The WHO's recommendations are set up as part of Prevention of Mother-to-Child HIV Transmission (PMTCT) strategies. In a way, Desclaux and Alfieri (2009, p. 822) point out, HIV-positive mothers are asked to consider two choices: replacement feeding (with breast milk substitutes) or exclusive breastfeeding with early weaning (see also WHO/UNICEF/UNFPA/UNAIDS 2007a, b). Of course, due to their likelihood to have better access to resources, nearly all HIV-positive women in developed countries could afford to choose replacement feeding. However, the option is more problematic for women in resource-poor nations where sanitary conditions and inappropriate use of formula may lead to diarrhea and dehydration in infants. As we have witnessed, these have been major causes of infant mortality in poor countries (UNICEF 2007). Additionally, insufficient adherence to preventative options may result in mixed feeding, and this in turn leads to a high risk for HIV transmission (Desclaux & Alfieri 2009).

For resource-poor nations, there have been debates regarding what should be the most appropriate option at a social group level (Coutsoudis, Coovadia et al. 2008). There is, however, as Desclaux and Alfieri (2009) suggest, an agreement for individual women to be able to select the feeding choice by taking into account their social, cultural, environment, economic, and medical situations (see also Chapters 10–12 in this volume).

However, according to international recommendations, women must be provided with sufficiently modified information that suits their living circumstances. This information should be provided by health professionals during counseling. This signifies an important role of health professionals in infant feeding practices and HIV/AIDS. Health professionals hold a crucial role because they could also provide not only guidance but also support to HIV-positive mothers. They should offer women counseling on infant feeding, 'specific guidance' and support to enable them to make an 'informed choice' between these options. Desclaux and Alfieri (2009, p. 822) contend that all HIV-positive mothers 'should receive counseling, which includes provision of general information about the risks and benefits of various infant feeding options, and specific guidance in selecting the option most likely to be suitable for their situation. Whatever a mother decides, she should be supported in her choice' (see Coutsoudis 2005; WHO/UNICEF/UNFPA/UNAIDS 2007b; see also Chapter 12 in this volume).

1.6 Authoritative Knowledge and the Health Professionals

The authoritative knowledge (Jordan, 1997), or privileged knowledge (Zeitlyn & Rowshan, 1997), of health professionals and particularly doctors are evidenced in the accounts regarding infant feeding practices among the women in many societies (see Manderson, 1985; Millard, 1990; Apple, 2006; Liamputtong 2007b). This is marked in relation to the promotion of 'correct' or 'proper' breastfeeding (see Lawrence 1995; Dykes 2005). In a more subtle way, as Zeitlyn and Rowshan (1997, p. 58) contend, the 'proper' breastfeeding promotion implicitly makes existing feeding patterns problematic, and hence 'require surveillance and correction by experts with privileged knowledge.' Zeitlyn and Rowshan (1997, pp. 56–57) also argue that despite the fact that breastfeeding is perceived as 'a natural activity,' it is also seen as one that could be improved with the assistance of experts including doctors and other health professionals. In the Bangladeshi context, Zeitlyn and Rowshan (1997, p. 66) argue, 'the legitimacy of professional experts is supported by claims of privileged knowledge about breast-feeding and the right of professionals to define what is 'natural' for infants and their mothers.' I contend that current discourses on breastfeeding provide health professionals with a venue for expressing changing ideas about motherhood in addition to confirming their authority.

As I have indicated earlier that many mothers would discard colostrum due to a belief that colostrum is harmful to the newborn infant's health. This belief is pervasive in many traditional societies (see Jellife &Jellife 1978; Morse 1984, 1985; Conton 1985; Dettwyler 1987; King & Ashworth 1987; Fernandez & Popkin 1988; Fishman et al. 1988; Morse et al. 1990; Gunnlaugsson & Einarsdottir 1993; Liamputtong Rice 2000). But, we have also seen that women can change their attitudes toward colostrum. In my own study with Thai women in northern Thailand (Liamputtong 2007b), for example, women, both rural poor and urban educated women, believed strongly in the benefit of colostrum. It appears that this changed knowledge and perceptions of colostrum derived from the advice of doctors and other health professionals including nurses at hospitals or health care centers. Not only the knowledge of breastfeeding was passed on by health professionals but also the 'right' or 'proper' way of feeding their infants. Doctors always gave women advice regarding how to breastfeed their infants.

Feeding on schedule is a clear example of authoritative knowledge of health professionals. Feeding on schedule was recommended by health professionals in many societies. Millard (1990) asserts, women are educated to make distinctions between 'on-demand feeding' and 'by-the-clock' feeding. Millard (1990, p. 217) contends, 'the clock has assumed a central location in breastfeeding advice.' This is 'a symbol of science, discipline, and the coordination of human effort.' In her analysis of pediatric advice on breastfeeding, Millard (1990, p. 211) concludes that 'the concept of scheduled feedings dominates as a consistent, central concern. Despite the fact that today's advice is to breastfeed on demand, the clock continues to occupy a central location.' This trend continues to be observed in maternity hospitals due to the medicalisation of childbirth in many societies. Often, women would be told to feed their infants every three or four hours. This was evidenced in my own research in northern Thailand (Liamputtong 2007b).

Millard (1990, p. 211) suggests that feeding on schedules force women to pay their attention to the clock and advice from professionals, and this implies that 'their own bodily signals, the behaviour of their infants and other lay women are not to be trusted' in their attempts to breastfeed. But, this attempt may be too costly for mothers. As Apple (1987) notes, this 'proper' feeding involves 'rigid schedules' and all too often mothers fail to sustain adequate milk supplies. Millard (1990) also points out that feeding on schedule would reduce milk supplies and increase infant hunger. This often discourages women to continue to breastfeed. Not only that, any irregular pattern of breastfeeding may also have a real physiological effect (Woolridge 1995; Dykes 2005, p. 2287).

Millard (1990, p. 212) provides a good historical perspective on the authority of medical professions, at least in the Western context like America. Around the twentieth century, the upper middle-class women sought and welcomed advice on motherhood from professionals, mainly physicians. Childrearing was seen as their primary work and they attempted to apply 'the science of mothering' (Margolis 1984) in order to emphasise 'regularity, punctuality, cleanliness and discipline' (see also Dykes 2005). This is the result of the medicalisation discourse, which encouraged 'receptivity to biomedical advice on breastfeeding' that women experienced after childbirth. As we have witnessed, physicians continue to regulate and control childbirth and infant feeding (Martin 1992; Davis-Floyd 1992; Dykes 2005; Apple, 2006; Liamputtong 2007b). Women are, therefore, encouraged to follow advice of health professions and adhere to hospital practices. They are advised to listen to measurements taken by health professions and machines, and to treat any signals from their own bodies as 'irrelevant or misleading.' Millard (1990, p. 212) puts it bluntly:

> Women come to breastfeeding with a recent intense experience in ignoring their own bodily signals, which have been redefined as problems instead of guides to action. In this situation, they may not need convincing that in breastfeeding, their own and their infant's bodily signals are to be ignored in favour of a schedule imposed by biomedical personnel. Biomedical advice and practice have the potential to disrupt breastfeeding right from the start in the hospital, when new mothers are most under biomedical control, most reliant on advice about breastfeeding, and most precarious in their transition to motherhood.

The scientific discourses concerning infant feeding at the turn of the twentieth century is a reflection of the Enlightenment principle (Dykes 2002, 2005; Palmer 2009). The Enlightenment, which began in Western Europe in the seventeenth century, revolutionised objective science to be an ultimate source of authoritative knowledge (Crotty 1998). As such, Dykes (2005, p. 2285) contends, within the medicalisation of childbirth, it has led to 'the growing medical imperative to supervise and regulate women's bodies' in order to minimise the threat of chaos (Carter 1995; Blum 1999). As the twentieth century progressed, we saw more scheduling and placing of rigid time controls on every aspect of the breastfeeding relationship (Millard 1990; Dykes 2005). And this is what we still see nowadays.

1.7 Conclusion

Whether women breastfeed or not does not have a straightforward answer. Indeed, as Dykes (2005, p. 2292) concludes:

> Breastfeeding is a complex relationship between mother and baby, the wider family and community. It is a fluid, literally and metaphorically, ever-changing activity influenced by the counterbalancing effects of past events, the daily lived experience and future plans.

As I have discussed in this chapter, infant feeding practice is a contentious issue. There are many factors that dictate whether mothers will breastfeed their infants or not. Some may be due to their social positions and cultural beliefs. Others are influenced by their employment outside their homes. And there are those who are affected by their health problems, in particular HIV/AIDS. Whatever choice (or lack of choice) that women make, health professionals also play an important role in women's decisions. It is crucial that we, as health professionals, researchers, and health educators/promoters, take many of these issues into account in working with women in all corners of the world so that women will have a better chance to deal with their infant feeding choices properly.

Note

1. WIC is the Special Supplemental Nutrition Program for Women, Infants and Children (WIC), and is responsible for the improvement of nutritional health of vulnerable mothers and children. WIC provides supplemental foods, infant formula, and advice on infant feeding and health care referrals for mothers from low-income but diverse groups of mothers (Cricco-Lizza 2005). In 2000, 37% White women enrolled in WIC clinic, 35% were Hispanic, and 22% were Black non-Hispanic mothers (Fox, McManus, & Schmidt 2003)

References

Apple, R. (1987). *Mothers and medicine: A social history of infant feeding, 1890–1950.* Madison: University of Wisconsin Press.

Apple, R. (2006). *Perfect motherhood: Science and childrearing in America* New Brunswick: Rutgers University Press.
Baumslag, N., & Michels, D. L. (1995) *Milk, money, and madness: The culture and politics of breastfeeding*. Westport, CT: Bergin & Garvey.
Beal, A. C., Kuhlthau, K., & Perrin, J. M. (2003). Breastfeeding advice given to African American and White women by physicians and WIC counsellors. *Public Health Reports, 118*, 368–376.
BHITS (2004). Late postnatal transmission of HIV-1 in breast-fed children: An individual patient data meta-analysis. *Journal of Infectious Diseases, 189*, 2154–2166.
Blum, L. M. (1999). *At the breast: Ideologies of breastfeeding and motherhood in the contemporary United States*. Boston: Beacon.
Brent, N. B., Redd, B., & Dworetz, A. (1995). Breast-feeding in a low-income population. *Archives of Pediatrics and Adolescent Medicine, 149*, 798–803.
Buskens, I., Jaffe, A., & Mkhatshwa, H. (2007). Infant feeding practices: Realities and mind sets of mothers in southern Africa. *AIDS Care, 19*(9), 1101–1109.
Buxton, K. E., Gielsen, A. C., Faden, R. R., & Brown, H. C. (1991). Women intending to breastfeed: Predictors of early infant feeding experiences. *American Journal of Preventive Medicine, 7*, 101–106.
Callen, J., & Pinelli, J. (2004). Incidence and duration of breastfeeding for term infants in Canada, United States, Europe, and Australia: A literature review. *Birth, 31*(4), 285–292.
Carter, S. (1995). Boundaries of danger and uncertainty: An analysis of the technological culture of risk assessment. In J. Gabe (Ed.), *Medicine, health and risk: Sociological approach* (pp. 133–150). Oxford: Blackwell.
Chisenga, M., Kasonka, L., Makasa, M., Sinkala, M., Chintu, C., Kaseba, C., et al. (2005). Factors affecting the duration of exclusive breastfeeding among HIV-infected and -uninfected women in Lusaka, Zambia. *Journal of Human Lactation, 21*, 266–275.
Conton, L. (1985). Social, economic and ecological parameters of infant feeding in Usino, Papua New Guinea. In L. B. Marshall (Ed.), *Infant care and feeding in the South Pacific* (pp. 97–120). New York: Gordon and Breach.
Coutsoudis, A. (2005). Breastfeeding and the HIV positive mothers: The debate continues. *Early Human Development, 81*, 87–93.
Coutsoudis, A., & Rollins, N. (2003). Breast-feeding and HIV transmission: The jury is still out. *Journal of Pediatric Gastroenterology and Nutrition, 36*(4), 434–442.
Coutsoudis, A., Pillay, K., Spooner, E., Kuhn, L., & Coovadia, H. M. (1999). Influence of infant-feeding patterns on early mother-to-child transmission of HIV-1 in Durban, South Africa: A prospective cohort study. South African Vitamin A Study Group. *Lancet, 354*, 471–476.
Coutsoudis, A., Pillay, K., Kuhn, L., Spooner, E., Tsai, W. Y., & Coovadia, H. M. (2001). Method of feeding and transmission of HIV-1 from mothers to children by 15 months of age: Prospective cohort study from Durban, South Africa. *AIDS, 15*, 379–387.
Coutsoudis, A., Coovadia, H. M., & Wilfert, C. M. (2008). HIV, infant feeding and more perils for poor people: new WHO guidelines encourage review of formula milk policies. *Bulletin of the World Health Organization, 86*(3), 210–214.
Cricco-Lizza, R. (2004). Infant feeding beliefs and experiences of Black women enrolled in a New York metropolitan area WIC clinic. *Qualitative Health Research, 14*, 1197–1210.
Cricco-Lizza, R. (2005). The milk of human kindness: Environmental and human interactions in a WIC clinic that influence infant-feeding decisions of black women. *Qualitative Health Research, 15*(4), 525–538.
Crotty, M. (1998). *The foundations of social research*. Sydney: Allen and Unwin.
Cunningham, A., Jelliffe, D. B., & Jellife, E. F. (1991). *Breastfeeding and health in the 1980s*. New Jersey: Prentice-Hall.
Davis-Floyd, R. E. (1992). *Birth as an American rite of passage*. Berkeley: University of California Press.
Del Rio, C. (2005). AIDS: The second wave. *Archives of Medical Research, 36*, 682–688.

Deschamps, M.-M., Devieux, J. G., Théodore, H., Saint-Jean, G., Antillus, L., Cadot, L., et al. (2009). A feeding education program to prevent mother-to-child transmission of HIV in Haiti. *AIDS Care, 21*(3), 349–354.

Desclaux, A., & Alfieri, C. (2009). Counseling and choosing between infant-feeding options: Overall limits and local interpretations by health care providers and women living with HIV in resource-poor countries (Burkina Faso, Cambodia, Cameroon). *Social Science and Medicine, 69*, 821–829.

Dettwyler, K. A. (1987). Breastfeeding and weaning in Mali: Cultural context and hard data. *Social Science and Medicine, 24*, 633–643.

Dewey, K., Nommsen-Rivers, L., Heinig, M., & Cohen, R. (2003). Risk factors for suboptimal infant breastfeeding behaviour, delayed onset of lactation, and excessive neonatal weight loss. *Pediatrics, 112*, 607–619.

Doherty, T., Chopra, M., Nkonki, L., Jackson, D., & Persson, L. (2006). A longitudinal qualitative study of infant feeding decision making and practices among HIV-positive women in South Africa. *Journal of Nutrition, 136*, 2421–2426.

Duncan, S., Edwards, R., & Reynolds, T. (2003). Motherhood, paid work and partnering: Values and theories. *Work, Employment & Society, 17*(2), 309–330.

Durongdej, S. (1991). *An innovation approach on promotion of breastfeeding in urban communities*. Bangkok: Department of Nutrition, Faculty of Public Health, Mahidol University.

Dykes, F. (2002). Western marketing and medicine-construction of an insufficient milk syndrome. *Health Care for Women International, 23*(5), 492–502.

Dykes, F. (2005). 'Supply' and 'demand': Breastfeeding as labour. *Social Science & Medicine, 60*, 2283–2293.

Eckhardt, K. W., & Hendershot, G. E. (1984). Analysis of the reversal in breast feeding trends in the early 1970s. *Public Health Reports, 99*, 410–414.

Family Health Division (1994). *A study of breastfeeding situation*. Bangkok: Family Health Division, Ministry of Public Health, Thailand.

Fernandez, M. E. L., & Popkin, B. M. (1988). Prelacteal feeding patterns in the Philippines. *Ecology of Food and Nutrition, 21*, 303–314.

Fikree, F. F., Ali, T. S., Durocher, J. M., & Rahbar, M. H. (2005). Newborn care practices in low socioeconomic settlements of Karachi, Pakistan. *Social Science and Medicine, 60*(5), 911–921.

Fishman, C., Evans, R., & Jenks, E. (1988). Warm bodies, cool milk: Conflicts in post partum food choice for Indochinese women in California. *Social Science and Medicine, 11*, 1125–1132.

Foster, F., Lader, D., & Cheesbrough, S. (1997). *Infant feeding 1995*. London: The Stationery Office.

Fox, H. B., McManus, M. A., & Schmidt, H. J. (2003). WIC reauthorization: Opportunities for improving the nutritional status of women, infants, and children. Washington: National Health Policy Forum, George Washington University. Retrieved 20 March 2007, from http://www.nhpf.org/pdfs_bp/BP_WIC2_8-03.pdf

Gabriel, A., Gabriel, K. R., Lawrence, R. (1986). Cultural values and biomedical knowledge: Choices in infant feeding. *Social Science & Medicine, 23*(5), 501–509.

Galtry, J. (2003). The impact on breastfeeding of labour market policy and practice in Ireland, Sweden and the USA. *Social Science & Medicine, 57*, 167–177.

Giugliani, E. R. J., Caiaffa, W. T., Vogelhut, J., Witter, F. R., & Perman, J. A. (1994). Effect of breastfeeding support from different sources on mothers' decisions to breastfeed. *Journal of Human Lactation, 10*, 157–161.

Gunnlaugsson, G., & Einarsdottir, J. (1993). Colostrum and ideas about bad milk: A case study from Guinea-Bissau. *Social Science Medicine, 36*, 283–288.

Guttman, N., & Zimmerman, D. R. (2000). Low-income mothers' views on breastfeeding. *Social Science & Medicine, 50*, 1457–1473.

Hills-Bonczyk, S. G., Avery, M. D., Savik, K., Potter, S., & Duckett, L. J. (1993). Women's experiences with combining breast-feeding and employment. *Journal of Nurse Midwifery, 38*(5), 257–266.

Hull, V., Thapa, S., & Pratomo, H. (1990). Breast-feeding in the modern health sector in Indonesia: The mother's perspective. *Social Science & Medicine, 30*(5), 625–633.

Iliff, P., Piwoz, E., Tavengwa, N. V., Zunguza, C. D., Marinda, E. T., & Nathoo, K. J. (2005). Early exclusive breastfeeding reduces the risk of postnatal HIV-1 transmission and increases HIV-free survival. *AIDS, 19*, 699–708.

Institute of Medicine (1991). *Nutrition during lactation*. Washington: National Academy Press.

Jacobson, S. W., Jacobson, J. L., & Frye, K. F. (1991). Incidence and correlates of breastfeeding in socio-economically disadvantaged women. *Pediatrics, 88*, 728–736.

Jelliffe, D. B., & Jelliffe, E. E. P. (1978). *Human milk in the modern world*. Oxford: Oxford University Press.

Jordan, B. (1997). Authoritative knowledge and its construction. In R.E. Davis-Floyd & C. F. Sargent (Eds.), *Childbirth and authoritative knowledge: Cross-cultural perspectives* (pp. 55–79). Berkley, CA: University of California Press.

Kiarie, J. N., Richardson, B. A., Mbori-Ngacha, D., Nduati, R. W., & John-Stewart, G. C. (2004). Infant feeding practices of women in a perinatal HIV-1 prevention study in Nairobi, Kenya. *Journal of AIDS, 35*, 75–81.

King, J., & Ashworth, A. (1987). Historical review of the changing pattern of infant feeding in developing countries: The case of Malaysia, the Caribbean, Nigeria and Zaire. *Social Science and Medicine, 25*, 1307–1320.

Kistin, N., Benton, D., Rao, S., & Sullivan, M. (1990). Breastfeeding rates among black urban low-income women: Effect of prenatal education. *Pediatrics, 86*(5), 741–746.

Knodel, J., Chayovan, N., & Wongboonsin, K. (1990). Breast-feeding trends, patterns and policies in Thailand. *Asia-Pacific Population Journal, 5*(1), 135–150.

Kourtis, A. P., Butera, S., Ibegbu, C., Beled, L., & Duerr, A. (2003). Breast milk and HIV-1: Vector of transmission or vehicle of protection? *Lancet Infectious Diseases, 12*, 786–793.

Kurinij, N., Shiono, P. H., Ezrine, S. F., & Rhoads, G. G. (1989). Does maternal employment affect breast-feeding? *American Journal of Public Health, 79*(9), 1247–1250.

Lawrence, R. (1995). The clinician's role in teaching proper infant feeding techniques. *The Journal of Paediatrics, 126*(Suppl), 112–117.

Li, R., & Grummer-Strawn, L. (2002). Racial and ethnic disparities among United States infants: Third National Health and Nutrition Survey, 1988–1994. *Birth, 29*, 251–257.

Liamputtong, P. (2002a). Childrearing practices and child health among the Hmong in Australia: Implications for health services. *International Journal of Health Services, 32*(4), 817–836.

Liamputtong, P. (2002b). Infant feeding practices: The case of Hmong women in Australia. *Health Care for Women International, 23*(1), 33–48.

Liamputtong, P. (2006). Motherhood and "moral career": Discourses of good motherhood among Southeast Asian immigrant women in Australia. *Qualitative Sociology, 29*(1), 25–53.

Liamputtong, P. (2007a). On childrearing and infant care: A cross-cultural perspective. In P. Liamputtong (Ed.), *Childrearing and infant care issues: A cross-cultural perspective* (pp. 3–29). New York: Nova Science.

Liamputtong, P. (2007b). *The journey of becoming a mother amongst women in northern Thailand*. Lanham: Lexington Books.

Liamputtong, P., Yimyam, S., Parisunyakul, S., Baosoung, C., & Sansiriphun, N. (2004). When I become a mother!: Discourses of Motherhood among Thai women in Northern Thailand. *Women's Studies International Forum, 27*(5–6), 589–601.

Liamputtong Rice, P. (2000). *Hmong woman and reproduction*. Westport: Bergin & Garvey.

Liamputtong Rice, P., & Naksook, C. (2001a) Infant feeding practices: The case of Thai mothers in Australia. *Australian Journal of Primary Health – Interchange, 7*(1), 46–55.

Liamputtong Rice, P., & Naksook, C. (2001b) Breastfeeding practices among Thai mothers in Melbourne. *Midwifery, 17*(1), 11–23.

Manderson, L. (1985). To nurse and to nurture: Breastfeeding in Australian society. In V. Hull & M. Simpson (Eds.), *Breastfeeding, child health and child spacing* (pp. 162–186). London: Croom-Helm.

Margolis, M. L. (1984). *Mothers and such: Views of American women and why they changed.* Berkeley: University of California Press.

Martin, E. (1992). *The woman in the body: A cultural analysis of reproduction.* Boston: Beacon.

Millard, A. V. (1990). The place of the clock in pediatric advice: Rationales, cultural themes, and impediments to breastfeeding. *Social Science & Medicine, 31*(2), 211–221.

Mistry, Y., Freedman, M., Sweeney, K., & Hollenbeck, C. (2008). Infant-feeding practices of low-income Vietnamese American women. *Journal of Human Lactation, 24*(4), 406–414.

Moffat, T. (2007). Women's work and weaning: A case study from Periurban Kathmandu, Nepal. In P. Liamputtong (Ed.), *Childrearing and infant care issues: A cross-cultural perspective* (pp. 109–126). New York: Nova Science Publishers.

Morse, J. M. (1984). The cultural context of infant feeding in Fiji. *Ecology of Food and Nutrition, 14*, 287–296

Morse, J. M. (1985). The cultural context of infant feeding in Fiji. In L. B. Marshall (Ed.), *Infant care and feeding in the South Pacific* (pp. 287–296). New York: Gordon and Breach.

Morse, J. M., Bottorff, J. L., & Boman, J. (1989). Patterns of breastfeeding and work: The Canadian experience. *Canadian Journal of Public Health, 80*(3), 182–188.

Morse, J. M., Jehle, C., & Gamble, D. (1990). Initiating breastfeeding: A world survey of the timing of postpartum breastfeeding. *International Journal of Nursing Studies, 3*, 303–313.

Nadesan, M. H., & Sotirin, P. (1998). The romance and science of 'breast is best': Discursive contradictions and contexts of breast-feeding choices. *Text and Performance Quarterly, 18*, 217–232.

National Center for Health Statistics. (1996). *Healthy people 2000 review, 1995–96.* DHHS (PHS) Publication No. 96–1256. Hyattsville: Author.

O'Gara, C. (1989). Breastfeeding and maternal employment in urban Honduras. In J. Leslie & M. Paolisso (Eds.), *Women, work and child welfare in the Third World* (pp. 113–130). Colorado: Westview.

Omari, A. A. A., Luo, C., Kankasa, C., Bhat, G. J., & Bunn, J. (2003). Infant-feeding practices of mothers of known HIV status in Lusaka, Zambia. *Health Policy and Planning, 18*, 156–162.

Palmer, G. (2009). *The politics of breastfeeding* (3rd ed.). London: Pinter & Martin.

Philipona, J. (1994). L'allaitement maternel en Europe. *Les dossiers de l'obstetrique, 216*, 38–40.

Piwoz, E. G., Ferguson, E. O., Bentley, M. E., Corneli, A. L., Moses, A., Nkhoma, J., et al. (2006). Differences between international recommendations on breastfeeding in the presence of HIV and the attitudes and counselling messages of health workers in Lilongwe, Malawi. *International Breastfeeding Journal, 1*, 2. Retrieved 12 April 2006, from http://www.internationalbreastfeedingjournal.com/content/1/1/2

Podhisita, C., Havanon, N., Knodel, J., & Sittitrai, W. (1990). Women's work and family size in rural Thailand. *Asia-Pacific Population Journal, 5*(2), 31–52.

Quarles, A., William, P. D., Hoyle, D. A., Brimeyer, M., & William, A. R. (1994). Mother's intention, age, education and duration and management of breastfeeding. *Maternal-Child Nursing Journal, 22*(3), 102–107.

Reissland, N., & Burghart, R. (1988). The quality of a mother's milk and the health of her child: Beliefs and practices of the women of Mithila. *Social Science and Medicine, 27*(5), 461–469.

Richter, K., & Yoddumnern-Attig, B. (1992) Framing a study of Thai women's changing roles and statuses. In B. Yoddumnern-Attig, K. Richter, A. Soonthorndhada, C. Sethaput, & A. Pramualratana (Eds.), *Changing roles and statuses of women in Thailand: A documentary assessment* (pp. 1–7). Salaya: The Institute for Population and Social Research, Mahidol University.

Riordan, J. (1997). Cost of not breastfeeding: A commentary. *Journal of Human Lactation, 13*, 93–97.

Riordan, J. (2005). *Breastfeeding and human lactation* (3rd ed.). Sudbury: Jones and Bartlett.

Robinson, J. B., Hunt, A. E., Pope, J., & Garner, B. (1993). Attitudes toward infant feeing among adolescent mothers from a WIC population in northern Louisiana. *Journal of American Diet Association, 93*, 1311–1313.

Rollins, N., Meda, N., Becquet, R., Coutsoudis, A., Humphrey, J., Jeffrey, B., Kanshana, S., Kuhn, L., Leroy, V., Mbori-Ngacha, D., Mcintyre, J., & Newell, M-L. (2004). Preventing postnatal transmission of HIV-1 through breastfeeding: Modifying infant feeding practices. *Journal of AIDS, 35*, 188–195.

Romito, P., & Saurel-Cubizolles, M.-J. (1996). Working women and breast-feeding: The experience of first-time mothers in and Italian town. *Journal of Reproductive & Infant Psychology, 14*, 145–156.

Ross Laboratories (1995). *Ross Laboratories mothers' survey: 1986–1994*. Unpublished report, Ross Laboratories, Columbus, OH.

Ryan, A. S., & Martinez, G. A. (1989). Breast-feeding and the working mothers: A profile. *Pediatrics, 83*(4), 524–531.

Ryan, A. S., Rush, D., Krieger, F. W., & Lewandowski, G. E. (1991). Recent declines in breastfeeding in the United States, 1984–1989. *Pediatrics, 88*, 719–727.

Scavenius, M., van Hulsel, L., Meijer, J., Wendte, H., & Gurgel, R. (2007). In practice, the theory is different: A processual analysis of breastfeeding in northeast Brazil. *Social Science and Medicine, 64*, 676–688.

Scott, J. A., & Binns, C. W., (1999). Factors associated with the initiation and duration of breastfeeding: A review of literature. *Breastfeeding Reviews, 7*, 5–16.

Selvaratnam, S. (1988). Population and status of women. *Asia-Pacific Population Journal, 3*(2), 3–23.

Semenova, G. (2001). Breastfeeding and weaning practices of mothers and infants in Uzbekistan. *Food and Nutrition Bulletin, 22*(2), 190–203.

Spisak, S., & Gross, S. S. (1991). *Second follow-up report: The surgeon general's workshop on breastfeeding and human lactation*. Washington: National Centre for Education in Maternal and Child Health.

Timbo, B., Altekruse, S., Headrick, M., & Klontz, K. (1996). Breastfeeding among black mothers: Evidence supporting the need for prenatal intervention. *Journal of Social Pediatrics and Nursing, 1*(1), 35–40.

Tsianakas, V., & Liamputtong, P. (2007). Infant feeding practices and Afghan immigrant women in Australia. In P. Liamputtong (Ed.), *Childrearing and infant care issues: A cross-cultural perspective* (pp.249–273). New York: Nova Science.

UNAIDS (2008). *Report on the global AIDS epidemic*. UNAIDS.

UNICEF (2007). *The state of the world's children 2008. Child survival*. New York: UNICEF. Retrieved 28 November 2008, from http://www.unicef.org/publications/index_42623.html

United Nations Children's Fund/Joint United Nations Program on HIV/AIDS/World Health Organization (1998). *HIV and infant feeding: a guide for health care managers and supervisors*. Geneva, Switzerland: World Health Organization.

Van Esterik, P. (1988). The cultural context of infant feeding. In B. Winikoff, M. A. Castle, & V. H. Laukaran (Eds.), *Feeding infants in four societies: Causes and consequences of mothers' choices* (pp. 187–202). New York: Greenwood.

Van Esterik, P., & Greiner, G. (1981). Breastfeeding and women's work: Constraints and opportunities. *Studies in Family Planning 12*(4), 184–197.

Van Esterik, P., & Menon, L. (1996). *Being mother-friendly: A practical guide for working women and breastfeeding*. Penang: World Alliance for Breastfeeding Action.

Vong-Ek, P. (1993) How popular beliefs influence breastfeeding practices in Northeast and Central Thailand. *Journal of Primary Health Care and Development, 6*, 61–76.

White, A., Freeth, S., & O'Brien, M. (1992). *Infant feeding 1990*. London: HMSO.

WHO Collaborative Study Team on The Role of Breastfeeding on the Prevention of Infant Mortality (2000). Effect of breastfeeding on infant and child mortality due to infectious diseases in less developed countries: A pooled analysis. *Lancet, 355*, 451–455.

WHO/UNAIDS/UNICEF/UNFPA (2004a). *HIV and infant feeding: Guidelines for decisions-makers*. Geneva: World Health Organization.

WHO/UNAIDS/UNICEF/UNFPA (2004b). *HIV and infant feeding: A guide for health care managers and supervisors*. Geneva: World Health Organization.

WHO/UNICEF/UNFPA/UNAIDS. (2007a). *HIV and infant feeding. New evidence and programmatic experience*. Report of a technical consultation. Geneva: World Health Organization.

WHO/UNICEF/UNFPA/UNAIDS. (2007b). *HIV and infant feeding*. Update. Geneva: World Health Organization. Retrieved 28 November 2008, from http://whqlibdoc.who.int/publications/2007/9789241595964_eng.pdf

Wiemann, C. M., DuBois, J. C., & Berenson, A. B. (1998). Racial/ethnic difference in the decision to breastfeed among adolescent mothers. *Pediatrics, 101*, E11.

Woolridge, M. (1995). Baby-controlled feeding: Biocultural implications. In P. Stuart-Macadam & K. Dettwyler (Eds.), *Breastfeeding: Biocultural perspectives* (pp. 168–217). New York: Aldine De Gruyer.

World Health Organization (1993). *Breastfeeding: The technical basis and recommendations for action*. Geneva: World Health Organization.

World Health Organization (2001). *New data on the prevention of mother-to-child transmission of HIV and their policy implications: Conclusions and recommendations*. WHO technical consultation on behalf of the UNFPA/UNICEF/WHO/UNAIDS Inter-agency Task Team on Mother-to-Child Transmission of HIV. Geneva: WHO; Report: WHO/RHR/01.28.

Wright, A. L., Clark, C., & Bauer, M. (1993). Maternal employment and infant feeding practices among the Navajo. *Medical Anthropology Quarterly, 7*, 260–280.

Yimyam, S. (1997). *Breastfeeding experiences among employed Thai women in Chiang Mai*. Unpublished doctoral thesis, Key Centre for Women's Health in Society, The University of Melbourne, Melbourne.

Yimyam, S., & Morrow, M. (1999). Breastfeeding practices among employed Thai women in Chiang Mai. *Journal of Human Lactation, 15*(3), 225–232.

Yimyam, S., & Morrow, M. (2003). Maternal labor, breast-feeding, and infant health. In Heymann, J. (Ed.), *Global inequalities at work: Work's impact on the health of individuals, families, and societies* (pp. 105–135). New York: Oxford University Press.

Yimyam, S., Morrow, M., & Srisuphan, W. (1999). Role conflict and rapid socio-economic change: Breastfeeding among employed women in Thailand. *Social Science & Medicine, 49*, 957–965.

Zeitlyn, S., & Rowshan, R. (1997). Privileged knowledge and mother's "perceptions": The case of breast-feeding and insufficient milk in Bangladesh. *Medical Anthropology Quarterly, 11*(1), 56–68.

Part I
Socio-cultural Perspective of Infant Feeding and Policy Framework

Chapter 2
Managing the Lactating Body: The Breastfeeding Project in the Age of Anxiety

Orit Avishai

Contents

2.1 Introduction

For most of human history, feeding infants at the breast was a fact of life. Although feeding practices varied widely (Maher 1992) with regards to the timing of weaning, the extent and variety of supplementary foods and the source of breast milk (maternal, maternal networks, or a hired wetnurse), infants depended on breast milk for survival in their first several months or years of life. The introduction of safe breast milk alternatives ('formula') in the twentieth-century rendered breastfeeding an increasingly less appealing option in Western countries until breastfeeding advocates and public health campaigns began to intervene to reverse the trend in the 1980s.

O. Avishai (✉)
Fordham University, 407 Dealy Hall, Rose Hill Campus, Bronx, New York, NY 10458, USA
e-mail: avishai@fordham.edu

P. Liamputtong (ed.), *Infant Feeding Practices*, DOI 10.1007/978-1-4419-6873-9_2,
© Springer Science+Business Media, LLC 2011

Public health campaigns are based on two premises: 'the breast is best' and breastfeeding as 'natural' (Kukla 2006; Wolf 2007). This chapter demonstrates that these premises are flawed. Like other parenting, reproductive, health and lifestyle choices, breastfeeding is an option framed by access to resources, corporate interests, public policy, competing ideas about science, motherhood and standards of infant care. Drawing on interviews with class-privileged American mothers, this chapter sheds light on how breastfeeding is shaped at the crossroads of moralised motherhood, public health campaigns and grass-roots activism, economic disparities and the commercialised, medicalised and professionalised contexts that characterise contemporary parenting. Specifically, I demonstrate that this group of women constructs the lactating body as a carefully managed site and breastfeeding as a mothering project – a task to be researched, planned, implemented and assessed, with reliance on expert knowledge, professional advice and consumption. The construction of breastfeeding as a maternal project sheds light on breastfeeding disparities ('successful' breastfeeders tend to be white, educated, older and heterosexually partnered mothers) and on the fallacy of the 'breast is best' and 'breastfeeding is natural' slogans.

2.2 Breastfeeding Trends in the United States

When breast milk alternatives were first introduced in the late 1800s, results were disastrous, spurring the first wave of breastfeeding campaigns (Apple 1987; Wolf 2006). As safer alternatives became widely available in the 1920s, breastfeeding rates began to decline worldwide and by the 1930s breastfeeding was viewed as a matter of choice in Western nations. Breastfeeding came under scrutiny in the 1950s, as part of the process that brought reproduction and parenting under the purview of experts. Many mothers were diagnosed with insufficient milk syndrome and advised to discontinue breastfeeding. According to Apple (1987) and Carter (1995), this syndrome was typically the by-product of hospital practices and child care advice that interfered with lactation mechanisms, such as maternal–infant separation in hospitals following childbirth and the promotion of strict breastfeeding schedules. In this climate, physicians and public health officials began to promote formula as a more convenient and nutritiously equivalent alternative to breast milk; formula was sometimes touted as a *superior* alternative (Apple 1987; see also Chapter 9 in this volume). Amidst this culture of scientific motherhood, in the 1950s a group of women in Chicago founded a breastfeeding advocacy and support organisation, La Leche League (see Gorham & Andrews 1990; Ward 2000; see also Chapter 7 in this volume).

By the early 1970s, breastfeeding initiation rates in the United States dropped to an all-time low of 25%, coinciding with the large-scale entry of mothers of young children to the workforce. Initially, breastfeeding rates declined most rapidly among privileged mothers, but by the 1970s all demographic groups exhibited low breastfeeding rates. In a trend that continues today, low-income, uneducated and

African-American mothers exhibited the sharpest declines in breastfeeding rates (Ryan 1997, Ryan, Wenjun, & Acosta 2002).

Since the late 1970s, breastfeeding rates have rebounded. By the mid-2000s, 70% of American mothers initiated breastfeeding, and about 35% of infants were receiving some breast milk at 6 months. Both rates are short of the goals of the United States Department of Health and Human Services (2000) and of the World Health Organisation (WHO). At the same time, breastfeeding has become even more stratified. Once associated with poor, immigrant and unsophisticated mothers, in Western nations breastfeeding has become a marker of privileged motherhood (Apple 1987; Blum 1999), where white, middle-class, educated, heterosexually partnered and older mothers are more likely to initiate breastfeeding, continue breastfeeding beyond the first few days and upon return to paid employment and breastfeed exclusively (Ryan et al. 2002; Ahluwalia, Morrow, Hsia, & Grummer-Strawn 2003). Given the emphasis that breastfeeding experts put on mothers' access to adequate nourishment, rest and a relaxing environment (Sears & Sears 1993; Huggings 1995), these disparities are hardly surprising. This chapter shows that this advice plays a key role in the construction of breastfeeding practices of 'successful' breastfeeding mothers.

Breastfeeding disparities are a product of two intersecting processes. First, public policies in the United States that privatise childrearing responsibilities offer little support to mothers whose short maternity leaves, inflexible schedules and work environments interfere with breastfeeding routines and are inhospitable to establishing pumping as an alternative. Mothers who take longer maternity leaves, work part time or on a flexible schedule and pump their breasts regularly while separated from their infants are able to breastfeed their infants longer (Avishai 2004). Countries that offer more generous support to new mothers such as New Zealand, Australia and Canada, exhibit higher breastfeeding rates across the population and less significant racial and socio-economic disparities.

These disparities are also a product of racialised and sexualised public discourses. Blum (1999) argues that the 'breast is best' frame creates a standard of good mothering that faults mothers who cannot comply with this standard or do not wish to comply with it. These mothers are usually poor, uneducated and minority women, some of whom resist what they see as imposition of white, middle-class mothering standards (see Ladd-Taylor & Umansky 1998; cf Chapter 9 in this volume).

2.3 'The Breast Is Best': Public Health Campaigns

Oblivious to breast milk and breastfeeding throughout much of the twentieth century, in the mid-1970s medical and nutrition scientists and practitioners began to investigate breast milk composition, lactation physiology and the correlation between breast milk and a range of medical and psychological conditions and diseases, including ear infections, asthma, gastrointestinal ailments, diabetes, allergies, intelligence, obesity, autism and infant death syndrome (AAP 2005). The cumulative data suggest that breast milk has a positive effect on various health conditions. This evidence is captured by the now-axiomatic notion that 'the breast is best' for infants, mothers, families, populations and the environment (AAP 2005). On the heels of this evidence, the WHO, national medical associations and international breastfeeding advocacy organisations (such as WABA, the World Alliance for Breast-Feeding Advocacy) recommend that infants be breastfed without any supplementary foods (including breast milk alternatives) during their first 6 months of life, followed by a combination of breastfeeding and complementary foods (excluding breast milk alternatives) up to age two (see policy statements and calls for action of the American Academy of Pediatrics, 1997, 2005; the Department of Health's 2000 Blueprint for Action on Breastfeeding; WHO 2002 Global Strategy on Infant Feeding).

These guidelines are accompanied by public health campaigns that tout breast milk as 'liquid gold', vital for the health, intelligence and emotional well-being of infants. These campaigns promote breastfeeding as a natural, medically informed, rational and responsible parenting choice (Kukla 2006; Wolf 2007). Supporting these campaigns, parenting books and magazines offer mothers expert advice as to why they should breastfeed ('*Why Breast is Best*'; '*The Secret to Quick Weight Loss*'; '*Avoid Ear Infections*') and how (exclusively and 'on demand', in response to the infants' needs rather than according to a pre-set feeding schedule (Sears & Sears 1993; Huggings 1995). Public health campaigns are further supported by grass-roots anti-corporate activists, advocates of natural parenting methods and, most recently, by feminist 'lactivists' (lactation activists; see Carpenter 2007).

Critics of the science of human lactation caution that the data are not unequivocal, especially with regards to the benefits of breastfeeding beyond the first few months and exclusive breastfeeding (Blum 1999; Law 2000; Wolf 2007). Some also argue that when formula feeding is sanitary and breastfeeding rates mirror class disparities, these benefits may be the product of confounding socio-economic effects. They further charge that contemporary breastfeeding campaigns that are framed by privatised risk, choice and moralism are divorced from the cultural and institutional realities that structure breastfeeding in Western nations that offer little support to parents and sexualise women's breasts (Kukla 2006; Wolf 2007). This very conversation suggests that breastfeeding is far from a natural practice, but rather one that needs to be understood in specific cultural contexts.

2.4 Breastfeeding at the Age of Anxiety: Expert and Consumerist Regimes

While *infant* feeding has been subject to expert and medicalised control for decades, breastfeeding was largely left unregulated by experts (Fildes 1986; Apple 1987). As physicians promoted 'formula' as the modern, responsible, scientific and 'American' way of feeding babies starting in the 1950s and legions of mothers were diagnosed with 'insufficient milk syndrome', mothers who persevered enjoyed a relatively expert-free cultural space; the description of breastfeeding as a counter-hegemonic, natural, symbiotic and simple practice in the 1973 version of *Our Bodies Ourselves* is instructive.

This has changed with the confluence of studies that establish the benefits of breastfeeding with feminist, anti-corporate and maternalist breastfeeding advocates' efforts to increase breastfeeding rates (Palmer 1988; Van Esterik 1989). In addition, a new profession – lactation consulting – emerged in the mid-1980s as an alternative to the free breastfeeding advice offered by La Leche League. Working within a clinical frame, this profession boasts formal training and certification procedures, a vibrant professional association, the International Lactation Consultant Association (ILCA),[1] and a peer reviewed journal (Spangler 2000; Bailey 2005). Breastfeeding is additionally supported by a vast market of goods and services, including lactation classes and books, nursing clothes, bras, pillows, chairs and breast pumps and related paraphernalia. Numerous websites also provide breastfeeding advice, support and merchandise.

To researchers conversant in the social history of reproduction and mothering and in theories of bodily disciplinary practices, the emergence of breastfeeding as a medicalised, expert, disciplinary and consumerist regime is hardly surprising. Such regimes govern health and reproduction (Davis-Floyd 1992; Martin 1992; Rapp 1999; Clarke, Mamo, Fishman, Shim, & Fosket 2003; Davis-Floyd 2004) and appearance (Bartky 1988; Bordo 1993; Gimlin 2002). The consumerist, technological, medicalised, professionalised and expert-reliant contexts that shape contemporary parenting and mothering are well documented (Hays 1996; Rapp 1999; Litt 2000; Hochschild 2003; Hulbert 2003; Lareau 2003; Taylor, Layne, & Wozniak 2004; Pugh 2005). Warner (2005) argues that this parenting context is indicative of an age of anxiety where parents and mothers, especially, are caught up in a ceaseless attempt to meet good mothering standards that render them exhausted and frustrated. It is within these multiple contexts that contemporary breastfeeding practices are forged (see also Chapters 6, 7, and 9 in this volume).

In what follows, I show how the women who participated in my study respond to good mothering standards defined by the number of ounces of breast milk produced. Analysing how they prepare for breastfeeding, the advice they seek and the gadgets they purchase, I show how these women produce the lactating body as a carefully managed site and breastfeeding as a 'project' – a task to be researched, planned, implemented and assessed. Analysis of the breastfeeding project demonstrates that breastfeeding is far from a natural practice.

2.5 The Study and Methods

This study is based on interviews with twenty-five first-time, educated, work-force-experienced and class-privileged mothers in the San Francisco Bay Area in

[1] Although the ILCA was formed by La Leche League, it quickly became an independent organisation.

1999–2000. I recruited half of the participants through a local virtual parents' organisation. Other women were recruited using a snowball technique that began with personal acquaintances, a mothers' groups' moderator and a lactation consultant. I also interviewed the latter two as informants. The focus on privileged women was motivated by data suggesting persistent racial, ethnic and class disparities in breastfeeding practices. I was interested in the experiences of women who from a statistical perspective achieved breastfeeding success.

Most of the women in my sample were in their thirties; they ranged in age from twenty-five to forty-one. Twenty were white, one was East-Indian, two were Latina and two were mixed-race (Asian/white). About one-half were native to the Bay Area or had local extended family support. All but one were in heterosexual marriages; one was a lesbian single mother who otherwise shared the group's cultural capital. All were college graduates and almost half held professional or graduate degrees. Before birth, they pursued careers in white-collar professions, such as law, medicine, accounting, engineering, management, nursing and teaching. Many of this group who returned to paid employment attempted to provide their babies with breast milk by pumping at work, with varying degrees of success (Avishai 2004). One-third decided not to return to paid employment for the time being. The babies' ages ranged from 6 months to 2 years. Interviews lasted between 2 and 3 h and were loosely structured, recorded and transcribed in full. Interview topics included pregnancy and birth experiences, childrearing ideologies, the breastfeeding decision process, breastfeeding and pumping practices, women's sources of breastfeeding information and advice, breastfeeding-related consumption, spousal and other support systems, perception of the maternal body and enjoyment of breastfeeding.

2.6 The Breastfeeding Project

2.6.1 Consulting the Books and Asking the Experts

Without exception, the women in my study subscribed to the 'breast is best' axiom (for similar findings in Britain and Australia see Murphy 2000; Schmied & Lupton 2001; see also Chapters 4, 6, and 7 in this volume). Therefore, 'breastfeeding wasn't much of a decision', one interviewee said, because 'the benefits are clear'. However, the effortless decision to breastfeed typically marks the beginning of a long, laborious and demanding process.

While study participants knew that their bodies were 'equipped' to breastfeed, many approached breastfeeding with awe: 'Is this going to work?' 'Is it supposed to be so painful?' 'Am I producing enough milk for him?' and 'Is she gaining enough weight?' Dykes (2005) notes similar anxieties among British women. They did not expect breastfeeding to just happen, nor did they trust their bodies to know intuitively what to do. Breastfeeding was both an art and a science, a skill to be learned and mastered by acquiring specialised knowledge and mobilising resources.

Diane, a 30-year-old engineer turned stay-at-home mom, was most fastidious in her preparation. Though she remarked that 'you didn't need to know much', she referred to over a dozen childbirth, breastfeeding and childrearing books. She also took pre- and post-natal breastfeeding classes and met with a lactation consultant. In contrast, Lara, a 34-year-old administrator thought that little preparation was necessary. She assumed she would just know how to breastfeed. 'What's there to it? The baby sucks on your breasts'. However, she encountered a host of difficulties in the first few months, including sore nipples and insufficient weight gain. In hindsight, she said she wished she 'had learned how to breastfeed'. Knowledge, she assumed, would have prevented these difficulties.

Experiences like Lara's circulate among expectant mothers through books, classes, doctors' offices, websites and informal networks, serving as cautionary tales which underscore the importance of adequate preparation. Accordingly, study participants were proactive. Starting early in their pregnancies, most women sought some information about breastfeeding, and most mentioned books of the 'how to' genre such as *The Nursing Mothers' Companion* (Huggings 1995), *The Baby Book* (Sears & Sears 1993) and the *What to Expect Series* (Eisenberg, Murkoff, & Hathaway 1996). Some supplemented reading with hands-on training in the form of breastfeeding preparation classes; two also met privately with a lactation consultant pre-natally, *anticipating* difficulties. In these classes, offered as stand-alone or as part of a birth preparation series, mothers-to-be and their partners learn breastfeeding techniques and practice with life-size dolls. Not surprisingly, they attributed post-birth breastfeeding success to a pre-natal preparation:

> I was extremely nervous, thinking, 'I am not going to get sore, I do not want to get sore.' I heard numerous stories from my girlfriends, how they were sore, how they were cracked, and stopped. I was so determined, 'I want the proper latch on'. That's the key, I heard. So I would start, and my husband would give directions: 'no, you're a little high, you probably want to do this direction.' That class was extremely useful. (Angela)

The quest for expert knowledge was more pronounced after childbirth, when many women felt insecure about breastfeeding techniques and breast milk production, or, in some cases, encountered significant difficulties. Most did not mobilise social networks to alleviate anxieties and problems (many accepted general advice from friends, but not hands-on instruction). It is important to remember that most of these women could not expect practical advice from older kin. As a result of the social history of breastfeeding in the United States, social, cultural and practical knowledge about breastfeeding had been lost over the past two generations (Gorham & Andrews 1990), eradicating the traditional role of older female kin as a resource for new mothers; geographical and emotional distance between family members exacerbates this process. Many women also felt that they could not expect much emotional support. The older generation of women were often critical of their daughters' or daughters'-in-law breastfeeding, and some baulked at the sight of breastfeeding 'in public' (which, in many cases, referred to breastfeeding in front of family members at home!) and criticised the practice of breastfeeding 'older' babies. In this social setting, an expert – the lactation consultant – fills the need for expertise and support.

Almost half of study participants had met with a lactation consultant at least once. While lay lactation experts, associated with La Leche League (LLL), have served American women since the 1950s, certified lactation consultants, who are health professionals, are a recent phenomenon. The women in my sample considered these experts more professional than LLL volunteers, and preferred to pay rather than utilise LLL's free assistance (visits cost between $50 and $100; some insurance companies partially cover the cost). In addition, many women associated LLL with radicalism or conservatism, both unappealing.

By their own accounts, only four women turned to these experts for assistance with conditions that the medical profession defines as potentially dangerous conditions that require professional intervention, such as poor infant weight gain, unbearable soreness, or infected nipples. The others primarily sought a professional stamp of approval or emotional support. In Melanie's case, the lactation consultant alleviated anxieties about the milk she could not see:

> I went twice to [a local lactation consultant]. When you're desperate, it's the obvious choice; it's like calling Jiffy Lube. I needed someone who knew a lot about breastfeeding to watch her breastfeed and say, 'yes, you're breastfeeding, it's working, she's doing fine.'

Melanie's insecurity highlights the ambivalence many women felt and which they thought could only be alleviated by an 'objective' professional. As in the case of pre-natal preparation, the aggregate message is that professional, quasi-scientific expertise is requisite in order to realise a 'natural' process – for those who can afford it.

Undoubtedly, lactation consultants are a vital resource for some breastfeeding mothers. Without their expert knowledge and practical advice, women who face painful or potentially life-threatening conditions, such as poor infant weight gain, would probably discontinue breastfeeding. Perceiving of the mother–infant unit as a patient, armed with clinical experience coupled with holistic and scientific approaches to lactation, these experts are better positioned to assist breastfeeding mothers than either paediatricians or obstetricians (medical professionals routinely refer their patients to lactation consultants). They teach women tricks of a newly rediscovered trade, and diagnose and treat a range of breastfeeding-related conditions. At the same time, these certified and paid professionals contribute to the construction of breastfeeding as a mothering project.

2.6.2 Setting Goals and Assessing the Product

The participants deployed other strategies to manage lactation: they set goals and strove to manage uncooperative lactating bodies. Both strategies emphasise the product, breast *milk*, over the process, breast*feeding*.

In accordance with the American Academy of Pediatrics' then-recent recommendation concerning exclusive breastfeeding (1997), the participants established breastfeeding targets, stated in terms of duration and quantities to be produced, and sought to avoid commercial formula during their babies' first year of life. To achieve exclusivity, a woman must supply *all* of her infant's nourishment needs until the age of 6 months, a period during which supplementation of any kind is discouraged, and all of her infants' milk requirements during at least the first year. (In 2003, 18% of American mothers met the first goal, and 11% met the second; Ross Mothers Survey 2003).[2]

My participants ceaselessly evaluated their 'success'. Employing the terms 'supply' and 'demand', they reported how much their infants drank each day and how this quantity measured against the amounts they were able to produce and/or pump (see Dykes 2005 for similar imagery among British women). Though more pronounced amongst women who pumped their breasts at work (Avishai 2004), the emphasis on 'making it' to the 1-year mark without introducing breast milk alternatives, and the focus on quantities pumped, was shared by most interviewees.

Consequently, while a handful viewed formula as liberation from full-time motherhood, formula feeding generated almost universal anxieties. Janine apologised to her baby when she first offered her a bottle of formula. Bridgett viewed formula as junk food – 'it's like feeding your baby potato chips'. Leslie, who suffers from severe migraines and occasionally could not nurse her daughter until her medication cleared out of her system, 'kept a backlog of milk in the freezer'. She felt nervous if she 'had fewer than eight 4-ounce bottles in the freezer. Because then what would I feed her?'

The emphasis on exclusivity resulted in constant monitoring and assessment of 'production' levels and the 'stash in the fridge', taking a heavy toll on many study participants. Stay-at-home mothers grappled with the '24/7 duty' entailed by their commitment to exclusivity, and resented the time spent at the pump (stay-at-home mothers often pump for emergencies, occasional breaks, and to mix with solid foods). Many experienced exclusivity as emotionally straining, and several were concerned that exclusivity would set in motion a gendered long-term family dynamic. For mothers who worked outside of their homes and were separated from their babies for several hours at a time, exclusivity entailed long hours of pumping at the work place; for these mothers, exclusivity was a physically draining enterprise. (Most of the working mothers in my sample were not able to pump sufficient amounts of milk; their babies' first birthday signified liberation from pumping; see Avishai 2004).

Many mothers remarked that exclusivity was irrational, ridiculous and unreasonable, insisting that 'formula fed babies do just fine'. Yet, in the context of breastfeeding as a middle-class mothering project, exclusivity makes rational sense: as goal-attaining individuals, these women were determined to meet a target, which happened to be stated in terms of ounces produced per day over a certain period of time. For these success-oriented, high-achieving women, a breastfeeding goal was no different than an educational, professional, or athletic goal. Accordingly, many mothers attributed 'success' to their mindsets and go-getter attitudes; 'failures' damaged their egos. Jennifer reflected:

[2] The notion of exclusivity itself is a relatively new construction (Maher 1992; Law 2000).

> We didn't supplement with formula until she was eight months old. I got the flu and it screwed up my production. I was bummed. It's irrational, but I felt like I failed. There was the ego thing. 'Oh look what I can do'. And I couldn't do it anymore.

Jennifer continued to spend an hour-and-a-half of her 9-h workday as an accountant at the pump until she reached the 1-year mark. She explained that pumping became 'like running a marathon. You just seem so close, why stop now? Then you can say, 'I did it for a year!' as opposed to wimping out at 8 months. I probably would have felt like I failed'.

Margaret, another working mother, did feel like a failure. Faced with a widening gap between supply and demand, Margaret described how she 'worked' on her milk production by increasing her food intake, adding late-night and early morning pumping sessions, and purchasing herbal supplements. The next section examines these and other strategies to increase production.

2.6.3 Managing the (Uncooperative) Lactating Body

In accordance with the breastfeeding goals they had set, the women in my study monitored their breast milk production. Melanie, a stay-at-home mother who pumped very little, was nevertheless anxious. She traced her anxieties to lactation experts' emphasis on 'numbers':

> The books made me upset. *The Nursing Mother's Companion* made me particularly unhappy. It has this table on calculating how much your baby should be eating. It always freaked me out, because I just never seem to be producing that much. I don't read it anymore. Part of me realised, 'why am I worried about this book and these numbers, everything is OK on this end.' I feel it's best not to ask too many questions, just accept that it's a system that works. It's better that your breasts aren't clear. [Blum's 1999 book cover provides a jarring illustration of the image Melanie alludes to: a woman with one-ounce marks on her bare breasts].

Yet, Melanie did not accept her body as 'a system that works'. 'Lacking' the one-ounce marks, her breasts were a source of anxiety. For other women, concerns about 'the numbers' bred ceaseless attempts to increase breast milk production. Although this was especially characteristic of women who encountered difficulties, or women who pumped their breasts at work, I found that almost everyone engaged in some form of body assessment, management and control.

Breastfeeding plans devised by lactation consultants to deal with poor infant weight gain or maternal pain represent an extreme form of body management. In some cases, lactation consultants merely provide clients with objective tools to assess levels of production, easing anxieties about milk that mothers cannot see. Bridgett described the breastfeeding chart she filled out 'religiously' after meeting with a lactation consultant, who taught her 'to write down how many times I fed, what time of day, how many diapers, how long did I feed, left, right. If I had to pump, how much came out of the pump'. These charts bear a resemblance to infant feeding charts favoured by mid-twentieth century doctors.

Lactation consultants also help clients work through physiological impediments. Janine turned to a lactation consultant due to insufficient weight. The consultant determined that her daughter was an 'inefficient nurser', and devised a breastfeeding plan, which Janine compared to a gym workout program. For several weeks, Janine was overwhelmed by the plan that had her 'nurse her for ten minutes, then pump and give her whatever was left. Then we would supplement with formula'. Heather's workout plan was more elaborate, and included a supplemental nursing system consisting of milk bottles that deliver formula through tubes attached to the nipples. This system teaches babies to nurse and 'jumpstarts milk production', without jeopardising the baby's health. This regimen was time-consuming.

> I would make formula, clean the apparatus, tape tube, have him latch on with the tube in the mouth. And it's hard, you keep having to adjust the apparatus. Then I would nurse for 15–20 minutes on each side, then pump again for 15 minutes, and clean. And by the time it was done, it was time to begin all over again!

These plans enabled Heather and Janine to supply their infants with *some* breast milk, though they were unable to breastfeed exclusively. However, their partial success came at a hefty price, as they were left drained, tired and upset about their failed bodies.

Though these are extreme cases, many interviewees had some qualms about their breast milk production which they attempted to increase, with varying degrees of success, by employing a variety of solutions, including drinking, eating and sleeping sufficiently and taking herbal supplements. Working mothers also added more pumping sessions and invested in a 'workhorse' of a pump.

The range of strategies deployed by the participants, including pre-marital preparation, 'workout plans' and 'working' on production, indicate that breastfeeding cannot be left up to nature. Breastfeeding can – and sometimes must – be actively assessed, controlled and managed. In addition, many women found that breastfeeding came with a hefty price tag.

2.6.4 Investing in Production Facilities

> I got the Madella [breast pump], a Boppy [nursing pillow], and the glider [nursing rocking chair] (Eva, a 30-year-old corporate lawyer)

Though most of the women in this study suggested that breast milk is produced by their bodies 'free of charge', and contrasted breastfeeding's 'simplicity' with the 'bagfuls of paraphernalia' associated with bottle-feeding, many of them were immersed in breastfeeding-related consumption, reflecting broader consumption trends that characterise privileged parenthood (Hays 1996; Lareau 2003; Taylor et al. 2004; Pugh 2005). Since the physiology of lactation assumes proper levels of nourishment and rest as well as maternal health – all stratified in the United States – the very construction of breast milk as 'free' by mothers and lactation experts masks social inequalities (Blum 1999; Law 2000). In addition, unlike the white, middle-class women in Blum's (1999) and Bobel's (2002) studies, whose understanding of breastfeeding as 'natural' entailed rejection of breastfeeding-related objects and technologies, participants in my study embraced the expanding market of nursing gear, gadgets and accessories. They invested in nursing bras (~ $40), nursing pads, breast pumps and related kits ($200–400), nursing pillows (~ $40) and nursing chairs (~$200). Some purchased herbal supplements to enhance their milk supply or acquired breastfeeding outfits. Bridgett, who said she 'didn't go into a lot of expenses', offered a list amounting to several hundred dollars.

> People think breastfeeding is natural. But you do have to expect [to spend money]. It's $150 to have the lactation consultant come to the hospital, and it's $50 for half-hour consultation. And the breast pump is like $200, and the nursing bras, and the lactation outfits are $30 each. I only have one... Oh, also, when we got home, I couldn't find the right chair in the house. We had an antique rocking chair, but the arms didn't work. So we bought the glider. And then the pillow....

Margaret's story about 'the chair' demonstrates the fetishised value that many study participants placed on specialty objects. Although she attributed her initial nursing difficulties to a variety of factors, including the physical conditions in a cold bedroom and her husband's family's breastfeeding purism, she associated alleviation of her difficulties with the purchase of a specialty breastfeeding glider:

> When he was about four weeks old I nursed him in another woman's rocking chair. I was like, 'it doesn't hurt! Is this what a chair could feel like?' Because here I am in a room that's too cold, with shrunken nipples, and a husband saying 'go breastfeeding, go breastfeeding, you know my mom is La Leche.' And my chair was too low! I thought: 'I've got to get one of those chairs. I don't care how much they cost'.... I drove out to [a baby store]. I walked in the door and I said: 'I want that chair, I want it now'. And the clerk said, 'well, we'll order it for you, it'll take...' 'No, I want the floor model'. And she said 'well, all right, what kind of car do you have?' 'Honda'. And she said 'it won't fit in your car, we'll have it delivered.' 'Take it apart.' She gets a screwdriver and takes the chair apart and puts it in the car. And I said 'how much is it'? 'Oh, this one is on sale.' 'Thank god! You could have charged me $5,000 for it, I would have paid it....' Because I was distraught. I was getting two hours of sleep at a time at night.... And that really changed things. After that it stopped hurting.

2.7 Conclusion

Public health and advocacy campaigns are based on the twin assumptions that 'the breast is best' and that breastfeeding is 'natural'. From a sociological perspective, human decisions, practices and experiences – including those that pertain to reproduction, health and parenting in general and infant feeding in particular – arise within specific historical, cultural, economic and political contexts. 'Best practices' are also constructs shaped by specific conditions, norms and customs. These conditions, norms and customs govern infant feeding decisions – breast milk or breast milk alternatives; who may feed the child at the breast – the mother, a paid wet-nurse, other mothers in a network of childcare; where breastfeeding is to occur – in public, at the workplace, in the presence of family members, or only in the privacy of one's home; how often breastfeeding should occur – according to a fixed schedule or 'on demand', in response to infant cues; how long breastfeeding should last – through early infancy or well into toddlerhood; how breastfeeding is to be learned – within the mother's informal kin and social networks or through specialised professionals; and how breastfeeding is experienced – as pleasurable and empowering or as a burden.

To demonstrate that breastfeeding practices are social constructs, this chapter has focused on the experiences of one particular group of women – class privileged American mothers, who, from a statistical perspective, achieve breastfeeding success. The chapter demonstrates that these women construct breastfeeding as a mothering project – a task to be researched, planned, implemented and assessed, with reliance on expert knowledge, professional advice and consumption. They do so in the context of discourses of health promotion, good outcome childrearing, science, rationality and the market; breastfeeding is but one of many informed decisions they make daily about their health, lifestyle and parenting (Hays 1996; Rapp 1999; Lareau 2003). Significantly, these women have access to the resources and gadgets which assist them in materialising these choices, including high-quality pre-natal and paediatric care, household help and relatively long maternity leaves, all positively associated with 'successful' breastfeeding. In the process, these women draw on – and create a market for – commercial resources, including nursing and childrearing books, lactation consultants, pre-natal and breastfeeding classes and mothers' support groups.

Analysis of the mothering project sheds light on the obstacles encountered by women who cannot mobilise such resources, which are no longer considered optional. Viewed in this light, the twin constructs of 'the breast is best' and 'breastfeeding is natural' are impoverished slogans that do not capture the extent to which both the science and the imagery of breastfeeding are shaped by normative assumptions and middle-class experiences.

I expect that some feminists will find the project frame troubling, as it contrasts with emphases on pleasure, embodied subjectivity, relationality and empowerment that characterise much of the breastfeeding literature across the humanities and social sciences (Baumslag & Michels 1995; Giles 2003; Hausman 2003; Bartlett 2005; Dykes 2005; the November 2004 issue of *Australian Feminist Studies*). Elsewhere (Avishai 2007), I note that my study participants negotiated the project frame with notions of pleasure, intimacy, and, as one interviewee put it, a 'romantic image of breast-feeding that you would probably have if you didn't read anything'. However, the project frame dominated their narratives.

To be effective, I believe that feminist analyses of infant feeding must distinguish between normative/political agendas and empirical realities. Framing breastfeeding as an embodied, feminist-maternalist, empowering and post-modern response to corporate, gendered and medicalised regimes is a fine goal – but it insufficiently accounts for ethnographic data that point to the ambivalences and chaos associated with breastfeeding (Balsamo, Mari, Maher, & Serini 1992; Blum 1999; Schmied & Lupton 2001; Avishai 2004; Dykes 2005; Avishai 2007). I suggest that rather than criticising the project frame (and mothers who describe their breastfeeding experiences in consumerist, rational and scientific terms), feminists understand this frame as a sensible solution to an otherwise potentially threatening, alien, or unintelligible practice. As Blum (1999) notes, privileging the sensual and relational aspects of breastfeeding may amount to coercive moralism (which is precisely the tone Kukla 2006 identifies in breastfeeding campaigns). Accordingly, my emphasis has been on how women approach breastfeeding within a specific social, cultural, political and historical context, with the understanding that breastfeeding is a cultural event shaped by institutional, historical, cultural, raced, gendered and sexualised arrangements.

References

Ahluwalia, I. B., Morrow, B., Hsia, J., & Grummer-Strawn L. M. (2003). Who is breastfeeding? Recent trends from the pregnancy risk assessment and monitoring system. *Journal of Pediatrics, 142*(5), 486–493.

American Academy of Pediatrics, Work Group on Breastfeeding. (1997). Policy Statement: Breastfeeding and the use of human milk. *Pediatrics, 100*, 1035–1039.

American Academy of Pediatrics, Section on Breastfeeding. (2005). Policy Statement: Breastfeeding and the uses of human milk. *Pediatrics, 115*, 496–506.

Apple, R. (1987). *Mothers and medicine: A social history of infant feeding, 1890–1950*. Madison: University of Wisconsin Press.

Avishai, O. (2004). At the pump. *Journal of the Association for Research on Mothering, 6*, 138–149.

Avishai, O. (2007). Managing the lactating body: The Breast-Feeding Project and privileged motherhood. *Qualitative Sociology, 30*(2), 135–152.

Bailey, D. (2005). ILCA: 20 years of building a profession. *Journal of Human Lactation, 21*(3), 239–242.

Balsamo, F., Mari, G. D., Maher, V., & Serini, R. (1992). Production and pleasure: Research on breastfeeding in Turin. In V. Maher (Ed.), *The anthropology of breastfeeding: Natural Law or social construct* (pp. 59–90). Oxford: Berg.

Bartky, S. L. (1988). Foucault, femininity, and the modernization of patriarchal power. In I. Diamond & L. Quinby (Eds.), *Feminism and Foucault: Reflections on resistance* (pp. 61–86). Chicago: Northern University Press.

Bartlett, A. (2005). *Breastwork: Rethinking breastfeeding*. Sydney: UNSW.

Baumslag, N., & Michels, D. L. (1995). *Milk, money, and madness: The culture and politics of breastfeeding*. Westport: Bergin & Garvey.

Blum, L. M. (1999). *At the breast: Ideologies of breastfeeding and motherhood in the contemporary United States*. Boston: Beacon.

Bobel, C. (2002). *The paradox of natural mothering*. Philadelphia: Temple University Press.

Bordo, S. (1993). *Unbearable weight: Feminism, Western culture, and the body*. Berkeley: University of California Press.

Boston Women's Health Book Collective (1973). *Our bodies, ourselves*. New York: Simon and Schuster.

Carpenter, F. C. (2007). "(L)Activists and lattes": Breastfeeding advocacy as domestic performance. *Women & Performance: A Journal of Feminist Theory, 16*(3), 347–367.

Carter, P. (1995). *Feminism, breasts and breast feeding*. New York: St. Martin's Press.

Clarke, A. E., Mamo, L., Fishman, J. R., Shim, J. K., & Fosket, J. R. (2003). Biomedicalization: Technoscientific transformations of health, illness, and U.S. biomedicine *American Sociological Review, 68*(April), 168–194.

Davis-Floyd, R. E. (1992). *Birth as an American rite of passage*. Berkeley: University of California Press.

Davis-Floyd, R. E. (2004). Consuming childbirth: The qualified commodification of midwifery care. In J. S. Taylor, L. L. Layne &, D. F. Wozniak (Eds.), *Consuming motherhood* (pp. 211–248). New Jersey: Rutgers University Press.

Department of Health and Human Services (2000). *HHS blueprint for action on breastfeeding*.

Dykes, F. (2005). 'Supply' and 'demand': Breastfeeding as labor. *Social Science and Medicine, 60*, 2283–2293.

Eisenberg, A., Murkoff, H. E., & Hathaway, S. E. (1996). *What to expect when you're expecting*. New York: Workman.

Fildes, V. (1986). *Breasts, bottles, and babies: A history of infant feeding*. Edinburgh: Edinburgh University Press.

Giles, F. (2003). *Fresh Milk: The secret life of breasts*. New York: Simon & Schuster.

Gimlin, D. (2002). *Body work: Beauty and self-image in American culture*. Berkeley: University of California Press.

Gorham, D., & Andrews, F. K. (1990). The La Leche League: A feminist perspective. In K. Arnup, A. Levesque, & R. R. Pierson (Eds.), *Delivering motherhood: Maternal ideologies and practices in the Nineteenth and Twentieth Centuries* (pp. 238–69). New York: Routledge.

Hausman, B. (2003). *Mother's milk: Breastfeeding controversies in American culture*. New York: Routledge.

Hays, S. (1996). *The cultural contradictions of motherhood*. New Haven: Yale University Press.

Hochschild, A. R. (2003). *The commercialization of intimate life: Notes from home and work*. Berkeley: University of California Press.

Huggings, K. (1995). *The nursing mothers' companion*. Boston: Harvard Commons Press.

Hulbert, A. (2003). *Raising America: Experts, parents, and a century of advice about children*. New York: Knopf.

Kukla, R. (2006). Ethics and ideology in breastfeeding campaigns. *Hypatia, 21*(1), 157–180.

Ladd-Taylor, M., & Umansky, L. (1998). *"Bad" Mothers: The politics of blame in Twentieth-century America*. New York: New York University Press.

Lareau, A. (2003). *Unequal childhoods: Class, race, and family life*. Berkeley: University of California Press.

Law, J. (2000). The politics of breastfeeding: Assessing risk, dividing labor. *Signs: Journal of Women in Culture and Society, 25*(2), 407–450.

Litt, J. S. (2000). *Medicalized motherhood: Perspectives from the lives of African-American and Jewish women*. New Brunswick: Rutgers University Press.

Maher, V. (1992). *The anthropology of breast-feeding: Natural law or social construct*. New York: Berg.

Martin, E. (1992). *The woman in the body: A cultural analysis of reproduction*. Boston: Beacon.

Murphy, E. (2000). Risk, responsibility, and rhetoric in infant feeding. *Journal of Contemporary Ethnography, 29*(3), 291–325.

Palmer, G. A. (1988). *The politics of breastfeeding*. London: Pondora.

Pugh, A. J. (2005). Selling compromise: Toys, motherhood, and the cultural deal. *Gender Society, 19*(6), 729–749.

Rapp, R. (1999). *Testing women, testing the fetus: The social impact of amniocentesis in America*. New York: Routledge.

Ross Products Division of Abbott (2003). *Breastfeeding trends—2003*. Columbus: Ross Products Division. Available from http://www.ross.com

Ryan, A. S. (1997). The resurgence of breastfeeding in the United States. *Pediatrics, 99*(4), e12.

Ryan, A. S., Wenjun, Z., & Acosta, A. (2002). Breastfeeding continues to increase into the new millennium. *Pediatrics, 110*(6), 1103–1109.

Schmied, V., & Lupton, D. (2001). Blurring the boundaries: Breastfeeding and maternal subjectivity. *Sociology of health and illness, 23*(2), 234–250.

Sears, W., & Sears, M. (1993). *The baby book*. Boston: Little, Brown.

Spangler, A. (2000). Lactation education in the 21st century: A retrospective. *Journal of Human Lactation, 16*(2), 129–131.

Taylor, J. S., Layne, L., & Wozniak, D. F. (2004). *Consuming motherhood.* New Jersey: Rutgers University Press.

Van Esterik, P. (1989). *Beyond the breast-bottle controversy.* New Jersey: Rutgers University Press.

Ward, J. (2000). *La Leche League: At the crossroads of medicine, feminism, and religion.* Chapel Hill: University of North Carolina Press.

Warner, J. (2005). *Perfect madness: Motherhood in the age of anxiety.* New York: Riverhead Books.

WHO (2002). *Infant and young child nutrition: Global strategy, Fifty-fifth world health assembly.* Geneva: WHO.

Wolf, J. H. (2006). What feminists can do for breast-feeding and what breast-feeding can do for feminists. *Signs, 31*(3), 397–424.

Wolf, J. B. (2007) Is the breast really best? Risk and total motherhood in the national breast-feeding awareness campaign. *Journal of Health Politics, Policy and Law, 32*(4), 595–635.

Chapter 3
Attitudes to Breastfeeding

Jane A. Scott

Contents

3.1 Introduction

Most research focussing on the determinants of breastfeeding outcomes, namely initiation and duration, have focussed on the relationship between breastfeeding and socio-demographic and biomedical factors. There is, however, evidence to suggest that maternal attitudes to breastfeeding are a stronger predictor of infant feeding decisions than socio-demographic factors (Losch, Dungy, Russell, & Dusdieker 1995). This is consistent with the Theory of Reasoned Action (Fig. 3.1) first proposed by Ajzen and Fishbein (1977), which attempts to explain human behaviour, in this case breastfeeding, that is under voluntary control. This theory asserts that the best predictor of behaviour is behavioural intention, which is thought to be influenced by attitudes towards the behaviour and social normative perceptions regarding the execution of the behaviour (Montano & Kasprzyk 2008).

Attitudes in turn are determined by the belief that a desired outcome will occur if the behaviour is performed and that the outcome will be beneficial. For example, in

J.A. Scott (✉)
School of Medicine, Flinders University, Adelaide, South Australia, Australia 5042
e-mail: jane.scott@flinders.edu.au

P. Liamputtong (ed.), *Infant Feeding Practices*, DOI 10.1007/978-1-4419-6873-9_3,
© Springer Science+Business Media, LLC 2011

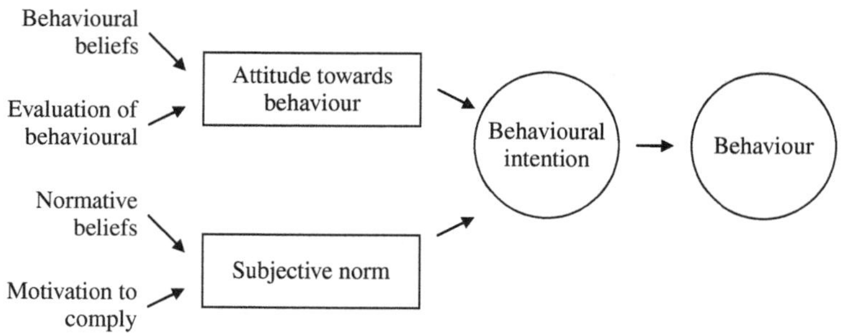

Fig. 3.1 Theory of Reasoned Action

the case of breastfeeding if a mother perceives that her breast milk will adequately nourish her infant and that breastfeeding is convenient and better for the health of her infant, then she will have positive attitudes towards breastfeeding. An individual's social normative perceptions, also referred to as social norms, relate to what that individual believes other people, in particular significant referent individuals (i.e. partners, family and peers) think he or she should do, and by an individual's motivation to comply with the wishes of others (Montano & Kasprzyk 2008). For instance, if a woman believes that most women breastfeed, then she would perceive there is a social norm that favours breastfeeding. Similarly, if she believes that her partner thinks she should breastfeed, then she is more likely to breastfeed. Conversely, if a woman has had limited exposure to positive breastfeeding role models and believes that breastfeeding in public is socially unacceptable, then she will be less likely to breastfeed.

Support for the Theory of Reasoned Action as a useful model to explain breastfeeding outcomes and underpin the planning of breastfeeding interventions is provided by Losch and colleagues (1995). They identify numerous studies that demonstrated a strong correlation between behavioural intentions prior to the birth of a child and subsequent infant feeding practices following birth. Similarly, a consistent association has been reported between intended duration of breastfeeding and actual duration (Cronenwett et al. 1992; Lawson & Tulloch 1995; Scott, Aitkin, Binns, & Aroni 1999). Quarles and colleagues (1995) reported that, after controlling for potentially confounding socio-demographic factors, intended duration was the strongest predictor of the actual duration of breastfeeding.

In this chapter, I will explore the association between maternal breastfeeding attitudes and breastfeeding outcome and factors that influence a woman's attitudes towards breastfeeding. The chapter will also consider how the attitudes of a woman's partner, family, peers and the broader community can influence her normative beliefs and motivation to breastfeed.

3.2 Mothers' Breastfeeding Attitudes

Maternal breastfeeding attitudes have been explored using a variety of quantitative (de la Mora, Russell, Dungy, Losch, & Dusdieker 1999; Shepherd, Power, & Carter

2000; Khoury, Moazzem, Jarjoura, Carothers, & Hinton 2005; Scott, Binns, Oddy, & Graham 2006a; Wagner et al. 2006) and qualitative techniques (Scott, Binns, & Arnold 1997; Dykes & Griffiths 1998; Hoddinott & Pill 1999; Scott, Mostyn, & the Greater Glasgow Breastfeeding Initiative Management Team 2003). Researchers employing quantitative techniques have in general attempted to control for maternal attitudes when exploring the strength and consistency of socio-demographic and biomedical determinants of breastfeeding outcomes. Other researchers have employed qualitative methods in order to gain a richer insight into, and understanding of, factors that influence a woman's decision to initiate and continue breastfeeding.

The Iowa Infant Feeding Attitude Scale (IIFAS) is a simple-to-use instrument developed to quantitatively measure infant feeding attitudes (de la Mora et al. 1999), and has been employed in studies of English-speaking women in the United States (de la Mora et al. 1999), Scotland (Scott, Shaker, & Reid 2004; Dungy, McInnes, Tappin, Wallis, & Oprescu 2008), Northern Ireland (Sittlington, Stewart-Knox, Wright, Bradbury, & Scott 2007) and Australia (Scott et al. 2006a). It has also been used to measure the infant feeding attitudes of a woman's partner (Shaker, Scott, & Reid 2004) and members of her social support network (Dungy et al. 2008). Most recently, it has been used to measure maternal infant feeding attitudes in a group of Romanian mothers (Wallis et al. 2008).

The IIFAS consists of 17 attitude questions covering a variety of domains (see Table 3.1) including nutrition (e.g. 'Breast milk is the ideal food for babies'), health (e.g. 'Babies fed breast milk are healthier than babies who are formula fed'), costs of infant feeding (e.g. 'Formula feeding is more expensive than breastfeeding'), convenience (e.g. 'Formula feeding is more convenient than breastfeeding') and infant bonding (e.g. 'Breastfeeding increase mother–infant bonding') (de la Mora et al.

Table 3.1 Iowa Infant Feeding Attitude Scale Items (IIFAS)

1. The benefits of breast milk last only as long as the baby is breast fed (R).	10. Breastfed babies are more likely to be overfed than formula-fed babies (R).
2. Formula feeding is more convenient than breastfeeding (R).	11. Fathers feel left out if a mother breasts feeds (R).
3. Breastfeeding increases mother infant bonding.	12. Breast milk is the ideal food for babies.
4. Breast milk is lacking in iron (R).	13. Breast milk is more easily digested than formula.
5. Formula-fed babies are more likely to be overfed than breastfed babies.	14. Formula is as healthy for an infant as breast milk (R).
6. Formula feeding is the better choice if the mother plans to go out to work (R).	15. Breastfeeding is more convenient than formula.
7. Mothers who formula feed miss one of the great joys of motherhood.	16. Breast milk is cheaper than formula.
8. Women should not breastfeed in public places such as restaurants (R).	17. A mother who occasionally drinks alcohol should not breastfeed her baby (R).
9. Breastfed babies are healthier than formula-fed babies.	

Items followed by (R) are reversed-scored before computing a total score.
de la Mora et al. (1999)

1999). Approximately, half of the items are worded in a manner favourable to breastfeeding and the remaining favourable to formula feeding. Participants are asked to respond to each individual item using a bipolar 5-point scale (strongly disagree–strongly agree). Items that favour formula feeding are reverse-scored (i.e. 1=5, 2=4, 4=2 and 5=1), and a total attitude score is computed via an equally weighted sum of responses to the individual items. Total attitude scores range from 17, reflecting positive formula feeding attitudes, to a high of 85 indicative of attitudes that favour breastfeeding. The IIFAS has been shown to have robust internal consistency when used among English-speaking groups with alphas ranging from 0.79 to 0.86 for mothers (de la Mora et al. 1999; Shaker et al. 2004), 0.77 for women's partners (Shaker et al. 2004), and 0.89 for their social network members (Dungy et al. 2008). It was shown to have adequate internal reliability ($\alpha = 0.50$ to 0.63) when translated into Romanian (Wallis et al. 2008).

There have been calls for the development of assessment tools to conduct epidemiological and socio-behavioural 'diagnosis' of infant feeding practices (Wallis et al. 2008). The IIFAS is potentially one such tool, having been shown to be a valid predictor of breastfeeding outcome in a variety of countries. That is, women with higher IIFAS scores were more likely to intend to breastfeed (de la Mora et al. 1999; Sittlington et al. 2007), to initiate breastfeeding (Scott et al. 2004; Sittlington et al. 2007) and to breastfeed for longer (Scott et al. 2006a) compared to women with lower scores. Scott and colleagues (2004), in a study of Scottish women, reported that the IIFAS was the strongest independent predictor of breastfeeding initiation after controlling for age, maternal education and level of social deprivation. When calculated for a 10-point difference in attitude score, a woman with an IIFAS score of 65, for instance, was more than 4 times more likely to breastfeed as a woman with a score of 55.

Wallis and colleagues (2008) identify a number of advantages in using the IIFAS to assess infant feeding attitudes.

1. It is easy to administer and score, making it a low-cost and effective means of gathering information.
2. It can be administered as a needs assessment tool to understand general attitudes or to pinpoint specific attitudes or gaps in knowledge through item analysis, thus allowing practitioners to shape breastfeeding promotion programs that specifically target relevant issues.
3. Once a program is implemented, it can be used as a pre/post-test or with comparison or control groups to measure program effectiveness.

While other researchers (Shepherd et al. 2000; Khoury et al. 2005; Wagner et al. 2006) have quantitatively measured and analysed maternal breastfeeding attitudes and beliefs, the psychometric properties of their instruments as a whole, and individual items, have not been reported to the same extent as the internal reliability and predictive validity of the IIFAS. Nor have their instruments been employed in such a wide variety of settings as the IIFAS. Nevertheless, they all include a number of items designed to identify maternal attitudes and beliefs that are similar to items in the IIFAS and shown to be predictive of infant feeding outcomes. For instance, Wagner and colleagues (2006) reported that of the 80.2% of mothers in their US study who agreed that breastfeeding was healthier than formula feeding, 74.5% initiated breastfeeding. While of the 19.8% who were neutral or disagreed with the statement, only one woman chose to breastfed. Similarly, of the 51.9% of mothers who agreed with the statement, 'Breastfeeding would be easy and convenient', 92.9% chose to breastfeed.

3.3 Embarrassment with Breastfeeding

Embarrassment with breastfeeding is frequently cited by women, particularly from Western cultures, as a reason for not breastfeeding. Focus group interviews of low-income women from a deprived area of Glasgow (Scott et al. 2003), recognised for its low breastfeeding rates, revealed that virtually all of the women interviewed were embarrassed with the prospect of breastfeeding in public and often went to great lengths to avoid having to do so. This included preparing for an away-from-home excursion by expressing milk at home to take with them when out, expressing milk or breast feeding in a toilet stall whilst out or giving the occasional supplementary formula feed (see also Chapter 2 in this volume). Similarly, Whelan and Lupton (1998), in an earlier study of low-income women in the South West of England, reported that many women viewed everyday activities such as shopping, visiting family and friends, and walking in the park, as being out of bounds with a breastfeeding baby, as they lacked the confidence to breastfeed out of the immediate vicinity of their home.

It appears that women embarrassed at the prospect of breastfeeding in public often will confine themselves to home or attempt to restrict their movement and length of time that they are away from home to avoid the need to nurse in public. However, this self-imposed confinement is not feasible in the long-term and women will often reach the stage when the immediate need to breastfeed their infant finally overrides their embarrassment and they will breastfeed in a public place. Usually, to discover that once they have overcome their initial embarrassment, they are less concerned about breastfeeding in public places and consider it to be other people's problem if they are offended (Scott et al. 1997; Scott et al. 2003; cf Chapter 2).

Most women's embarrassment with breastfeeding in public stems from how they perceive other people will react to them when they breastfed. In particular, they are fearful of other people commenting upon them breastfeeding, or even showing disapproval for breastfeeding. The study of Glaswegian women by Scott and colleagues (2003) revealed that while the majority of these women agreed that there was nothing 'shameful' or 'disgusting' about breastfeeding, they felt that other people often viewed it as something 'dirty' (see also Chapters 2 and 7 in this volume).

While most women anticipate a negative reaction from others to their breastfeeding in public, a study in Ontario, Canada (Sheeshka et al. 2001), suggested that this may not necessarily be the case. In this study, bottle-feeding and breastfeeding mothers made visits to family restaurants and shopping malls. The reaction of others when a woman from either group fed her infant in public were observed and evaluated by trained, independent observers. Although more total attention was paid to breastfeeding mothers, there was no difference in the amount of overtly negative or positive attention given during breastfeeding versus bottle-feeding. While the breastfeeding mothers acknowledged that they did not receive the undesirable attention that they anticipated they nevertheless felt vulnerable breastfeeding in public and admitted that they would be extremely embarrassed if someone complained.

Sheeshka and colleagues (2001) asked women what enabled them to breastfeed in public despite the stresses involved. Determination, confidence and commitment to breastfeeding were considered important. They also noted that becoming skilled at breastfeeding and having positive experiences feeding in public were important for building confidence.

3.4 Fathers' Breastfeeding Attitudes

As previously discussed, the Theory of Reasoned Action asserts that an individual's intention to perform a behaviour is influenced by his or her perceived social norms, which are determined by what that individual believes other people think he or she should do (Montano & Kasprzyk 2008). In keeping with this theory, fathers have been shown to participate in and influence the choice of infant feeding method by acting as key supports or deterrents to breastfeeding by the mother (Jordon & Wall 1993; see Chapter 12 in this volume). In Western cultures in particular, a father's feeding preference has been shown consistently to exert a significant influence over both the incidence (Black, Blair, Jones, & DuRant 1990; Giugliani, Caiaffa, Vogelhut, Witter, & Perman 1994b; Littman, VanderBrug Medendorp, & Goldfarb 1994; Scott, Oddy, Binns, & Graham 2006b) and duration of breastfeeding (Scott et al. 2006a).

In a Brazilian study, Giugliani and colleagues (1994b) reported that the father's opinion about breastfeeding was the most important factor related to breastfeeding, regardless of maternal age, educational level, ethnic group and marital status. Mothers who said that their partners favoured breastfeeding were significantly more likely to breastfeed, compared with mothers whose partners either preferred bottle-feeding or were ambivalent about infant feeding. Similarly, Birenbaum, Fuchs, and Reichman (1989) used multivariate analysis techniques to study the interdependence of factors influencing the initiation of breastfeeding and reported that husbands' opinions regarding breastfeeding appeared to be the major determinant for the initiation of breastfeeding in a population of Israeli women. More recently, Scott and colleagues, in an Australian study, reported that women who perceived that their partner preferred breastfeeding were significantly more likely to initiate breastfeeding (Scott et al. 2006b) and to breastfeed for longer (Scott et al. 2006a) compared to women who perceived their partner to either prefer formula feeding or be ambivalent as to how they fed their infant.

In most studies (Birenbaum et al. 1989; Scott et al. 2006b), the attitudes of fathers were not measured directly and the measure of paternal support for breastfeeding usually represented a woman's perception of her partner's attitudes. Obviously, her answers may be biased by her own decision. For instance, a mother who is herself feeling ambivalent about breastfeeding might influence and/or misinterpret her partner's attitudes. This argument is supported by the work of Freed, Fraley, and Schanler (1993) who showed in a US study that women were unable to accurately predict their partner's attitudes and opinions regarding breastfeeding, despite having reported that they had discussed infant feeding plans with their partner. A large number of women incorrectly predicted negative responses from fathers, raising the possibility that the father's negative influence on breastfeeding is based on the mother's inaccurate perceptions. Perception of a lack of spousal support may decrease enthusiasm for breastfeeding among women who had planned to initiate lactation. Alternatively, the mother may have accurately perceived her partner's attitude to breastfeeding due to her knowledge and comprehension of his attitudes to other aspects of her bodily and emotional life. This latter argument is supported by a study by Scott and colleagues (2004), which measured and compared the infant feeding attitudes of Scottish couples using the IIFAS. They found reasonable congruence of couple's total IIFAS scores and good congruence of attitudes for individual scale items. This suggests that a woman's perception of her partner's infant feeding attitude is a reasonable proxy of paternal attitudes when they cannot be measured directly.

The level or amount of support provided by the father will depend on his commitment to, and expectations of, breastfeeding (Gamble & Morse 1992). Freed, Fraley, and Schanler (1992) proposed that variations in support for breastfeeding among fathers might be explained by a lack of information or the harbouring of negative cultural perceptions. Previous studies have found that fathers of bottle-fed children were more likely to believe that breastfeeding is bad for the breasts, makes breasts ugly, interferes with sex, is painful, and that prevention of sore and cracked nipples is not possible (Freed et al. 1992; Giugliani et al. 1994a).When compared with fathers of breastfed infants, fathers of children who were bottle-fed were generally unaware of the benefits of breastfeeding for either their child or their partner and were comparatively less aware of how a father can provide practical and psychological support for breastfeeding (Freed et al. 1992; Giugliani et al. 1994a).

The last half century has seen dramatic changes in the parenting role of fathers. Fathers are now encouraged, and expected, to be present at the birth of the child and to participate in antenatal and parenting programs. Furthermore, they are expected by health care professionals to encourage and support breastfeeding. However, not all fathers will have positive reactions to breastfeeding. New fathers may experience negative and conflicting feelings such as jealousy, inadequacy, exclusion and sexual frustration (Waletzky 1979). Fathers (and their partners) often have an idealised picture of postpartum happiness and are unprepared for these negative feelings and unaware of the particular emotional problems that may relate to breastfeeding.

Fathers should be included in breastfeeding discussions, however, few opportunities exist for fathers to prepare themselves to offer the emotional and practical support required by their partners and health professionals should seek ways of including fathers in breastfeeding discussions. For instance, breastfeeding literature should not focus solely on the mother–infant pair, but should highlight the role that partners can play in supporting and encouraging the breastfeeding mother (Freed et al. 1992). Similarly, the content of antenatal and parenting classes should be expanded to allow time for explanation of the supportive roles fathers can play in the breastfeeding process. Losch and colleagues (1995) recommend that educational forums should include males and that they should occur before the birth of the baby and even as early as childhood and adolescence.

3.5 Societal Attitudes to Prolonged Breastfeeding

The World Health Organization recommends that a woman exclusively breastfeed her infant for the first 6 months and that she continues breastfeeding into the second year of life or longer (WHO/UNICEF 2003). While the practice of breastfeeding beyond 12 months may be common in traditional societies (Rao & Kanade 1992; Liamputtong Rice 2000; Tsianakas & Liamputtong 2007; see also Chapter 9 in this volume), it is relatively unusual in most Western cultures. For instance, in Australia and the United States, only one in four children are still receiving breast milk at 12 months of age (Donath & Amir 2005; Grummer-Strawn, Scanlon, & Fein 2008), while in Italy only one in ten children still receive breast milk at this age (Giovannini et al. 2004).

There appears to be a culturally approved age by which time a child should have been weaned from the breast. This is not necessarily measured in terms of chronological age, but is more related to a child's development. For instance, Scott and colleagues (1997) explored social attitudes to prolonged breastfeeding in a series of sex- and age-specific focus groups involving mothers, fathers, young male university students and adolescent girls. When shown a picture of what appeared to be a toddler wearing day clothes and shoes, there was a general consensus across all groups that the child was too old to still be breastfed. Of interest was that the photographed child was in fact less than 12-months-old but large for his age, being above the 95 percentile for both weight and height.

A large national survey of public attitudes to breastfeeding conducted in the United States reported that two in three adults think that babies should not be breastfed beyond 12 months of age (Li et al. 2004). This finding is consistent with the results of the Australian focus group interviews (Scott et al. 1997), which indicated that there was general consensus amongst the male university students that up to 12 months was an appropriate length of time for a child to be breastfed. After this age most expressed some concern over the appropriateness of breastfeeding toddlers, especially with regard to the effect that this might have on the psychological development of the child. Comments such as 'that poor kid's going to have an enormous lot of trouble' and 'missing a step in the maturity process' were common. Concern was also expressed by mothers and fathers that prolonged breastfeeding would make the child too dependent on the mother. There was almost unanimous agreement amongst the adolescent girls that the child was too old to be breastfed. Several thought that it would cause the child to be too dependent on the mother and were 'disgusted' at the possibility of a woman breastfeeding an older child in public. Most participants thought that by the time a child can walk, eat family foods or ask for the breast – in short becomes an aware person – that he or she should have been weaned.

3.6 Societal Attitudes to Breastfeeding in Public

Li and associates have attempted to quantitatively measure public attitudes and beliefs about breastfeeding in a series of studies in the United States (Li, Fridinger, & Grummer-Strawn 2002; Li et al. 2004; Hannan, Benton-Davis, & Grummer-Strawn 2005). They included a number of breastfeeding-related items in an annually conducted national mail survey. Participants in these surveys represent a demographically diverse sample of people, which is weighted to reflect the general population and as such the survey results reflect the social and cultural norms of Americans at the turn of the 21st century. While public perceptions were generally positive for the majority of items, just over one quarter (27%) considered breastfeeding in public 'embarrassing' (Li et al. 2002). In a subsequent survey, while 43.1% of American adults supported a woman's right to breastfeeding in public, only one in four adults (27.9%) thought it appropriate to show a woman breastfeeding her baby on television shows (Li et al. 2004). The work of Li and colleagues (2002) highlights the apparent contradiction between society's endorsement of breastfeeding as the best way to feed a baby while at the same time frowning on, or even prohibiting, breastfeeding in public (Glover, Manaena-Biddle, & Waldon 2007; and cf. Chapters 2, 7, and 15 in this volume).

While these days in Western society, the sight of bare breasts on our television and cinema screens and on the beach is viewed as commonplace, the act of breastfeeding in public is still viewed as being offensive or at least distasteful by some sections of society. This attitude to breastfeeding in public is influenced largely by the dichotomous role of the breast in Western society, namely the sexual, or what Natalie Angier (1999) calls the aesthetic role, and the functional or physiological role of the breast. It is the convergence of the functional and aesthetic role that Angier contends 'disturbs and irritates us'. See Chapter 2 in this volume.

3.7 Media Portrayal of Breastfeeding

The way in which breastfeeding is portrayed in the media both informs and reflects public attitudes towards breastfeeding. The common belief among Western women that breastfeeding in public is embarrassing and unacceptable (McIntyre, Hiller, & Turnbull 1999; Scott et al. 2003), is often reinforced by the negative portrayal of breastfeeding in the media, as evidenced by the caustic comment of a Scottish newspaper columnist in response to seeing a woman breastfeed in a public park. This comment, while more than 10-years-old, still represents the views of a section of Scottish and other Western societies (Li et al. 2002).

Alright, dear, we saw you. Now you can put it away. The exhibitionist mother who on Sunday selected a bench just inside the Royal Botanic Gardens to breast-feed her baby made everyone's day

Evening News
Edinburgh 19 July 1994

A newspaper item such as this will contribute to and reinforce a woman's perception of breastfeeding-related social norms in her community and conceivably influence her breastfeeding behaviour. On reading this item, she might perceive that breastfeeding in public is not socially acceptable and be dissuaded from doing so. If following the birth of her infant, she initiates breastfeeding but does not feel comfortable or confident enough to breastfeed in public because of perceived public disapproval, she must by necessity restrict her movements outside the home. While in the early postpartum period she may find this acceptable and even desirable, eventually she will wish, or need, to be absent from her home for longer periods of time during which time her infant likely will require feeding. In order to conform to her perceived social norms, she will be forced to bottle-feed her infant, either expressed breast milk (at best) or formula, or alternatively in the worst case will discontinue breastfeeding (see Chapters 2 and 7 in this volume).

Even in Australia, which has near universal breastfeeding initiation rates, the act of a breastfeeding mother being asked to leave a restaurant can cause a media furore and divided public opinion. This was seen as recently as April 2009 when a mother breastfeeding her infant in an upmarket restaurant in a five star hotel in Perth was asked by a staff member to leave the restaurant in order to breastfeed her infant elsewhere. The incident received wide media coverage with talk of the case being taken up by the Equal Rights Commission. In the days that followed, the management of the hotel involved offered a public apology to the woman, explaining that it was not hotel policy to prohibit breastfeeding in public areas of their establishment, but that this was an isolated incident in which an individual staff member had taken it upon themselves to ask the mother to breastfeed elsewhere. Even though the media coverage of this event was largely pro-breastfeeding, the publicity nevertheless will have evoked a range of reactions among breastfeeding women. For instance, the incident prompted a breastfeeding 'sit-in' by a group of mothers in the lobby of the hotel (at which time they were warmly welcomed by management and served morning tea). However, a less confident mother may have empathised with the woman at the centre of the incident and the embarrassment and perhaps shame at being asked to leave the restaurant, further undermining her confidence to breastfeed in public.

Of interest was a lively debate, primarily by males, which ensued on a football web chat forum. A representative sample of the range of opinions expressed in a total of 33 related postings on the forum (FootyGoss 2009) is provided in Table 3.2. Again, highly publicised incidences of this kind, no matter how uncommon, when reported in the media continue to promulgate the general impression that breastfeeding in public is socially unacceptable.

Foss and Southwell (2006, p. 2) argue that the mass media has often discouraged breastfeeding and encouraged the widespread adoption of breastfeeding alternatives.

Table 3.2 Representative example of comments posted on a football webchat forum after a well-publicised incident in which a breastfeeding woman was asked to leave a hotel restaurant

Negative comments	Supportive comments
The first comment Here we go again. A young mother gets her five minutes of fame and the attention off the Perth media all because she was asked to discreetly breastfeed her baby in the hotel restaurant.	The error lay with the Hyatt, fair and square. Their management admitted as much! . . . Next time you hear a little Squirt screaming for its meal in a restaurant, what would you have the lady do?
	Mutter under your breath, "For Christ's sake, feed the little brat (*sic*) will ya". "What's a bit of breast amongst customers?!"
One thing in the argument I don't get is the "it's natural, so it should be ok". Going to the toilet, spitting, copulation, etc. are all natural – but we don't want them happening next to us whilst at a restaurant.	There is nothing dirty or unhygienic about breastfeeding, unlike those other acts.
	I have no problem with it and if you are offended by it you are going to struggle in life. You rarely 'see' anything during the feeding and as someone rightly pointed out on the radio, when you ask the staff to heat a bottle they refuse. What other option is there? Are mothers with newborns not allowed to have a life while they are raising a kid?
	. . . for Gods sake if a baby needs a feed then what is the problem, I've never ever seen a woman flop the tit out in plain view of everyone, All women who breast feed throw a towel or cloth over their shoulder and shove the kid on the tit. I know I'd much prefer to see a woman do that than putting up with a screaming baby. And who cares where this happens, whether at the Hyatt or at McDonalds – if a baby needs a feed it needs a feed.
	Get over yourself . . . it's a natural part of life. To the idiot who said 'why can't they do it in toilet' are you a complete psycho??? Do u eat your food in a toilet . . .?

Source: FootyGoss (2009)

This is particularly the case with media advertising, which 'not only alerts the public to new merchandise but also teaches people why they need the product'. They contend that advertising contributed to the decline in breastfeeding that began in the 1950s by promoting the idea of 'scientific motherhood' and the modernity of infant formula. They analysed the relationship between the frequency of advertisements for hand feeding (which included infant formula/ cereal/solid food or hand feeding equipment) in a popular parenting magazine from 1972 to 2000 and breastfeeding initiation rates. Their content analysis demonstrated a negative correlation between the number of advertisements for hand feeding in a year and the reported breastfeeding rate in the subsequent year.

While the entertainment media, particularly medical dramas, have successfully been used to raise public awareness of important health issues and present health promotion messages (Langlieb, Cooper, & Gielen 1999), the media rarely present positive information on breastfeeding. For instance, Henderson, Kitzinger, and Green (2000) undertook a content analysis of all British television programs that made reference to infant feeding over a 1 month period. During the monitoring period, there were 235 references to infant feeding, 194 related to bottle-feeding and 41 to breastfeeding. Bottle-feeding was not only more commonly referenced than breastfeeding, it was more positively presented. Furthermore, breastfeeding was rarely shown (just one scene in a popular soap opera), with most references to breastfeeding being verbal. On the other hand, most references to bottle-feeding were visual (outweighing verbal references by 7:1). The way in which bottle-feeding and breastfeeding were portrayed was also very different. Bottle-feeding was portrayed as being less problematic than breastfeeding and was associated with ordinary families, whereas breastfeeding was associated with middle-class or celebrity women and references frequently highlighted potential problems or portrayed breastfeeding as a source of humour and embarrassment. Henderson and colleagues (2000, p. 1198) contend that the limited media coverage of breastfeeding 'may, of course, reflect the reality of what is publicly visible – that is, that many women do not breastfeed in public'. They further argue that the limited portrayal of breastfeeding 'may also help perpetuate a lack of acceptance of breastfeeding in public'.

The coverage of breastfeeding in the press media is no more encouraging. For instance, Henderson and colleagues (2000) reported that the majority of items in the British press related to problems associated with breastfeeding with few providing suggestions for how the problems might be resolved. Similarly, a discourse analysis of the way in which breastfeeding was represented in the Australian press and popular magazines over a 6 month period revealed mixed messages (Henderson 1999). While breastfeeding was seen as being natural and the best way to feed infants, it was nevertheless portrayed as being fraught with problems. Examples of problems included that breastfeeding was demanding and it was difficult to hold down a fulltime job and breastfeed, that many breastfeeding babies cry a lot and that it was necessary for mothers to make a number of lifestyle changes such as avoid caffeine, alcohol and smoking in order to successfully breastfeed.

One notable example of where television has been used successfully to promote breastfeeding is a 6 month mass media campaign conducted in Brazil in the early 1980s (Castello Branco 1990). A series of four television advertisements were developed based on qualitative research with the target audience, including extensive pre-testing. Each advertisement included a testimonial by a local celebrity appropriate to the theme of the message with the goal of providing popular and credible sources of the messages and role models. All advertisements were linked with the same slogan '*Breastfeeding – Six months that build up life*', to establish a common goal. An evaluation of the campaign 5 years later indicated that there was still recall of some of the television advertisements and that there had been significant and positive changes in the duration and prevalence of breastfeeding, which were at there highest when the campaign was at its peak. This campaign and the successful use of medical dramas and soap operas to present other health messages (Langlieb et al. 1999) highlight the potential for using television to positively promote breastfeeding as the optimal way to feed an infant and to increase the social acceptability of breastfeeding in public.

3.8 Conclusion

The Theory of Reasoned Action is a useful model for understanding how breastfeeding behaviour is influenced by both a woman's personal attitudes towards breastfeeding and what she perceives to be social normative perceptions regarding breastfeeding. If a woman perceives that those in her immediate social support network, in particular her partner or society in general, do not value or encourage breastfeeding, then she is unlikely to choose to breastfeed. In Western society, while breastfeeding is generally acknowledged as the optimal way to feed an infant, there still remains a belief amongst sectors of the population that it is inappropriate for a woman to breastfeed in public and may even be considered pornographic. Individuals may disapprove of a woman breastfeeding in public, because in Western cultures the female breast has a dichotomous role and individuals may be unable to dissociate the sexual or aesthetic role from the functional or physiological role.

The media both informs and reflects societal attitudes to breastfeeding. The fact that breastfeeding is seldom portrayed in the entertainment media may be a reflection of real life, and that in Western cultures many women are too embarrassed to breastfeed in public and will often go to great lengths to avoid doing so. On the other hand, the limited and often negative portrayal of breastfeeding on television may be a reflection of, and contribute to, a societal attitude that breastfeeding in public is unacceptable. The positive portrayal of breastfeeding on television and film and in other public arenas will go a long way towards making it 'normal' in our society, positively influencing a woman's perception that breastfeeding is the social norm when it comes to feeding her infant. In turn, as more women have positive attitudes towards and experience with breastfeeding, society itself will change and become more baby friendly.

References

Ajzen, I., & Fishbein, M. (1977). Attitude-behaviour relations: A theoretical analysis and review of empirical research. *Psychology Bulletin, 84*, 888–918.

Angier, N. (1999). *Woman: An intimate geography*. Melbourne: Scribe Publications.

Birenbaum, E., Fuchs, C., & Reichman, B. (1989). Demographic factors influencing the initiation of breast-feeding in an Israeli urban population. *Pediatrics, 83*, 519–523.

Black, R. F., Blair, J., Jones, V. N., & DuRant, R. (1990). Infant feeding decisions among pregnant women from a WIC population in Georgia. *Journal of the American Dietetic Association, 90*(2), 255–259.

Castello Branco, H. (1990). Breastfeeding on prime-time in Brazil. *Development Communication Report, 71*, 4–7.

Cronenwett, L., Stukel, T., Kearney, M., Barrett, J., Covington, C., Del Monte, K., et al. (1992). Single daily bottle use in the early weeks postpartum and breastfeeding outcomes. *Pediatrics, 90*(5), 760–766.

de la Mora, A., Russell, D. W., Dungy, C. I., Losch, M., & Dusdieker, L. (1999). The Iowa Infant Feeding Attitude Scale: Analysis of reliability and validity. *Journal of Applied Social Psychology, 29*(11), 2362–2380.

Donath, S. M., & Amir, L. H. (2005). Breastfeeding and the introduction of solids in Australian infants: Data from the 2001 National Health Survey. *Australian & New Zealand Journal of Public Health, 29*(2), 171–175.

Dungy, C., McInnes, R., Tappin, D., Wallis, A., & Oprescu, F. (2008). Infant feeding attitudes and knowledge among socioeconomically disadvantaged women in Glasgow. *Maternal and Child Health Journal, 12*(3), 313–322.

Dykes, F., & Griffiths, H. (1998). Societal influences upon initiation and continuation of breastfeeding. *British Journal of Midwifery, 6*(2), 76–80.

FootyGoss (2009). Breastfeeding at the Hyatt. Retrieved 12 November 2009, from http://www.footygoss.com/index.php/forums/viewthread/11275/

Foss, K. A., & Southwell, B. G. (2006). Infant feeding an the media: The relationship between *Parents' Magazine* content and breastfeeding, 1972–2000. *International Breastfeeding Journal, 1*,10. Available from http://www.internationalbreastfeedingjournal.com/content/1/1/10

Freed, G. L., Fraley, J. K., & Schanler, R. J. (1992). Attitudes of expectant fathers regarding breastfeeding. *Pediatrics, 90*(2), 224–227.

Freed, G. L., Fraley, J. K., & Schanler, R. J. (1993). Accuracy of expectant mothers' predictions of fathers' attitudes regarding breast-feeding. *Journal of Family Practice, 37*(2), 148–152.

Gamble, D., & Morse, J. M. (1992). Fathers of breastfed infants: Postponing and types of involvement. *International Journal of Gynecology and Obstetrics, 22*(4), 358–365.

Giovannini, M., Riva, E., Banderali, G., Scaglioni, S., Veehof, S., Sala, M., et al. (2004). Feeding practices of infants through the first year of life in Italy. *Acta Paediatrica, 93*, 492–497.

Giugliani, E. R. J., Bronner, Y., Caiaffa, W. T., Vogelhut, J., Witter, F. R., & Perman, P. A. (1994a). Are fathers prepared to encourage their partners to breast feed? A study about fathers' knowledge of breast feeding. *Acta Paediatrica, 83*, 1127–1131.

Giugliani, E. R. J., Caiaffa, W. T., Vogelhut, J., Witter, F. R., & Perman, J. A. (1994b). Effect of breastfeeding support from different sources on mothers' decisions to breastfeed. *Journal of Human Lactation, 10*(3), 157–161.

Glover, M., Manaena-Biddle, H., & Waldon, J. (2007). Influences that affect Maori women breastfeeding. *Breastfeeding Review, 15*(2), 5–14.

Grummer-Strawn, L. M., Scanlon, K. S., & Fein, S. B. (2008). Infant feeding and feeding transition during the first year of life. *Pediatrics, 122*(Suppl 2), S36–S42.

Hannan, A., Li, R., Benton-Davis, S., & Grummer-Strawn, L. (2005). Regional variation in public opinion about breastfeeding in the United States. *Journal of Human Lactation, 21*(3), 284–288.

Henderson, A. (1999). Mixed messages about the meanings of breast-feeding representations in the Australian press and popular magazines. *Midwifery, 15*, 24–31.

Henderson, L., Kitzinger, J., & Green, J. (2000). Representing infant feeding: content analysis of British media portrayals of bottle-feeding and breast feeding. *British Medical Journal, 321*, 1196–1198.

Hoddinott, P., & Pill, R. (1999). Nobody actually tells you: A study of infant feeding. *British Journal of Midwifery, 7*, 558–565.

Jordon, P. L., & Wall, V. R. (1993). Supporting the father when an infant is breastfed. *Journal of Human Lactation, 9*(1), 1993.

Khoury, A., Moazzem, S., Jarjoura, C., Carothers, C., & Hinton, A. (2005). Breast-feeding initiation in low income women: Role of attitudes, support, and perceived control. *Women's Health Issues, 15*, 64–72.

Langlieb, A., Cooper, C., & Gielen, A. (1999). Linking health promotion with entertainment television. *American Journal of Public Health, 89*(7), 1116–1117.

Lawson, K., & Tulloch, M. I. (1995). Breastfeeding duration: Prenatal intentions and postnatal practices. *Journal of Advanced Nursing, 22*, 841–849.

Li, R., Fridinger, F., & Grummer-Strawn, L. (2002). Public perceptions on breastfeeding constraints. *Journal of Human Lactation, 18*(3), 227–235.

Li, R., Hsia, J., Fridinger, F., Hussain, A., Benton-Davis, S., & Grummer-Strawn, L. (2004). Public beliefs about breastfeeding policies in various settings. *Journal of the American Dietetic Association, 104*(7), 1162–1168.

Liamputtong Rice, P. (2000). *Hmong woman and reproduction*. Westport: Bergin & Garvey.

Littman, H., VanderBrug Medendorp, S., & Goldfarb, J. (1994). The decision to breastfeed. The importance of fathers' approval. *Clinical Pediatrics, 33*(4), 214–219.

Losch, M., Dungy, C., Russell, D., & Dusdieker, L. (1995). Impact of attitudes on maternal decision regarding infant feeding. *The Journal of Pediatrics, 126*, 507–514.

McIntyre, E., Hiller, J., & Turnbull, D. (1999). Determinants of infant feeding practices in a low socio-economic areas: Identifying environmental barriers to breastfeeding. *Australian and New Zealand Journal of Public Health, 23*, 207–209.

Montano, D. E., & Kasprzyk, D. (2008). Theory of reasoned action, theory of planned behaviour, and the integrated behavioural model. In K. Glanz, B. K. Rimer, & K. Viswanath (Eds.), *Health behavior and health education: Theory, research, and practice* (pp. 67–96). San Francisco: Jossey-Bass.

Quarles, A., Williams, P. D., Hoyle, D. A., Brimeyer, M., & Williams, A. R. (1995). Mothers' intention, age, education and the duration and management of breastfeeding. *Maternal-Child Nursing Journal, 22*(3), 102–108.

Rao, S., & Kanade, A. N. (1992). Prolonged breast-feeding and malnutrition among rural Indian children below 3 years of age. *European Journal of Clinical Nutrition, 46*, 187–195.

Scott, J., Binns, C., & Arnold, R. (1997). Attitudes towards breast-feeding in Perth, Australia: Qualitative analysis. *Journal of Nutrition Education, 29*, 244–249.

Scott, J., Aitkin, I., Binns, C., & Aroni, R. (1999). Factors associated with the duration of breastfeeding amongst women in Perth, Australia. *Acta Paediatrica, 88*, 416–421.

Scott, J., Mostyn, T., & the Greater Glasgow Breastfeeding Initiative Management Team (2003). Breastfeeding in a bottle-feeding culture. *Journal of Human Lactation, 19*, 270–277.

Scott, J., Shaker, I., & Reid, M. (2004). Parental attitudes toward breastfeeding: Their association with feeding outcome at hospital discharge. *Birth, 31*(2), 125–131.

Scott, J. A., Binns, C. W., Oddy, W. H., & Graham, K. I. (2006a). Predictors of breastfeeding duration: evidence from a cohort study. *Pediatrics, 17*, e646–e655.

Scott, J. A., Oddy, W. H., Binns, C. W., & Graham, K. I. (2006b). Temporal changes in the determinants of breastfeeding initiation. *Birth, 33*, 37–45.

Shaker, I., Scott, J., & Reid, M. (2004). Infant feeding attitudes of expectant parents: Breastfeeding and formula feeding. *Journal of Advanced Nursing, 45*(3), 260–268.

Sheeshka, J., Potter, B., Norrie, E., Valaitis, R., Adams, G., & Kuczynski, L. (2001). Women's experiences of breastfeeding in public places. *Journal of Human Lactation, 17*, 31–38.

Shepherd, C., Power, K., & Carter, H. (2000). Examining the correspondence of breastfeeding and bottle-feeding couples' infant feeding attitude. *Journal of Advanced Nursing, 31*(3), 651–660.

Sittlington, J., Stewart-Knox, B., Wright, M., Bradbury, I., & Scott, J. A. (2007). Infant-feeding attitudes of expectant mothers in Northern Ireland. *Health Education Research, 22*(4), 561–570.

Tsianakas, V., & Liamputtong, P. (2007). Infant feeding practices and Afghan immigrant women in Australia. In P. Liamputtong (Ed.), *Childrearing and infant care issues: A cross-cultural perspective* (pp. 249–273). New York: Nova Science Publishers.

Wagner, C. L., Wagner, M. T., Ebeling, M., Chatman, K. G., Cohen, M., & Hulsey, T. C. (2006). The role of personality and other factors in a mother's decision to initiate breastfeeding. *Journal of Human Lactation, 22*(1), 16–26.

Waletzky, L. R. (1979). Husbands' problems with breast-feeding. *American Journal of Orthopsychiatry, 49*(2), 349–352.
Wallis, A. B., Brînzaniuc, A., Razvan Chereche, F., Oprescu, F., Eirlincan, E., David, I., et al. (2008). Reliability and validity of the Romanian version of a scale to measure infant feeding attitudes and knowledge. *Acta Paediatrica, 97*(9), 1194–1199.
Whelan, A., & Lupton, P. (1998). Promoting successful breastfeeding among women with a low income. *Midwifery, 14*, 94–100.
WHO/UNICEF (2003). *Global strategy for infant and young child feeding*. Geneva: World Health Organization.

Chapter 4
The Imperative to Breastfeed: An Australian Perspective

Athena Sheehan and Virginia Schmied

Contents

4.1 Introduction

Australia is considered to have a high breastfeeding initiation rate. Research has demonstrated that the main reason that many women choose to breastfeed their baby is based on their understanding that 'breast is best'. This is not surprising given that the benefits of breastfeeding are broadly promoted and a number of strategies have been deliberately employed globally, nationally and locally to actively support and promote breastfeeding. In this chapter, we argue that in Australia there is now a well-constructed cultural imperative to breastfeed. The message of 'breast is best'

A. Sheehan (✉)
Faculty of Nursing and Health, Avondale College, 185 Fox Valley Rd, Wahroonga, Australia 2076
e-mail: athena.sheehan@avondale.edu.au

P. Liamputtong (ed.), *Infant Feeding Practices*, DOI 10.1007/978-1-4419-6873-9_4,

© Springer Science+Business Media, LLC 2011

is powerful and is transmitted through public health and professional discourses and increasingly within the broader social and cultural context influencing the personal decisions and experiences of women. Most women in Australia make the decision to initiate breastfeeding, yet many women abandon the practice within the first 6 weeks following the birth of their baby. It appears that personal commitment, prenatal preparation and support to initiate breastfeeding is not always enough to sustain breastfeeding. In this chapter, we assert that the current investment in promoting and supporting women to initiate breastfeeding in Australia is having little impact on the longevity of breastfeeding and, for many women, appears to be causing a high level of emotional distress. We argue that the current public health policy, professional and social investment in breastfeeding initiation may be better directed at providing appropriate support in the weeks following birth for women who wish to breastfeed (see also Chapter 5 in this volume).

The purpose of this chapter is twofold. Firstly, we describe public health policies promoting breastfeeding in Australia and, consider how these policies may be impacting on the practice of midwives and nurses who have a key role in providing effective support for breastfeeding women. Second, we will use findings from a grounded theory study conducted by the first author that explored women's experiences of infant feeding in the first 6 weeks post-birth, to present women's responses to the cultural imperative to breastfeed in Australia. Specifically, this chapter aims to articulate from an Australian perspective the current imperative to breastfeed and the impact this has on women's experiences and decisions to breastfeed.

4.2 The Benefits of Breastfeeding

Exclusive breastfeeding for the first 6 months has been identified as the superior method of feeding infants with advantages encompassing health, social, economic, and environmental benefits for both infant and mother (Oddy 2001; Gartner, Morton, & Lawrence 2005). Infants who are not exclusively breastfed for the first 6 months are more likely to suffer from gastroenteritis, respiratory infections, otitis media, urinary tract infections, necrotising enterocolitis, atopic disease in families where there is a history of this and diabetes mellitus (Oddy 2001; Marild, Hansson, & Jodal 2004; Sadauskaite-Kuehne, Ludvigsson, Padaiga, Jasinskiene, & Samuelsson 2004; Quigley, Kelly, & Sacker 2007). A recent systematic review and meta-analysis of evidence of the long-term effects of breastfeeding among older children and adults found evidence that individuals who were breastfed had lower mean blood pressure and total cholesterol, and the prevalence of obesity and type-2 diabetes were also lower among those who had been breastfed (WHO 2007).

In Australia, whether a woman chooses to formula feed or breastfeed, it has been demonstrated that they are knowledgeable about the benefits of breastfeeding with many of the benefits cited as important reasons why women choose to breastfeed (Schmied, Sheehan, & Barclay 2001; Sheehan, Schmied, & Barclay 2010). It can be argued that current breastfeeding initiation rates are reflective of this knowledge. The Longitudinal Study of Australian Children (Australian Institute of

Family Studies, 2008) found initiation of breastfeeding rates among 5,000 infants at 92%. Despite this high rate of breastfeeding initiation, exclusive breastfeeding rates dropped each month until at 6 months they were at a low 14%. New South Wales (NSW) statistics are lower than these with 87% of infants ever breastfed and a gradual decline in exclusive breastfeeding until at 6 months only 18.1% of infants are exclusively breastfed (NSW Health 2006).

4.3 International and National Strategic and Policy Responses

Breastfeeding initiation and duration rates differ significantly between and within countries, as well as social and cultural groups (Homer, Sheehan, & Cooke 2002; Hawkins, Lamb, Cole, & Law 2008). In 1974, the World Health Assembly (WHA) formally noted a decline in breastfeeding, and considered this to be largely due to the inappropriate promotion of breast milk substitutes. Consequently, the WHO recommended member countries review sales promotion of these products and introduce legislation to remedy the decline of breastfeeding (WHO 1981). This concern for the support and promotion of breastfeeding and the inappropriate sales promotion of artificial infant formulas continued to be an issue for both WHO and UNICEF. In 1979, a meeting organised by WHO and UNICEF resulted in a statement on infant feeding, endorsed by the World Health Assembly in 1980. Amongst its recommendations and of particular note was that there should be an international code of marketing of infant formula and other products used as breast milk substitutes (WHO, 1981, pp. 6–7). In 1981, the International Code of Marketing of Breastmilk Substitutes was adopted by the World Health Assembly (WHO 1981). Since this time, a number of global policy statements have continued to be developed including: Protecting, Promoting and Supporting Breastfeeding: the special role of maternity services (WHO 1989); the Innocenti Declaration (WHO & UNICEF 1991a), the Baby Friendly Hospital (now Health) Initiative (WHO & UNICEF 1991b) and most recently, the Global Strategy for Infant and Young Child Feeding (WHO & UNICEF 2003). The Global Strategy renews the WHO and UNICEF commitment to the BFHI recommending developing approaches and tools for expanding BFHI into the community and making Baby Friendly Health Care health system wide (WHO & UNICEF 2003). Research suggests the BFHI is effective in increasing breastfeeding initiation rates, and in the past 15 years 15,000 hospitals in 134 countries have received BFHI accreditation (UNICEF 2009)

Australia is a signatory to the WHO's International Code of Marketing of Breast milk substitutes and, in response to this, a code of conduct known as the MAIF agreement was signed between manufacturers and importers of infant formula and the Australian Government. The MAIF Agreement is authorised under the Trade Practices Act 1974 (Australian Government 2009). Although the MAIF agreement is voluntary and self-regulatory, and therefore, not legally binding, an Advisory Panel on the Marketing in Australia of Infant Formula (APMAIF) has been established to monitor compliance with the agreement. Breaches of the agreement are published in the annual report of the APMAIF (Australian Government 2009) and tabled in Parliament (McVeigh 2005). There are some, however, who consider the MAIF agreement does not sufficiently support the WHO Code (McVeigh 2005). The Australian Breastfeeding Association (ABA), for example, would like Australia to implement the WHO code in its entirety and make it legally binding (Australian Breastfeeding Association 2007).

Australia has continued to acknowledge the importance of breast milk to the health and well-being of Australians through a number of policies and strategies. In June 1982, the Dietary Guidelines for Australians was developed and recommended breastfeeding, and in 1995 the first edition of Infant Feeding Guidelines for Health Workers was produced (Australian Government 2008). The National Health and Medical Research Council (NHMRC) have continued to recommend breastfeeding in their updated policies, and in the revised NHMRC Dietary Guidelines for Australians incorporating the infant feeing guidelines for health workers recommends exclusive breastfeeding for the first 6 months of life (NHMRC 2003). In addition to these recommendations, in 1993 a document 'Goals and Targets for Australia's Health in the year 2000 and beyond' was developed and included recommendations to increase the percentage of children being breastfed following discharge from hospital to 90% and up to 50% fully breastfeeding and 80% partially breastfeeding at 6 months of age (Nutbeam, Wise, Bauman, Harris, & Leeder 1993).

Between 1996 and 2001, the Australian Government funded the 'National Breastfeeding Strategy' as part of its *Health Throughout Life* policy statement for 2 million dollars. This money funded nine breastfeeding projects (Commonwealth Department of Health and Aged Care 2001). A further 15 projects to the value of two million dollars were also funded through the National Child Nutrition Program (Department of Health and Aging 2006) and the Australian Government supports the Australian Midwives Association to lead the implementation of the BFHI in Australia.

In 2006, the Australian Government launched the Breastfeeding Inquiry, and as a result 22 recommendations were made (Commonwealth of Australia 2007). Included in these recommendations is 'that the Department of Health and Ageing fund the Australian College of Midwives to run the Baby Friendly Hospital Initiative in Australia, to facilitate the accreditation of all maternity hospitals'; 'that the Department of Health and Ageing work with the Australian Council on Healthcare Standards (and/or equivalent accreditation organisation) towards including Baby Friendly Hospital status as part of the accreditation process; 'that the Department of Health and Ageing adopt the World Health Organisation's International Code of Marketing of Breast-milk Substitutes and subsequent World Health Assembly resolutions' (Commonwealth of Australia 2007, pp. xix–xx).

In New South Wales too, promoting breastfeeding is one of five public health nutrition priority areas identified for action in *Eat Well NSW, NSW Health's Strategic Directions for Public Health Nutrition 2003-2007* (NSW Health 2004). In addressing the priority areas identified in Eat Well NSW, the report, 'Overview of recent interventions to promote and support breastfeeding' (Hector, King, & Webb 2004) was produced as reference material. This document identified that much of the available evidence relating to interventions 'relates to educational and support strategies designed to promote mother's personal skills and health service strategies (including training of health professionals) to implement hospital practices conducive to breastfeeding' (Hector et al. 2004, p. vi).

Following on from this in 2006, NSW released a policy on breastfeeding 'Breastfeeding in NSW: Protection Promotion and Support' (NSW Health 2006). Although the importance of breastfeeding has been acknowledged and promoted in other NSW Health Circulars reports and a special edition of the NSW Health Bulletin devoted to breastfeeding in 2005, this is the first comprehensive breastfeeding policy since 1989 (NSW Health 2006, p. 13). The policy was developed 'to assist personnel to increase support for breastfeeding within the NSW Health system and thereby contribute to improved population breastfeeding rates' (2006, p. ii). The policy is based on the following considerations: the health benefits of breastfeeding to both mothers and infants, the revised NHMRC Infant feeing guidelines for health workers (NHMRC 2003), a demonstrated need to improve NSW breastfeeding rates and recent systematic reviews of the evidence on effective interventions by health services (NSW Health 2006). Compliance with this policy is mandatory according to the webpage (NSW Department of Health 2006b). Although what aspects of the policy are mandatory are not made clear, one point in strategy 4 is to approach the National Accreditation Standards body for Maternal and Infant Care services to assess the feasibility of including BFHI standards in ACHS EQuIP Accreditation. This strategy is in line with a previous document by ABA Australian Breastfeeding Leadership Plan (ABLP) (ABA 2004) linking public funding of maternity hospitals to BFHI accreditation by 2014 and with the Commonwealth Parliamentary Inquiry into Breastfeeding (Commonwealth of Australia 2007).

The NSW policy has a large target audience, including senior management; maternity; child and family health; paediatric and neonatal services; other NSW Health services which come in contact with pregnant women, mothers and their infants such as hospital departments; outpatient clinics, parenting education services, community health; family and youth support services, nutrition services, oral health programs and NSW Health child care centres; employees relations, because the policy addresses issues associated with combining breastfeeding and work; workforce development; and health promotion, particularly with regard to facilitating collaborative action with service providers and external groups. In addition to these, the policy acknowledges other stakeholders such as 'tertiary institutions, private hospitals, Divisions of General Practice and general practitioners, professional representative bodies, research organisations, local government, the Australian Breastfeeding Association, Aboriginal Community Controlled Health Services and consumer organisations (such as playgroups) and other key groups (NSW Health 2006, p. ii).

The goals of the policy are to at least maintain current breastfeeding initiation rates, increase exclusive breastfeeding rates to 6 months and increase breastfeeding duration rates. Five strategic areas for action include: organisational support for an enhanced and coordinated effort across the NSW Health Sector; workforce development and provision of breastfeeding friendly workplaces; provision of evidence-based health services; intersectoral collaboration with organisations outside the NSW Health System and monitoring of breastfeeding rates. Under each of these strategic areas, there are 21 recommended strategies and corresponding actions. The WHO policies are a major factor in the NSW policy. There is a particular emphasis on the BFHI with a strategy to encourage Area Health Services to implement the BFHI across services (NSW Health 2006).

4.4 The Professional Perspective

Midwives and other professionals are knowledgeable about the benefits of breastfeeding (Cantrill, Creedy, & Cooke 2003), and in principle in Australia appear to support public health policies identified above including the implementation of BFHI. We have recently completed a study exploring health professionals' perceptions and experience of the implementation of the BFHI in one Area Health Service in NSW (Schmied et al. 2009a). Without question, midwives, neonatal nurses and child and family health nurses acknowledged and agreed with the value of promoting and supporting breastfeeding and spoke of the numerous health and economic benefits of breastfeeding as well as the importance of breastfeeding to the developing relationship between the mother and her baby. Although implementing BFHI was perceived as hard work, particularly '*getting everyone on board*', the participants considered it would return higher breastfeeding duration rates, it was well worth doing and doing now. Yet, these health professionals also spoke of the tension they experienced in practice around the implementation of BFHI.

Some participants believed that some women '*don't know*' and or resist the health promotional messages about breastfeeding stating that women are 'doing their own things, whatever their mother was taught or whatever ...' that some women lack antenatal preparation, have grandmothers giving poor advice and that there are cultural barriers such as lying in and not wanting to give colostrum. Midwives also experienced significant workplace stress and were concerned that they were limited in the time they were able to offer support to women. Ultimately, the steps that midwives find a little easier or more straightforward to implement are those that can be controlled, for example, offering no dummies, formula, and implementing skin to skin contact that they feel they are achieving, suggesting the creation of a new set of rules. Yet, these are the steps not necessarily proven to be effective in resource-rich countries in promoting breastfeeding duration and are at odds with women's perceptions of breastfeeding support identified in a recent meta-synthesis, which highlighted the importance of relationship building (Schmied et al. 2009b).

Lack of time and resources are themes identified by others as impacting on the ability of midwives to appropriately support women to breastfeed (Furber & Thomson 2007; Moore, Gauld, & Williams 2007) and implement the BFHI effectively (Furber & Thomson 2007; Moore et al. 2007). The small number of midwives in the study by Schmied and colleagues (2009a), who reflected on the way that BFHI impacted on the clinical area, were concerned that they were, or may be, becoming prescriptive in their approach and advice to women, and that this could be perceived as putting pressure on women because they do not have the time to give women what they need and it is rare that they have the opportunity to build a relationship with the woman.

It has been recognised, however, that a standardised approach to care based on rigid implementation of policies is likely to dominate because of the time constraints of midwives (Hauck, Langton, & Coyle 2002). Given these time constraints, it is not surprising that midwives have been found to 'focus on the 'rules', and the 'stuff I'll get the rap for' rather than on women's needs (Kirkham, Stapleton, Thomas, & Curtis 2002). In such a climate, 'truly individualised care, while central to the rhetoric, can be seen as deviance' (Kirkham et al. 2002, p. 449). Recently, it has been identified that in Australia, workloads and ways of measuring workloads for nurses is problematic (Duffield, Roche, & Merrick 2006). The implication here is that proper assessment of the time needed to deliver appropriate support needs to women needs to be undertaken and the workloads of midwives may need to be adjusted accordingly.

4.5 Women's Experiences of the Public Health, Professional, Social and Personal Imperative to Breastfeed

In this section, we present findings that are drawn from a constructionist grounded theory study that explored women's infant feeding experiences in the first 6 weeks post-birth (Sheehan 2006). This section of the chapter draws specifically from two major categories from this study 'It's really best to breastfeed' and 'It's not the only thing going on' to demonstrate how, from the perspective of the women, there is an imperative to breastfeed. See Box 4.1 for a brief overview of this study.

Box 4.1 Complex Decisions, Deconstructing Best: A Grounded Theory Study of Infant Feeding Decisions in the First 6 Weeks Post-birth

Aim: To explore and describe the experiences of women making infant feeding decisions in the first six weeks post-birth.

Methodology: A constructionist grounded theory methodology was used to collect and analyse data.

Data Collection: Data were collected through in-depth interviews with 37 women. The women were theoretically sampled in accordance with the principles of grounded theory.

Findings: Four main categories emerged from the data that described what women deemed important to their infant feeding decisions. These categories were 'it's really best to breastfeed', 'it's the unknown', 'its not the only thing going on' and 'everybody's best is different'. The Basic Social Process, which was also the core category, was labelled 'deconstructing best'. The core category 'deconstructing best' linked the categories in a process of decision-making that the women embarked on during this period.

Conclusions: The findings demonstrate that women's infant feeding decisions in the first 6 weeks post-birth are multifactorial. In contrast to this, hospital policies as well as health professionals' understandings and practices are generally embedded in the concept that breast is best.

In the category 'it's really best to breastfeed', there were three main subcategories. These subcategories were 'knowing breast is best', 'feeling the pressure', and 'it's really more acceptable to breastfeed'. The subcategory 'knowing breast is best' describes what the women knew about breastfeeding and how this was disseminated and responded to by the women. The subcategory 'feeling the pressure' describes how the women believed health professionals responded to and used the information that breast is best to influence and affect women's decisions and how this impacted on them. The subcategory 'it's really more acceptable to breastfeed' is not so much about the benefits of breastfeeding, but what happens when information about the benefits of breastfeeding is absorbed into the social realm. This subcategory describes how this knowledge is interpreted and played out in everyday society/life and, consequently, the impact this has on the women's infant feeding decisions and experiences. Finally, in the category 'it's not the only thing going on' we draw specifically from a subcategory 'establishing the maternal identity' to demonstrate how the imperative to breastfeed is also driven from within the women themselves and how this affects their experiences and decisions.

4.5.1 Knowing Breast Is Best

Although breastfeeding rates have not changed significantly in recent years, findings from our study suggest the promotion of breastfeeding has been successful. This study demonstrated that whether a woman chooses to breast or formula feed, she is well aware that breastfeeding is the recommended method of infant feeding. Women talked about how breastfeeding is marketed and promoted through infant care books, hospitals, midwives and antenatal classes as 'the best way' to feed their baby. As one woman described it, 'the media, everywhere, everywhere, hospital, you see it on the TV, breastfeed' (Sally).

What the findings of our research also demonstrated is that when women discuss breastfeeding, they commonly use the words 'natural' and 'best'. This, too, is not surprising given that in Australia, the words 'best' and 'natural' have formed the dominant themes in the promotion of breastfeeding with slogans such as 'breast is best'. Books such as *Breastfeeding Naturally*, and posters saying 'Breastfeeding Natural, Healthy, Loving' (Australian Breastfeeding Association 2004). Many women were able to list numerous health benefits of breastfeeding and although mention was made of the health benefits to women, what appeared to be of particular and of more pressing importance to the women were the health benefits of breast milk for the baby. Women who planned to breastfeed generally couched their decisions around the health benefits of breastfeeding, referring particularly to the health benefits for the baby, a finding similar to others (Coreil, Bryant, Westover, & Bailey 1995; Blum 1999; Hoddinott & Pill 1999; Murphy 1999; Lupton 2000; Shakespeare, Blake, & Garcia 2004; Dykes 2005).

The effect of the 'breast is best' mantra also meant that many women believed that by breastfeeding their baby, they were giving their baby the 'best start ', and therefore, this information was crucial to their plans to initiate breastfeeding. There was also an inference that by giving their baby the best start they were doing the right thing: 'You want to do the right, what you think is the right thing by them you know umm and give them the best possible start' (Bronte).

For a number of women in the study, the breast is best message was so powerful that they did not simply view breastfeeding as 'best', they viewed formula feeding as second-best or, even worse, detrimental to the health of their baby with the potential to cause life long damage.

> I think my biggest fear of stopping now is if someone said in ten years' time or discovered that if I'd have breastfed longer your son wouldn't have this if or you know if you gave your child formula we've now discovered formula is linked to this. I think that's my biggest fear (Emily).

This fear that formula feeding could be dangerous and cause future health problems was also reported by Murphy (2000) in the United Kingdom. Murphy (2000) found the techno-scientific risk discourse was a reference point for mothers from all the occupational classes and age groups she sampled, regardless of when formula milk was introduced.

It can be claimed that women view these messages in this manner because health promotion messages in Western industrialised nations are generally couched in risk discourse, with an increasing focus on reducing lifestyle risks (Lupton 1993). As opposed to the original mathematical definition of risk, which is considered neutral and refers to probability, in public health discourse risk is synonymous with danger and is largely weighted heavily in favour of disaster and anxiety rather than peace of mind (Lupton 1993).

Also embedded within the understanding of the benefits of breastfeeding was the notion that breastfeeding was the 'right' thing to do and that being a 'good' mother and breastfeeding are linked.

> I suppose I was just so convinced that she had to have breast milk that it had to come from me and that I had to be the good mother (Lucy).

It was believed that a good mother would breastfeed because it's the 'best' and consequently, a 'good' mother would only want to do the 'best' for her baby, as Rachel remarked: 'Just knowing all the positives of what's in breast milk why wouldn't you give you know if you could give your baby the best'. Wall (2001, p. 595) argues that breastfeeding being bound up in the moral construction of motherhood is related to 'the moralization of pregnancy that has accompanied the subjectification of the foetus and the neoliberal preoccupation with individual responsibility, individual self-enhancement, and the cost of social programs'. It has been argued that risk discourse associated with breastfeeding draws on the assumption good mothers will want to maximise their child's physical and psychological health outcomes (Murphy 1999; see also Chapters 7 and 9 in this volume). Contemporary Western notions of a good mother demand she will privilege the needs of her children above her own (Blum 1999; Murphy 1999; Schmied & Lupton 2001). This pre-eminence of the infant's needs over the mother's needs has been clearly identified in the promotional messages around breastfeeding (Wall 2001).

4.5.2 Feeling the Imperative to Breastfeed

With health promotional messages around breastfeeding given such pre-eminence, it is not surprising that a number of women also talked about a pressure to breastfeed from professionals, society in general and also from within themselves.

4.5.2.1 Professional Pressure

Women talked about experiencing a pressure to breastfeed particularly from professionals: 'the medical profession, I find really puts a lot of pressure on you to breastfeed' (Erin). The pressure from professionals was experienced in both overt and covert ways, with women stating formula feeding was not mentioned: 'They don't really talk about the bottle up there much, you sort of have to ask for it more' and 'every time I mentioned a bottle oh no, no, no, keep trying' (Sarah). Even when requested, information about bottle-feeding was withheld from some women. Tess elaborated on this:

> Every time I rang the ...or ... or even the health-care nurse, the early childhood nurse, would say no, keep going, come on, you can keep going. They wouldn't really give me any information on weaning and they weren't forthcoming with it. I'd ask the question okay, can you tell me how to wean and they'd say look just try this one more thing and then you can think about weaning. So then I started to get frustrated. Well, all I want to know is how to do it, so in the back of my mind I know what to do, but no-one would give me the information either.

Some of the women felt the pressure to breastfeed exerted on them by professionals extended to breastfeeding at all costs, regardless of what the woman herself was experiencing or her specific needs: 'The judgment was to continue to breastfeed regardless of all these problems' (Anna). For some women, the pressure to breastfeed at all costs impacted on them as a person. This meant they felt they were expected to put aside any personal discomforts or needs in preference to the baby's needs, which, given the superiority of breast milk, always meant breastfeeding. As a result of this, some of the women felt that their individual needs were disregarded: 'It was like, well, you just put up with pain' (Nanette). As a person, they became insignificant: 'It's almost like you as a person are gone and we need your body and we need those breasts and we need those nipples out' (Sheehan, Schmied, & Cooke 2003, p. 263).

The knowledge of the benefits of breastfeeding along with the pressure to breastfeed impacted on those women who felt they did not want to breastfeed. The pressure that women should do the 'best' for their baby was so powerful that for some women, despite preferring to bottle-feed, they ultimately felt coerced to breastfeed: 'I gave it a go because there was so much pressure'. This professional preference for and pressure to breastfeed also meant that some women who planned to bottle-feed feared they would be sanctioned: 'If I were to have said I want to bottle-feed him, they would have actually looked down on you. You could see it' (Melanie).

These findings are in line with other research that have identified how some women feel pressured to breastfeed by professionals (see Blum 1999; Carter 1995; Hoddinott & Pill 2000b; Shakespeare et al. 2004). In Murphy's (2000) study, the women talked about being challenged and criticised by health professionals. These women reported how health professionals tried to block their decision to formula feed. Also occurring in the Australian context was the study by Hauck and colleagues (2002), which found women reported they received information that was strongly biased towards breastfeeding or intolerant of bottle-feeding. The strength of this perceived bias and professional preference for breastfeeding experienced by some women was illustrated in a quote from Shakespeare et al.'s (2004, p. 257) study, where one of the women felt the health professionals at the breast clinics 'would be bestowing the virtues of breastfeeding and how, you know, people who bottle feed are the devil's spawn and I just felt awful'.

Given the perceived pressure from professionals, the results of our study would support the findings of Murphy (1999, p. 187) who argues the 'breast is best' message underpins policy and professional practice and 'is part of the context in which women decide how to feed their babies and in turn how they display and defend their decisions'. Women in our study, as well as others, were clearly knowledgeable of the health professionals' preference for breastfeeding over any other form of infant feeding, with some women feeling they were expected to breastfeed at all costs. It has been demonstrated in this study and other studies that professional pressure to breastfeed increases levels of distress in women during this early period (Blum 1999; Hoddinott & Pill 2000b; Murphy 2000; Shakespeare et al. 2004; see also Chapters 2 and 5 in this volume).

Although Murphy (2000) suggests that the power of expertise did not force the women in her study to feed their babies in ways they did not choose, findings of our research and also a study by Hoddinott and Pill (2000b) suggest pressure to breastfeed did mean that some women initiated and or continued breastfeeding despite not wanting to. In our study, as well as other studies, women have described how they felt coerced to breastfeed (Blum 1999; Hoddinott & Pill 2000b) and/or hid their decision to bottle-feed (Maushart 1997; Sheehan et al. 2003). Despite breastfeeding being referred to as a choice, this research supports the argument put forward by Bartlett (2005) that when it comes to infant feeding, there is quite obviously a right and wrong choice. Lupton (1993) argues that the discourse of risk contributes to this because seemingly the discourse of risk gives people a choice, but the rhetoric in which choice is couched leaves no room for manoeuvre.

Given that these mothers felt pressured to breastfeed and, therefore, the act of breastfeeding was not volitional may explain in part some of the early decline in breastfeeding rates. Experiencing a pressure to breastfeed may also help explain why some research has shown that providing specific antenatal breastfeeding education, particularly to groups who are least likely to breastfeed such as teenage mothers or women from culturally and linguistically diverse (CALD) groups can increase initiation rates but not duration rates (Rossiter 1994; Greenwood & Littlejohn 2002; see also Chapter 21 in this volume)

4.5.2.2 Societal Pressure to Breastfeed 'Its Really More Acceptable to Breastfeed'

Just as some women believed there was a professional pressure to breastfeed, many of the women also talked about a societal pressure to breastfeed believing that there was a general societal belief that 'it is really more acceptable to breastfeed' (Anna). At one level, the fact that it was really more acceptable to breastfeed was quite ethereal, something out there that they could not necessarily put their finger on: 'It was just like even though people don't actually say it you just know breast is, you know breast is best'(Katie.). They made comments such as 'I think everyone assumed I would breastfeed' (Bronte). This expectation was not always understated either, as one woman described it: 'You find a lot of strangers in the street that you're talking to and they say "oh are you breastfeeding?" and I'd go "no" and they'd go "oh you should be, you know"' (Erin). Not surprisingly, this powerful societal expectation meant many of the women themselves also just assumed they would breastfeed after the baby was born. 'I just assumed I'd breastfeed' (Serena), and 'I never really considered using the bottle, I always just assumed I'd breastfeed' (Joanna).

Not surprisingly, given the above statements, there were clear moral overtones around the infant feeding decision. Some women felt the expectation to breastfeed and its relationship to being a 'good' mother was so overt that if they chose to bottle-feed, they needed a good reason to do so: 'If you can breastfeed you're giving your child the better option and really, unless you've got a good reason for not breastfeeding, I get the impression you should' (Anna). These societal expectations were confirmed by the fact that a number of women in this research also held these views, as Lucy argues:

> I think that as mothers we produce milk for a reason and I think it's because that's what's best for our baby and if there is no actual physical or medical reason as to why we can't feed or umm, yeah, I just I think that's what should be done.

Or, as Mariam expressed it more strongly:

> If there's something wrong that's okay, but if there's not, they should have tried harder.

To this end, the women were aware that if someone chose to bottle-feed, she risked being judged and looked down on. They talked about women who bottle-fed being viewed as 'copping out', lazy and not doing their job as a mother: 'People sort of look down on you if you bottle-feed. . .that you're not as good of a mother or you are a bit lazy or, you know, didn't want to put in the effort' (Jane). Some of the women themselves admitted they judged other women who did not breastfeed, saying: 'Like you see a brand new newborn in a shopping centre being bottle-fed and you think God that's lazy or oh that's awful, that baby should be breastfed, knowing how good it is for the baby' (Miriam).

That a woman could be judged if she did not breastfeed influenced some women's decisions and experiences, because they were concerned that they would be viewed as not being a good mother: 'I was also worried initially about what other people would think if I chose not to breastfeed ... that people would judge me, that they would, you know, think I was not doing the right thing by the baby (Bronte). In fact, one of the women in this study did say she felt she was made to feel like a bad person for not breastfeeding: 'It made me feel like I was the bad person by not giving her my breast milk. By people saying that it was always better' (Carly). See also Chapter 9 in this volume.

Given that the women were aware they could be judged or sanctioned, the women in this study used a number of protective strategies including, justifying, hiding, shielding, toughing it out and clarifying. Justifying was an almost universal response to formula feeding.

> Well I just feel like I've got to justify like I felt like I needed to even justify to that lady at the shop and explain. . . I've even got to tell this stranger who's just stopped and talked to me like oh, I don't breastfeed because . . . I feel like I just can't say no, I'm bottle-feeding' (Anna).

In their discussions about justifying, the women discussed what was deemed appropriate as justification for formula feeding, including citing a bad experience as useful in defending their desire to wean or not breastfeed their baby: 'I don't know, getting the mastitis probably for me was probably like good in a way, 'cause then it gave me a reason to put her on the bottle' (Sally).

As well as justifying, the women hid their decisions: 'I was not game to tell the staff at the hospital that I wanted to bottle-feed, so I persevered that time in hospital and continued to breastfeed and express and give the bottle when they said to bottle-feed but changed in the car' (Anna).

Shielding was another protective strategy used by the women to avoid sanction. Shielding involved using others to support and defend their decision.

> When I went in to have my second son I said to the obstetrician I was going to bottle-feed and if it is possible could he please speak to the midwives first, because I was fairly worried about their attitude and how I was going to be accepted (Anna).

Finally, some women chose to protect themselves from being judged by toughing it out, making statements such as: 'I don't care what anyone says or if they don't like me at the hospital. I'm bottle-feeding' (Sally), and 'I had already decided that I would not be swayed' (Zara).

What was also illustrated in this study was that the fear of being judged and or sanctioned for formula feeding was so powerful that it extended beyond just giving formula. Even if women were giving expressed breast milk (EBM) in a bottle, they felt they needed to clarify this to avoid judgment.

> I do actually think I'd feel a bit ashamed to bottle, feed bottle-feed there and I do actually think if it was breastmilk in the bottle I'd have to tell them it was breastmilk ... because I think breast is best and I don't want them looking down on me because they think I'm giving the baby formula (Emily).

It is clear that breastfeeding is seen as a 'highly accountable matter' (Murphy 1999). This can explain why some women feel a sense of failure when they do not breastfeed (Hailes & Wellard 2000) and why Murphy (1999) argues that women in her study were accepting the fact that having failed at breastfeeding was deviant behaviour. It can also explain the societal expectation that a woman breastfeed, as found in our research as well as other studies (Maushart 1997; Murphy 1999). It has been highlighted by other researchers and commentators such as Maushart (1997), who describes in her book *The Mask of Motherhood* how in certain groups of women it is almost unacceptable to relate why one stopped breastfeeding. In this study, women who were bottle-feeding were fearful they would be judged as less than acceptable mothers. See also Chapter 9 in this volume.

4.5.2.3 Internal Pressure 'Breastfeeding Is Meant to Be'

The pressure to breastfeed, however, was not always external. Different from the societal construct and expectation that a good mother breastfeeds, for some women this belief and pressure to breastfeed came from within. Making the decision to breastfeed for these women was more than just simply deciding that breastfeeding was best and that is what they would do or even that it was more appropriate to breastfeed (as powerful as these may have been for them). For these women, the decision process was affected by feelings and emotions they found difficult to describe or even understand: 'There's probably things wells from within me that I just want to do it naturally' (Serena). These powerful feelings impacted on their experiences and decisions. Breastfeeding for these women just 'felt like the natural thing to be doing' (Elise) and was integral to their role as a mother 'that (breastfeeding) was part and parcel of being a mother' (Lucy)

Not only was breastfeeding viewed as integral to the maternal role, it was viewed as essential to creating a bond with their baby. For these women, there was a sense that a relationship with their baby could only be fully developed if they breastfed: 'I really felt that for me to have the best bonding experience with him ... I needed to breastfeed' (Nanette). For these women, breastfeeding not only enhanced the bonding experience but also created a closeness and connection with their child that was enjoyed by both mother and baby: 'When he feeds he is close, he's just really close to me and it's just really enjoyable' (Rachel).

Given that these women felt breastfeeding was integral to their maternal identity and their connection with their baby, they talked about a pressure that came from within them to achieve their goal of breastfeeding: 'On a subconscious level

I was so determined to do it' (Elise). These women talked about being 'devastated if I couldn't have breastfed' (Rachel); and if they experienced difficulties, they responded by saying: 'I've got to make this work' (Nanette). These findings correlate with findings from two earlier studies that demonstrated the intense commitment to breastfeeding by some women who undertook extraordinary physical and emotional work to achieve their goal as a breastfeeding mother (Schmied et al. 2001). As in these earlier studies, when these women could not breastfeed due to insurmountable difficulties, they felt a deep sense of failure as a mother: 'I still felt that I'd failed as a mother, not being able to breastfeed' (Kylie), and talked about letting their child down: 'No matter what happens you still think that you are not providing for your baby' (Miriam). Not surprisingly, they also talked about their grief at not being able to breastfeed: 'There is a lot of grief over it' (Nanette).

These findings complement the quantitative findings of another study by Cooke and colleagues (2007), who also identified that women with strong beliefs about the importance of breastfeeding for their maternal identity and who stopped breastfeeding were more likely to be categorised as distressed (Cooke, Schmied, & Sheehan 2007). The strong sense of maternal identity these women associated with breastfeeding is consistent with other findings that have found some women will persist with breastfeeding regardless of difficulties (Bottorff 1990; Schmied et al. 2001; Hauck et al. 2002), and that there is an association with increased breastfeeding duration where maternal identity and breastfeeding are linked (Leff et al. 1994; Riordan et al. 1994; Cooke et al. 2003; Cooke et al. 2007).

Schmied and Barclay (1999) demonstrated the embodied dimension of the breastfeeding experience. Schmied et al.'s study, originally focussing on mothering, identified that breastfeeding was central to women's experience of motherhood in the first 6 months post-birth. Their work also highlighted the relationship between being a 'good' mother and breastfeeding. More than this, however, it also demonstrated a dichotomy in women's embodied experiences with some women expressing a connected and harmonious experience while others talked about an experience that was both disruptive and distorting of their known self (Schmied & Barclay 1999).

Expanding on these findings, our study demonstrated a continuum of feelings that interrelated with choices around infant feeding and maternal identity. At one end of the continuum, there were women as described above whose maternal identity was inextricably linked to breastfeeding, and at the other end, there were women whose sense of self was distorted by breastfeeding. At a middle point on the continuum, there were women who wished to and intended to breastfeed because they believed it was best for their baby. For these women, breastfeeding in and of itself did not appear to be integral to their maternal identity, they simply did it because they considered it best for their baby, breastfeeding did not create any great emotional rushes, but neither did they experience any particularly negative emotions. These women talked about connecting to their baby in a way that was not so much about their feelings, but achieving a role that was focused on meeting the needs of the baby. Primarily, these women breastfed because it was considered best and they could.

4.6 The Need for Strategies That Support Women Who Are Breastfeeding

In the final section of this chapter, we examine the tensions and possible contradictions that arise within the public health, professional, social and personal discourses of breastfeeding. While current public health policy focuses on the promotion of the benefits of breastfeeding and strategies to assist breastfeeding initiation, this appears to take little account of women's personal experience. We argue that far more effort needs to be placed on supporting women to breastfeed using strategies identified by women themselves to achieve their breastfeeding goals in the weeks and months following birth.

4.6.1 Prioritising Breastfeeding as a Public Health Issue

Arguably, the imperative to breastfeed, evident in public health policies, focuses on the immunological and biological benefits for infant health. It is important to recognise that these benefits are reported at the population level, and that the risks for individual infants and mothers will be highly variable. However, the frequently cited public health benefits pay little attention to the individual lives and experience of women. As noted in the Federal government Senate Inquiry into breastfeeding in 2007 (Commonwealth of Australia 2007), there is little research on the socio-cultural influences on infant feeding decisions in Australia, nor the relational and emotional aspects that underpin breastfeeding success (WHO & UNICEF 2003). If women are not breastfeeding or initiating and not continuing to breastfeed, we need to understand why.

Decisions about infant feeding are embedded (and are continuously being made) within a woman's social and cultural context (Dykes 2006). Attitudes, social norms and cultural opinion about infant feeding are also shaped by the media (e.g. books, magazines, television, videos and the Internet) (Bartlett 2005). For example, a culture which focuses on body image and which sees breasts as sexual organs (Dykes & Griffiths 1998) can have a detrimental impact on a woman's willingness to breastfeed in public (Hoddinott & Pill 1999). An indication of the impact of culture on decision making is seen in new migrants who breastfeed long term in their culture of origin, but who shorten breastfeeding duration as they acculturate to infant feeding norms in Australia (Rossiter 1992; Tsianakas & Liamputtong 2007; see also Chapter 21 in this volume).

4.6.2 Is BFHI the Answer?

Although the Australian Government recommends the implementation of BFHI in all maternity services, the BFHI Australia website confirms only 67 hospitals in Australia have been accredited as Baby Friendly, and only nine of these are in NSW (http://www.bfhi.org.au/text/bfhi_hospitals.html). Currently, there is only limited research in Australia on BFHI, and Fallon, Crepinsek, Hegney, and O'Brien (2005) argue that there is little evidence to suggest the implementation of the BFHI into Australian hospitals will have any effect on breastfeeding duration rates. Pincombe and associates (2008) further question the relationship between the adherence to some of the steps in the BFHI and the duration of breastfeeding in first-time mothers. Their findings demonstrated that duration of breastfeeding did not appear to be associated with 'initiation of breastfeeding within 1 h after birth, with breastfeeding on demand, or with the mother and baby staying together 24 h a day (rooming in). Overall, their work revealed limited support for the BFHI as a whole, querying also step six, the use of no other food or drink apart from breast milk, and step nine, the use of dummies as detrimental to breastfeeding. These steps have also been questioned by other international researchers (Hill, Humenick, Brennan, & Woolley 1997; Kramer et al. 2001; Benis 2002; Schwartz et al. 2002; Ullah & Griffiths 2003). Limited international research also suggests barriers to the implementation of BFHI including lack of fidelity to components of the strategy, limited resources and resistance to abandon ineffective practices. Consequently, the success of some of the strategies can be considered equivocal and the implementation of BFHI challenging.

4.6.3 The Preferences and Practices of Health Professionals

Murphy (1999, p. 187) argues the 'breast is best' message underpins policy and professional practice and 'is part of the context in which women decide how to feed their babies and in turn how they display and defend their decisions'. Women in our study were clearly knowledgeable of the health professionals' preference for breastfeeding over any other form of infant feeding, with some women feeling they were expected to breastfeed at all costs. It has been demonstrated in our study as well as others studies that professional pressure to breastfeed increases levels of distress in women during this early period (Blum 1999; Hoddinott & Pill 2000b; Murphy 2000; Shakespeare et al. 2004).

Policies need to acknowledge that women need individualised care (Sheehan et al. 2010). Currently, policies and practices are entrenched in the concept that 'breast is best' and focus on the needs of the infant, regardless of the needs of the women. Further to this, it is suggested that these policies and practices are being applied rigidly (Schmied et al. 2001; Stein, Dykes, & Bramwell 2000).

The experiences that women report are powerful and often very distressing (Hoddinott 2000; Schmied et al. 2001; Cooke et al. 2007). With the potential to undermine a woman's perception of her capacity to mother. Although breastfeeding has been purported to give women freedom over their body (Palmer 1993), results from the study by Sheehan (2006) and others indicate that through the promotion of and education about breastfeeding, the subject positions of women can become restrictive (Blum 1999; Law 2000; Wall 2001). Strategies that promote breastfeeding based on information about the benefits of breastfeeding assume women will choose to breastfeed on the basis that 'breast is best'. This, however, fails to take the wider socio-cultural factors into account and also undermines a woman's concern for her baby's well-being (Gerrard 2001; see also Chapters 7, 8, and 9 in this volume).

Given the restricted subjectivity available to women, a number of authors have highlighted the paucity of feminist critique of breastfeeding promotion (Blum 1999; Carter 1995; Schmied et al. 2001). It has been argued that this lack of feminist debate around the assumptions underlying the growing biomedical and public health policy concern with increasing breastfeeding rates has occurred predominantly because it coincided with exposure of the exploitation of women in third-world countries by formula companies (Wall 2001). While there is an understanding that formula companies have exploited women, women can also feel restricted by rules that govern breastfeeding (Wall 2001). Wall (2001, p. 599) further claims the reluctance to acknowledge the range of difficulties that can accompany breastfeeding is because to do so would put breastfeeding into 'a negative light and feeding into ideas that have been used to promote infant formula as the better option'. Ultimately, women feel they bear the brunt of a failure to breastfeed by midwives and nurses who may imply that a woman is not doing her best.

A recently completed meta-synthesis of women's perceptions of breastfeeding support emphasised the importance of person-centred communication skills and of relationships in supporting a woman to breastfeed (Schmied et al. 2009b). Authentic presence, one of the major themes arising from the synthesis, is best supported by building a trusting relationship, demonstrating empathy, listening and being responsive to a woman's needs. Organisational systems and services that facilitate continuity of carer and time spent with the woman, for example, continuity of midwifery care or peer support models, are more likely to facilitate an authentic presence. McInnes and Chambers (2008) also suggest the need to increase opportunities to offer women across all social groups' access to peer support.

Yet, it can be argued midwives are caught in a bureaucratic system that does not acknowledge the temporal or embodied nature of breastfeeding (Dykes 2006), but rather enforces a production line process to 'get' women to breastfeed. Attaching funding to breastfeeding outcomes, as is suggested in a number of reports without committing to the structural changes required to provide the type of care women need and want, will only reinforce this process.

4.7 Conclusion

This chapter has focused on two dimensions of the breastfeeding experience. First, the public health policy and professional approach to breastfeeding promotion and support were described, and second, we reported on a study that examined the personal experiences of Australian women in the first 6 weeks following birth. We have argued that infant feeding decisions in Australia are currently influenced by an imperative to breastfeed, and that this raises a number of tensions across the personal, social, professional and public health dimensions of breastfeeding. In the final section of this chapter, we examined these tensions and possible contradictions and have argued that current public health policy is focused on the promotion of the benefits of breastfeeding and strategies to assist breastfeeding initiation to the neglect of women's personal experience and strategies demonstrated to support women to achieve their breastfeeding goals in the weeks and months following birth.

References

Australian Breastfeeding Association. (2004). *Australian breastfeeding leadership plan*. Australian Breastfeeding Association, Glen Iris, Australia.

Australian Breastfeeding Association. (2007). Submission by the Australian Breastfeeding Association to the Parliamentary Inquiry into Breastfeeding. Retrieved 1 May 2009, from http://www.breastfeeding.asn.au/advocacy/bfinquiryabaofficiallsubmission2007final.pdf

Australian Government. (2008). Breastfeeding. Retrieved 13 August 2009, from http://www.health.gov.au/internet/main/publishing.nsf/Content/health-pubhlth-strateg-brfeed-about.htm

Australian Government. (2009). *Advisory panel on the marketing in Australia of infant formula (APMAIF)*. Retrieved 5 June 2009, from http://www.health.gov.au/internet/main/publishing.nsf/Content/health-pubhlth-strateg-foodpolicy-apmaif.htm

Australian Institute of Family Studies. (2008). Growing up in Australia: The longitudinal study of Australian children: 2006–07 annual report, 2008. Retrieved 27 June 2008, from http://www.aifs.gov.au/growingup/pubs/ar/annualreport2006-07.pdf

Bartlett, A. (2005). *Breastwork*. Sydney: University of New South Wales Press.

Benis, M. M. (2002). Are pacifiers associated with early weaning from breastfeeding. *Advances in Neonatal Care, 2*(5), 259–266.

Blum, L. M. (1999). *At the breast*. Boston: Beacon Press.

Bottorff, J. (1990). Persistence in breastfeeding: A phenomenological investigation. *Journal of Advanced Nursing, 15*, 201–209.

Cantrill, R., Creedy, D., & Cooke, M. (2003). An Australian study of midwives' breast-feeding knowledge. *Midwifery, 19*, 310–317.

Carter, P. (1995). *Feminism, breasts and breast-feeding*. Basingstoke: Macmillan.

Commonwealth Department of Health and Aged Care. (2001). National breastfeeding strategy summary report [Electronic Version], 26. Retrieved 5 June 2009, from http://www.ranzcog.edu.au/publications/endorsedstatements/national-breastfeeding-strategy-summary.pdf.

Commonwealth of Australia. (2007). *The best start: Report on the inquiry into the health benefits of breastfeeding*. Canberra: Commonwealth of Australia

Cooke, M., Sheehan, A. & Schmied, V. (2003). A description of breastfeeding experiences, breast-feeding satisfaction and weaning in the first three months after birth. *Journal of Human Lactation, 19*(2), 145–156.

Cooke, M., Schmied, V., & Sheehan, A. (2007). An exploration of the relationship between post-natal distress and maternal role attainment, breastfeeding problems and breastfeeding cessation in Australia. *Midwifery, 23*(1), 66–76.

Coreil, J., Bryant, C. A., Westover, B. J., & Bailey, M. A. (1995). Health professionals and breastfeeding counselling: Client and provider views. *Journal of Human Lactation, 11*(4), 265–271.

Department of Health and Aging. (2006). Breastmilk makes Australia stronger. Retrieved 3 August 2010, from www.health.gov.au/internet/ministers/publishing.nsf/Content/health-mediarel-yr2006-cp-pyn050.htm

Duffield, C., Roche, M., & Merrick, E. T. (2006). Methods of measuring nursing workload in Australia. *Collegian, 13*(1), 16–22.

Dykes, F. (2005). 'Supply' and 'demand': Breastfeeding as labour. *Social Science and Medicine, 60*, 2283–2293.

Dykes, F. (2006). *Breastfeeding in hospital: Mothers, midwives and the production line*. London: Routledge.

Dykes, F., & Griffiths, H. (1998). Societal influences upon initiation and continuation of breastfeeding. *British Journal of Midwifery, 6*(2), 76–80.

Fallon, T., Crepinsek, M., Hegney, D., & O'Brien, M. (2005). The Baby- Friendly Hospital Initiative and breastfeeding duration: Relating the evidence to the Australian context. *Birth Issues, 14*(3), 90–95.

Furber, C. M., & Thomson, A. M. (2007). Midwives in the UK: An exploratory study of providing newborn feeding support for postpartum mothers in the hospital. *Journal of Midwifery and Women's Health, 52*(2), 142–147.

Gartner, L., Morton, J., & Lawrence, R. A. (2005). Breastfeeding and the use of human milk. *Pediatrics, 115*(2), 496–506.

Gerrard, A. (2001). Breast-feeding in Norway: Where did they go right? *British Journal of Midwifery, 9*(5), 294–295.

Greenwood, K., & Littlejohn, P. (2002). Breastfeeding intentions and outcomes of adolescent mothers in the Starting Out program. *Breastfeeding Review, 10*(3), 19–23.

Hailes, J. F., & Wellard, S. J. (2000). Support for breastfeeding in the first postpartum month: Perceptions of breastfeeding women. *Breastfeeding Review, 8*(3), 5–9.

Hauck, Y. L., Langton, D., & Coyle, K. (2002). The path of determination: Exploring the lived experience of breastfeeding difficulties. *Breastfeeding Review, 10*(2), 5–12.

Hawkins, S., Lamb, K., Cole, J., & Law, C. (2008). Influence of moving to the UK on maternal health behaviours: Prospective cohort study. *British Medical Journal, 336*(7652), 1052–1055.

Hector, D., King, L., & Webb, K. (2004). *Overview of recent interventions to promote and support breastfeeding*. Retrieved June 18, 2009, from http://www.health.nsw.gov.au/pubs/2004/pdf/bf_interventions.pdf

Hill, P. D., Humenick, S. S., Brennan, M. L., & Woolley, D. (1997). Does early supplementation affect long-term breastfeeding? *Clinical Pediatrics, 36*(6), 345–350.

Hoddinott, P., & Pill, R. (1999). Qualitative study of decisions about infant feeding among women in East End of London. *British Medical Journal, 318*(7175), 30–34.

Hoddinott, P., & Pill, R. (2000). A qualitative study of women's views about how health professionals communicate about infant feeding. *Health Expectations, 3*, 224–233.

Homer, C., Sheehan, A., & Cooke, M. (2002). Initial infant feeding decisions and duration of breastfeeding in women from English, Arabic and Chinese-speaking backgrounds in Australia. *Breastfeeding Review, 10*(2), 27–32.

Kirkham, M., Stapleton, H., Thomas, G., & Curtis, P. (2002). Checking not listening: How midwives cope. *British Journal of Midwifery, 10*(7), 447–450.

Kramer, M. S., Barr, R. G., Dagenais, S., Yang, H., Jones, P., Ciofani, L., et al. (2001). Pacifier use, early weaning, and cry/fuss behavior: A randomized controlled trial. *JAMA, 286*(3), 322–326.

Law, J. (2000). The politics of breastfeeding: Assessing risk, dividing labor. *Signs: Journal of Women in Culture and Society, 25*(2), 407–450.

Leff, E. W., Gagne, M. P. & Jefferis, S. C. (1994). Maternal perceptions of successful breastfeeding. *Journal of Human Lactation, 10*(2), 99–104.

Lupton, D. (1993). Risk as moral danger: The social and political functions of risk discourse in public health. *International Journal of Health Services, 23*(3), 425–435.

Lupton, D. (2000). 'A love/hate relationship': The ideals and experiences of first-time mothers. *Journal of Sociology, 36*(1), 50–63.

Marild, S., Hansson, S., & Jodal, U. (2004). Protective effect of breastfeeding against urinary tract infection. *Acta Paediatrica, 93*(2), 164–168.

Maushart, S. (1997). *The mask of motherhood.* Sydney: Vintage.

McInnes, R.J., & Chambers, J.A. (2008). Supporting breastfeeding mothers: qualitative synthesis. *Journal of Advanced Nursing,* 62(4), 407–427.

McVeigh, P. (2005). The World Health Organization code of marketing of breastmilk substitutes and subsequent resolutions (The WHO Code). *The NSW Health Bulletin, 16*(3–4), 67–68.

Moore, T., Gauld, R., & Williams, S. (2007). Implementing Baby Friendly Hospital Initiative Policy: The case of New Zealand public hospitals. *International Breastfeeding Journal, 2*(8). Retrieved from http://www.internationalbreastfeedingjournal.com/content/2/1/8

Murphy, E. (1999). 'Breast is Best': Infant feeding decisions and maternal deviance. *Sociology of Health & Illness, 21*(2), 187–208.

Murphy, E. (2000). Risk, responsibility and rhetoric in infant feeding. *Journal of Contemporary Ethnography, 29*(3), 291–325.

NHMRC. (2003). *The dietary guidelines for children and adolescents in Australia incorporating the Infant Feeding Guidelines for Health Workers*. Canberra: NHMRC.

NSW Department of Health. (2006). Breastfeeding in NSW: Promotion, Protection and Support. Retrieved 13 August 2009, from http://www.health.nsw.gov.au/policies/pd/2006/PD2006_012.html

NSW Health. (2004). Eat Well NSW, NSW Health's strategic directions for public health nutrition 2003–2007. Retrieved 13 August 2009, from http://www.health.nsw.gov.au/pubs/2002/pdf/eatwellnsw.pdf

Nutbeam, D., Wise, M., Bauman, A., Harris, E., & Leeder, S. (1993). *Goals and targets for Australia's health in the Year 2000 and beyond*. Canberra: Australian Government Publishing Service.

Oddy, W. H. (2001). Breastfeeding protects against illness and infection in infants and children: A review of the literature. *Breastfeeding Review, 9*(2), 11–18.

Palmer, G. (1993). *The politics of breastfeeding*. London: Pandora.

Pincombe, J., Baghurst, P., Antoniou, G., Peat, B., Henderson, A., & Reddin, E. (2008). Baby Friendly Hospital Initiative practices and breast feeding duration in a cohort of first-time mothers in Adelaide, Australia. *Midwifery, 24*(1), 55–61.

Quigley, M., Kelly, Y., & Sacker, A. (2007). Breastfeeding and hospitalization for diarrheal and respiratory infection in the United Kingdom Millennium Cohort Study. *Pediatrics, 110*(4), e837–e842.

Riordan, J. M., Woodley, G. & Heaton, K. (1994). Testing validity and reliability of an instrument which measures maternal evaluation of breastfeeding. *Journal of Human Lactation, 10*(4), 231–235.

Rossiter, J. C. (1992). Attitudes of Vietnamese women to baby feeding practices before and after immigration to Sydney, Australia. *Midwifery, 8*, 103–112.

Rossiter, J. C. (1994). The effect of a culture specific education program to promote breastfeeding among Vietnamese women in Sydney. *International Journal of Nursing Studies, 31*(4), 369–379.

Sadauskaite-Kuehne, V., Ludvigsson, J., Padaiga, Z., Jasinskiene, E., & Samuelsson, U. (2004). Longer breastfeeding is an independent protective factor against development of type 1 diabetes mellitus in childhood. *Diabetes/Metabolism Research and Reviews, 20*(2), 150–157.

Schmied, V., & Barclay, L. (1999). Connection and pleasure, disruption and distress: women's experience of breastfeeding. *Journal of Human Lactation, 15*(4), 325–334.

Schmied, V., & Lupton, D. (2001). Blurring the boundaries: Breastfeeding and maternal subjectivity. *Sociology of Health & Illness, 23*(2), 234–250.

Schmied, V., Sheehan, A., & Barclay, L. (2001). Contemporary breast-feeding policy and practice: Implications for midwives. *Midwifery, 17*, 44–54.

Schmied, V., Gribble, K., Sheehan, A., Dykes, F., Cioffi, J., & Taylor, C. (2009a). *The problem of breastfeeding in implementation of WHO/UNICEEF BFHI.* Paper presented at the Nutrition and Nurture in Infancy and Childhood: Bio-Cultural Perspectives Conference, Grange over Sands, Cumbria, 8–10 September 2009.

Schmied, V., Beake, S., Sheehan, A., McCourt, C., & Dykes, F. (2009b). *A meta-synthesis of women's perceptions and experiences of breastfeeding support.* (No. SR208). Adelaide: Joanna Briggs Institute.

Schwartz, K., D'Arcy, H. J. S., Gillespie, B., Bobo, J., Longeway, M., & Foxman, B. (2002). Factors associated with weaning in the first 3 months postpartum. *The Journal of Family Practice, 51*(5), 439–444.

Shakespeare, J., Blake, F., & Garcia, J. (2004). Breast-feeding difficulties experienced by women taking part in a qualitative interview study of postnatal depression. *Midwifery, 20*, 251–260.

Sheehan, A. (2006). *Complex decisions: Deconstructing best. A grounded theory study of infant feeding decisions in the first six weeks post-birth.* Unpublished PhD thesis, University of Technology, Sydney, Australia.

Sheehan, A., Schmied, V., & Cooke, M. (2003). Australian women's stories of their baby-feeding decisions in pregnancy. *Midwifery, 19*, 259–266.

Sheehan, A., Schmied, V., & Barclay, L. (2010) Complex decisions: Theorizing women's infant feeding decisions in the first 6 weeks after birth. *Journal of Advanced Nursing, 66*(2), 371–380.

Stein, J., Dykes, F., & Bramwell, R. (2000). Breast-feeding: Midwives meeting mothers in the middle. *British Journal of Midwifery, 8*(4), 239–245.

Tsianakas, V. & Liamputtong, P. (2007). Infant feeding beliefs and practices among Afghan women living in Melbourne, Australia. In P. Liamputtong (Ed.), *Childrearing & infant care issues: A cross-cultural perspective* (pp. 249–273). New York: Nova Science Publishers.

Ullah, S., & Griffiths, P. (2003). Does the use of pacifiers shorten breastfeeding duration in infants? *British Journal of Community Nursing, 8*(10), 458–463.

UNICEF (2009). The Baby-Friendly Hospital Initiative. Retrieved 14 August 2009, from www.unicef.org/programme/breastfeeding/baby.htm

Wall, G. (2001). Moral constructions of motherhood in breastfeeding discourse. *Gender & Society, 15*(4), 592–610.

World Health Organization (1981). *International code of marketing of breast-milk substitutes.* Unpublished manuscript, Geneva: World Health Organization.

World Health Organization (1989). *Protecting, promoting and supporting breast-feeding: The special role of maternity services*. Geneva: World Health Organization.

World Health Organization (2007). *Evidence on the long-term effects of breastfeeding: Systematic reviews and meta-analysis*. Geneva: World Health Organization.

World Health Organization & UNICEF. (1991a). *Innocenti Declaration. On the protection, promotion and support of breastfeeding*. Florence: UNICEF.

World Health Organization & UNICEF (1991b). *Take the Baby Friendly Initiative!* New York: UNICEF.

World Health Organization & UNICEF. (2003). *Global strategy for infant feeding and young child feeding*. Retrieved July 4, 2009, from http://whqlibdoc.who.int/publications/2003/9241562218.pdf

Chapter 5
Infant Feeding and the Problems of Policy

Ellie Lee

Contents

5.1 Introduction

> Breastfeeding is a major public health issue. A decision to breastfeed, especially if sustained for the first six months of a baby's life, can make a major contribution to infant health and development. Moreover, research indicates that cancers and coronary heart disease, and particularly childhood obesity, three of the Government's priority areas for health improvement, could be positively affected by increasing breastfeeding rates. Breastfeeding is also an important equality issue. The Infant Feeding Survey 2000 demonstrated that women from disadvantaged communities were significantly less likely to breastfeed.
>
> (Melanie Johnson, Minister for Public Health, Foreword, '*Good Practice and Innovation in Breastfeeding*', Department of Health 2004a).

How a mother feeds her baby is, formally, a decision for her to make. Yet, infant feeding is surrounded by conventions and precepts about appropriate maternal decisions (Blum 1999). British women feed their babies in a context dominated by a clear message: they should decide to breastfeed. This message is communicated by many agencies including the British Government. Recent years have seen the publication of a raft of policy statements (over 20 since 2000) that promote breastfeeding.

E. Lee (✉)
University of Kent, Canterbury, Kent CT2 7NF, United Kingdom
e-mail: e.j.lee@kent.ac.uk

P. Liamputtong (ed.), *Infant Feeding Practices*, DOI 10.1007/978-1-4419-6873-9_5,

© Springer Science+Business Media, LLC 2011

The above extract illustrates the key messages of British policy. Policy is unequivocal; no ambivalence is associated with attaching breastfeeding to important benefits for individual children, mothers, and the wider society. Thus, breastfeeding is a 'major public health issue' not only contributing to 'infant health and development' but also, we are told, to the health of the wider population, as rates of disease later in life could be 'positively affected' by the practice. Additionally, changing the infant feeding behaviour of specific groups of mothers – those in lower social classes who are the least likely to breastfeed – is represented in official discourse as a very important task as it is a route to their 'equality'.

Breastfeeding promotion programmes are also more and more justified on a third ground. Infant feeding has become part of policies concerning 'parenting'. The notion central to the concept 'parenting' is that the quality of the relationship between the parent and the child – in particular its emotional quality – is uniquely important in determining the course of a person's life. *Every Child Matters* (Department for Education and Sills (DfES) 2003, p. 26) states: 'The period from conception through to the start of school is critical to later life chances'. It continues that 'the bond between the child and their parents *is the most critical influence* on a child's life' (DfES 2003, p. 39, my emphasis). Breastfeeding promotion is included in the programmes developed on this basis to 'support parents'. *Every Child Matters* advocates 'universal parenting services', which include 'specialist parenting support', 'including home visiting services consisting of frequent visits to parents in the pre- and post-natal period, supporting breastfeeding and the detection and management of post-natal depression' (DfES 2003, p. 41).

Social scientific research indicates that the presumptions of policy are to some extent widely shared; assessments of mothers' attitudes to infant feeding show they mostly also make reference to benefits of breastfeeding cited in policy discourse when they are asked about how they think it is best to feed babies (Lee & Furedi 2005; Department of Health 2007). The Department of Health's most recent Infant Feeding Survey (IFS) published in 2007 found that over eight in ten mothers said they were aware of the health benefits of breastfeeding and most were able to spontaneously give at least one benefit. Yet, practice departs greatly from official advice. The Government has surveyed British mothers' feeding practices since the 1970s, and figures from the 2007 IFS show only 2% follow advice on exclusive breastfeeding (that babies should be exclusively breastfed for 26 weeks) and only one quarter breastfeed at all by 26 weeks. Most women do not breastfeed for anywhere near the recommended time. Seventy-six per cent of women initiate breastfeeding (defined as any contact between mother's nipple and baby's mouth following birth), an increase in the rate since the 2000 survey. However, by 6 weeks after birth, 52% of these mothers have stopped breastfeeding, meaning from this point the majority of mothers feed their baby formula milk at least in part. Twenty-five per cent of women exclusively formula feed from the outset (Department of Health 2007).

One interpretation of these statistics is that, in practice, mothers are more ambivalent about the benefits of breastfeeding than in the abstract. Policy, as it is currently formulated however, gives no indication that maternal experience may be characterised by ambiguity about how best to feed babies. This interpretation suggests there may be an important tension between policy presumptions and mothers' actual experience of feeding their babies.

Research utilising social scientific methods has largely not concerned itself with exploring maternal ambiguity and ambivalence. Rather, the paradigm informing the majority research about infant feeding practices is a public health perspective (Van Esterick 2002). Most studies, thus, explore why women do not initiate breastfeeding or do not breastfeed for the recommended length of time, and suggest interventions to change maternal behaviour. This work can perhaps be most accurately considered advocacy research as its purpose is to give additional weight to arguments for devoting more Government resources to breastfeeding promotion. A small number of studies have, however, utilised social science methods to generate important insights about the tensions between policy and maternal practice and experience. The purpose of this chapter is to summarise findings of this work.

My reading suggests an important critique of infant policy emerges from this research, and three major themes appear to be central to that critique: breastfeeding promotion and the individualisation of social problems; 'scientisation' and the effacing of maternal choice; and moralisation and the problem of moral jeopardy. I discuss each of these themes, and conclude by summarising the implications of this work and areas that require further socio-cultural investigation. Most of the research I discuss considers Britain, but some work (especially North American) is also referred to where its insights are important for British experience.

5.2 Breastfeeding Promotion and the Individualisation of Social Problems

As indicated by the quotation above, policy strongly associates breastfeeding with strategies to address social problems, including ill health and inequality. Research about Britain emphasises, first, there is a longstanding tendency for policy to individualise these social problems, through its claims and programmes about infant feeding. Some accounts have explored how in the late 19th and early 20th centuries, for example, wet nursing became a focus of concern, and the education of 'ignorant' mothers, especially those from the working classes, who did not breastfeed, was represented as the route to improving the health of the nation (Carter 1995; Murphy 2004). According to Murphy (2004, p. 205), this sort of approach, while 'politically expedient', rendered 'other sources of infant morbidity and mortality less visible'. The contemporary phase of policy development emerges in the 1970s, and historical continuity in official thinking about infant feeding has been detected. There are very obvious differences with the past – infant morality and malnutrition were no longer the scourges in the late 20th century that they were in the 19th and early 20th centuries. Practices such as wet nursing or feeding babies diluted condensed milk had been replaced by infant feeding with formula milk as alternatives to breastfeeding. However, suppositions informing policy that individualise social problems, it has been suggested, appear in some ways similar.

Carter (1995, p. 61) notes how the 1980s saw the rise of 'health inequality' as a policy concern and breastfeeding featured in discussion of this problem:

> The political agenda around nutrition has become increasingly polarised between those who see structural and material causes of poor diet, and those who see these things as a result of the of the 'carelessness and ignorance' beloved of policy makers earlier in the century. Although non breast-feeders are not explicitly labelled as ignorant breast-feeding must nevertheless be seen as a relatively safe political issue. . . .Instead of focusing on these broader health issues the policy agenda is limited to feeding habits and attitudes.

This analysis suggests breastfeeding promotion constitutes an important example of the resolution of the debate about the causes of ill health, in favour of an approach that prioritises 'habits and attitudes' over structural and material factors. Even if the language used by the 1980s was no longer explicit, the contention here is that relatively worse health among poorer sections of society came to be considered to be caused by the behaviour of poorer mothers, as measured by their relative failure to breastfeed.

Analysis of policy in the contemporary context has focussed on the account it offers of differential rates of breastfeeding by social and economic class. Hence, a second theme in the literature is a critique of the so-called problem of 'equality'. As Carter (1995) notes, the overtly pejorative language of the past was no longer apparent in official accounts of these differentials by 1980s. It has latterly been entirely replaced by reference to the need direct 'awareness' campaigns, 'information' and 'support' at women who are less likely to breastfeed (Murphy 2004). It has been argued however, that these contemporary approaches remain fundamentally consistent with the past in that they leave material and structural conditions unaffected. Murphy (2004, p. 207) argues that 'such support is generally just verbal encouragement and advice'. Set against this, she contends, a mother's ability to meet the demands of exclusive breastfeeding over many weeks 'is inextricably linked to the availability of human and material resources', which include someone else taking on running the home, looking after other children, and giving the mother time to rest (cf. Chapters 8 and 9 in this volume). Murphy (2004, p. 207) argues: 'Breastfeeding is a form of work to which a mother may not be able to readily commit herself if it conflicts with her other responsibilities'. Powerful structural and material factors shape the experience of motherhood, and these, it is argued, contextualise both low rates of exclusive breastfeeding and differentials among social groups.

Others point to cultural norms as way of explaining differential breastfeeding rates in the current context. On the basis of interviews with mothers, Pain, Bailey, and Mowl (2001, p. 313, my emphasis) suggest that 'there is . . . an *expectation* that middle-class women will choose to breastfeed'. This expectation links to powerful mores about sexuality, masculinity, and parenting, which work to validate breastfeeding as part of middle-class social life. For example, 'the middle class men in the study expressed relaxed attitudes to their partners' breastfeeding in front of others', note Pain and colleagues (2001, p. 267), and they highlight how this was considered one outcome of 'emotional correctness' within middle-class peer groups. The implication of this analysis, if it is correct, is that breastfeeding 'decisions' require, apart from material resources, a type of culturally validated lifestyle orientation.

Material and cultural explanations for infant feeding practices are posited in this way as more convincing than those informing policy. However, it does not follow that material and cultural resources lead to 'successful' breastfeeding as defined by policy as exclusive breastfeeding for 6 months. Government statistics show that most mothers in the higher social classes do not feed their babies this way, and it is notable that the 'expectation' that such mothers will breastfeed has been shown to co-exist with fairly widespread experience of breastfeeding 'failure' and concomitant feelings of guilt and anxiety (Bailey & Pain 2001; Lee 2007a). Thus, neither does it follow that the experience of motherhood in the context of a cultural 'expectation' in favour of breastfeeding is always positive.

One strikingly honest contribution illustrating this point comes from Crossley (2009). She uses her own experience to draw attention to how internalised cultural expectations regarding breastfeeding can work themselves out. She describes the ordeal of accepting her 'failure' as a mother by formula feeding, in the face of her baby consistently failing to gain enough weight over 12 weeks' exclusive breastfeeding. Her account includes important insights about how this 'failure' made her feel. She draws the conclusion that for some women breastfeeding has become an activity, 'fraught with tension', a 'normalised moral imperative', and a practice that can detrimentally impact on relations between mothers. Crossley (2009, p. 82) recounts: 'It is not surprising that I felt that the other women in my [National Childbirth Trust] group would think of me as a failure. After all this is how I had privately judged others who had failed in their attempt to breastfeed'. Others have also noted how mothers covertly (and sometimes overtly) make judgements about each other based on how they feed their babies (Lee 2007b).

One important outcome of individualisation presently associated with breastfeeding promotion, this suggests, is that some mothers have come to consider feeding babies as not only a *task* but as a *project* closely bound up with the development of their identity as a certain sort of 'good' mother. Some have internalised the idea that how babies are fed is a legitimate measure of motherhood, and they consciously or unconsciously judge other mothers accordingly. Thus, departing in feeding practice from what is 'best' – breastfeeding – is not experienced as acceptable and uncontroversial on pragmatic grounds, but as somehow symptomatic of an individual woman's failure as a mother (Murphy 1999; see also Chapters 6, 7, and 9 in this volume).

5.3 'Scientisation' and the Effacing of Maternal Choice

The most influential basis for current policy is the association of breastfeeding with better health. A simple logic is put forward; since evidence shows that formula feeding is harmful to health relative to breastfeeding, the promotion of breastfeeding by policy is obviously necessary and right. Socio-cultural research has told a different story, however.

Hausman (2003, p. 197) states that some writings from this perspective 'refute scientific claims to the health benefits of breastfeeding, at least in the developed world, so as to argue that breastfeeding promotion is largely political having most to do with certain kinds of mothering'. My reading of literature indicates that the degree to which 'the evidence' for the superiority of breastfeeding is contested varies. Recent important (mostly North American) contributions have generated controversy, arguing that, in contrast to the certainty with which many associate formula feeding with a large range of health problems, in many areas (for example, obesity, IQ, and psychological development) the evidence is varied and highly inconclusive (Wolf 2007; Rosin 2009). A consensual point in socio-cultural analysis is that the claim that how babies should be fed is to be determined by 'scientific evidence' is itself a cultural product. Wider social and cultural concerns have come to be expressed in medical and scientific language (Lee 2008). The rise of breastfeeding promotion based on 'the science' has been viewed, in particular, as one aspect of a culture of 'intensive' or 'total' motherhood (Wall 2001; Wolf 2007; Lee & Bristow 2009); it is a reflection of a 'broader child-centred mothering ideology', explains Knaak (2005, p. 201).

These terms describe a culture that defines successful childrearing as that which is 'child-centred', requiring that the parent – the mother especially – takes individual responsibility for maximising her child's physical and mental health, by avoiding risk at all costs. Culture holds out the promise of child-centred mothering as a rich source of personal fulfilment. However, intensive mothering ideology also constructs mothering as activity that, because of its significance for the development of the child, demands that serious attention be paid to scientific and expert guidance about 'parenting' and the reduction of risks to child health and welfare (Hays 1996). Contemporary culture is, therefore, one that requires parents to agree – even if ambiguously – that they will always put the child first, but also that they do not 'know best' about what makes children thrive (Furedi 2008). Providing parents with expert guidance has become central to modern 'parenting'. This culture, argue most, is historically continuous (Pain et al. 2001). The scientisation of infant feeding is 'just one aspect of the growing involvement of professional experts in all aspects of childrearing and family life throughout the twentieth century' (Murphy 2004, p. 207). The rules governing parenting have, however, become more extensive in recent years, and policy in particular has sought to play a far larger role in shaping parental behaviour (Gillies 2005a, b; Furedi 2008).

One policy concept associated with the rise of scientism is 'informed choice' (Knaak 2006; Lee & Bristow 2009). Analysis of this concept has suggested that while 'choice' has become a watchword of policy, in the form of 'informed choice' its content is modified considerably. Many have noted how public health policy in general has recently developed in particular way, so as to emphasise 'choice' (Burrows, Nettleton, & Bunton 1995; Nettleton 1995, 2004). 'Choosing Health', for example, is the title of a major document setting out the current British Government's public health policy (Department of Health 2004b). The reasons for this emphasis on 'choice' have been analysed as reflecting the ascendance of particular conceptualisation of causes of ill health, compared to that of the past. The approach will be familiar to any reader, so little detail is required. In summary, ill health is no longer considered misfortune of nature, to be addressed by medical care when it occurs. Rather, illness is a state that can be fostered or imperilled by individuals through their lifestyles and behaviour.

It has been argued that in general, the meaning of 'choice' embedded in this approach is very particular. To 'choose' is not to pick between two valid options each with advantages. Rather, it is to opt to live life in a way deemed manifestly superior by expert 'evidence' or to decide to continue living in a way that encourages illness and early death. In policy terms, the rise of what is termed 'informed choice' means a choice made in the full light of expert assessments of the risks associated with certain behaviours (Murphy 2004; Nettleton 2004). Studies of infant feeding policy have suggested that the meaning of 'choice' has evolved in a similar way.

Policies regarding 'informed choice' should, according to Wray (2005), mean that women are provided with a fair and honest account of alternatives, to assist the individual to come to a decision about a course of action. 'Informed choice' in infant feeding, it has been argued, is more and more defined differently, as a choice made only when women fully appreciate that formula milk use is a health risk for babies (Knaak 2006; Lee & Bristow 2009). Thus, 'choice' in infant feeding methods is not defined as something that is 'actual', meaning individual mothers might legitimately decide between two alternatives each with benefits. There is, rather, a context of 'constrained choice' because the alternative to breastfeeding is predominantly represented in very negative ways (Knaak 2005). For this reason, in the 21st century, breastfeeding promotion has been viewed as 'emblematic of the way in which risk discourses dominate a wide range of political programmes and professional practices' (Murphy 2004, p. 201). A one-sided emphasis on risk in North American breastfeeding promotion programmes has been the subject of important critiques (Kukla 2006; Wolf 2007). Risk-based promotion of breastfeeding is less overt in Britain, but is nonetheless more and more embedded in policy and practice (Murphy 2004; Lee 2007b).

A range of problems has been associated with the influence of scientism, and the associated redefinition of choice. Some have detected, first, that research about infant feeding has become insufficiently open-ended, and thus insensitive in this context. Studies often take for granted the claim that infant feeding practices are a problem because they do not match with what 'the evidence' deems best (Maclean 1988). Bowes and Domokos (1998 online) note: 'There is a tendency to look for deterministic explanations of breastfeeding'. They continue that 'research...has been preoccupied with the search for single factors ... generally in an attempt to discover why rates of breastfeeding are low or less low in different areas, social classes or ethnic categories'. This is a deficit that recent research, especially that using qualitative approaches, has sought to address. It has been found that the lived reality of motherhood is complex and contradictory, and contrasts with the image of that experience provided by studies that purport to find ways to 'fix' the 'problem' of low breastfeeding rates (Miller, Bonas, & Dixon-Woods 2007).

A second area of discussion emanating from such qualitative studies concerns the gap between expert opinion and the lived reality of feeding babies for mothers. A scientised approach, it is argued, is one-sided and effaces issues mothers might take into account. Knaak (2006, p. 413) explains: 'In general there is a failure to appropriately contextualise risk and benefit'. The overriding emphasis is on the drawbacks for young babies of formula feeding, with almost no consideration given to '[mothers'] many other health and mothering considerations' (2006, p. 413). British studies have done much to illuminate these 'health and mothering considerations' by making mothers' own accounts of infant feeding the starting point of research. They draw attention to a set of factors unrecognised by current policy.

The experience of the physical reality of breastfeeding – including pain, discomfort, and tiredness – features prominently in accounts of mothers' decisions to formula feed (Bowes & Domokos 1998; Murphy 1999; Murphy, Parker, & Phipps 1999; Bailey & Pain 2001; Lee 2007a, b; Stapleton, Fielder, & Kirkham 2008). Mothers being unsettled by their actual experience of what breastfeeding demands of them is also highlighted, and one theme in the literature along these lines is the gap between expectation and reality, which is highly disorienting for some mothers (Pain et al. 2001; Bailey, Pain, & Aarvold 2004; Lee 2007a; Miller et al. 2007). Bailey and Pain (2001) emphasise how the image of breastfeeding mothers often have is markedly at odds with the pain and discomfort that characterises actual experience, and which often persists despite professional support and help in breastfeeding techniques. The counter position of 'commitment to breast-feeding and high expectations of success', with 'unexpected difficulties' also featured in commentary on postnatal depression (Shakespeare, Blake, & Garcia 2003). Stories of women persisting and struggling to breastfeed in the face of pain and deterioration of maternal well-being, in order to do 'what is best', also appear. Notably, a sort of coercion or pressure to breastfeed generated in peer groups, as well as through force of expert pronouncements, has been identified as important in generating this experience (Bailey & Pain 2001; Crossley 2009).

A more or less overt conflict between the imperative to breastfeed and other cultural norms valued by many mothers is another theme in the literature. Official discourses, if they discuss mothers, represent breastfeeding as better for mothers than formula feeding in regard of both physical health and 'well-being' (with breastfeeding routinely represented as potent source of pride, as mothers can know they have decided to do what is best). Formula feeding is discussed by mothers in a way simply not recognised in these representations; it is described by mothers as means of 'getting back to normal' and 'having freedom' from the baby, and re-establishing their identity as 'non-mothers' (Bailey & Pain 2001; Earle 2002; Stewart-Knox, Gardiner, & Wright 2003). 'Convenience', 'ease', 'sharing feeding', 'getting my body back', 'getting back to normal' were all terms used by women in my own study (Lee 2007a, b) of reasons for formula feeding. Employment also shapes mothers' decisions with returning to work associated with stopping breastfeeding (Stewart-Knox et al. 2003; Sloan, Sneddon, Stewart, & Iwaniec 2006). Going back to work quite soon after birth is described as a necessity for many working-class mothers, making formula feeding from a fairly early point after birth appear to be an inevitability (Pain et al. 2001), but some studies also report a very positive identification with work on the part of mothers. Formula feeding is considered a valued means to an end, facilitating the transition back to work, and the restoration of an important part of 'normality' for mothers (Lee 2007b).

Male partners' involvement in feeding babies is also a theme in the literature and it is apparent that a lived reality of shared parenting, increasingly validated in culture and society, does shape feeding decisions (Pain et al. 2001; see also Chapter 3 in this volume). Fathers have been identified by mothers as being, in part, 'involved' in infant feeding in order to assist with the hard work of baby care (Earle 2000). Paternal involvement through formula feeding is also identified, however, as a positive and pleasurable aspect of maternal experience. Sharing baby care is deemed to matter a great deal by parents, and paternal involvement and 'bonding' is discussed as a source of pleasure for both mothers and fathers (Earle 2000; Bailey & Pain 2001; Pain et al. 2001; Lee 2008; Schmidt 2008).

Experience of the regime of 'informed choice' forms a third important discussion point. Commentaries about maternal experience emphasise worry and anxiety generated by an increasing emphasis on the risks of formula feeding (Lee 2007b). Some also note how worries of this sort impel mothers to carry on attempting to breastfeed, although their health or that of their babies appears to others to be clearly imperilled by them doing so (Stapleton et al. 2008; Crossley 2009). It has also been suggested that 'informed choice' is associated with mothers becoming less likely to know how best to formula feed babies. Based on a reading of information provided by health professionals, Wall (2006, p. 81) makes the strong claim that despite formula feeding being a majority practice, 'mothers are often denied information on an appropriate formula to use, how to prepare formula correctly or how to sterilise and store bottles of formula or expressed breast milk'. Cairney and Barbour (2007) concur counter posing the attention paid to informing and supporting women about breastfeeding to the lack of activity surrounding formula feeding. Studies have suggested that mothers report being not provided with information about bottle-feeding (Lee 2007a; Crossley 2009) and concerns have been raised about the practical effects of this development for the health of bottle-fed babies (Cairney & Alder 2001; Wall 2006; Cairney & Barbour 2007).

Other effects of a lack of information about formula feeding are also discussed. From my own work (Lee 2007a, p. 12), I contend that some mothers, who found health professionals unwilling or unable to discuss formula feeding with them, 'appeared to experience this as a slight to their identity as mothers who wanted to "do their best"'. The particular contribution of not being provided with information about this feeding strategy appeared to be the encouragement of 'guilty behaviour'. Some mothers reported they lied to health professionals about how they were feeding their babies in response to experiencing the absence of any official recognition that their behaviour was legitimate (2007a, p. 10).

The difficulties of a regime of 'informed choice' for health professionals are also highlighted by some studies. Cairney and Barbour (2007, p. 30) state that 'as a consequence of the lack of published evidence about bottle-feeding, health professionals may feel uncomfortable about, or lack knowledge in, providing assistance to bottle-feeding mothers'. This point of view appears reflected in findings of some work about midwives' experiences. According to Miller and colleagues (2007), some better qualitative work draws attention to dilemmas faced by health-care professionals, midwives especially, charged with responsibility for increasing breastfeeding rates but confronted with the reality of maternal experience. In their research with midwives, Furber and Thomson (2005, p. 365) detected 'a management strategy termed 'breaking the rules' for supporting mothers with baby feeding. The concept 'breaking the rules' represented practices that were 'not congruent with evidence-based, baby-feeding policy and recommendations'. Stapleton and associates (2008, p. 10) note that 'contemporary midwives are in a difficult position with regard to advising childbearing women', note since not only they must encourage breastfeeding but also 'strive to be "with" women (and the "bad" choices they make)'. Some studies highlight how midwives contravene what is considered good practice and help mothers to formula feed (Miller et al. 2007). Mirroring mothers' sense of deviance when they formula feed, midwives want to help alleviate tiredness and pain, but are aware that in doing so they are contradicting what is deemed 'best' (Cloherty, Alexander, & Holloway 2004).

5.4 Moralisation and the Problem of Moral Jeopardy

Policy today, unlike the past, eschews the use of categories to describe mothers who use formula milk that could be accused of stigmatising mothers or moralising about their behaviour. The scientised agenda of risk avoidance formally presents mothers as currently insufficiently 'supported', or in need of greater 'empowerment' by programmes to promote breastfeeding, rather than selfish or ignorant (Lee & Bristow 2009). Contemporary breastfeeding promotion has, nonetheless, been conceptualised as a moralised enterprise.

This case has been made through analysis of the new public health, of which breastfeeding promotion forms a part. It has been argued that regardless of the emphasis on support and empowerment to enable the individual to reduce risk and choose health, behaviour is strongly moralised in contemporary culture. 'Health' has come operate as a 'moral framework' for society, emphasising 'individual responsibility and ... compliance with the appropriate medically sanctioned standard of behaviour' (Fitzpatrick 2001, p. 70). The moral imperative to avoid risk, it is argued, has most purchase, however, where risk that might be taken impacts on another person. Following the socio-cultural approach to risk developed by Mary Douglas, Murphy (2004) suggests for this reason that actions that are considered risky for the health of *another person* have attained special significance. They even constitute the contemporary equivalent of sinful behaviour with the person put 'at risk' considered 'sinned against'. It is for this reason, since mothers have a particular responsibility for caring for children, that the moralisation of health has a special power and import for maternal experience.

Empirical studies documenting mothers' experience of feeding babies attest to the moralising force of breastfeeding promotion. Thus, Miller and associates (2007) suggest that a dominant theme which emerges from the qualitative literature is that infant feeding is often experienced by mothers as a moral problem. Infant feeding attitudes and practices are experienced as a measure of motherhood: 'The literature suggests that perceived societal and peer pressure, the expectations of health professionals, and feelings of guilt and concern over the need to be a "good" mother profoundly shape not only the decisions and practices of women but also the accounts they offer of these' (Miller et al. 2007, p. 216). Pain and colleagues (2001, p. 265) note that the mothers in their study 'felt under pressure to live up to certain ideas about good mothering. Frequently they felt judged by others, including heath professionals, friends, family members and strangers'. The evidence 'points to the struggles that women engage in to maintain their status as "good mothers" which lead them to produce accounts of infant feeding aimed at protecting the moral defensibility of their decisions and practices, regardless of what these are' (Miller et al. 2007, p. 224).

These 'struggles' have been documented in some detail. Murphy (1999) describes mothers' struggles to defend their status as identity work. The force of expert advice that defines how best to feed babies is not, she suggests, in 'compelling women to conform'. Rather, it is 'in the way it sets the moral context within which women negotiate their identities as mothers' (Murphy 2004, p. 209). It is important to note that the need to perform identity work to uphold moral status pertains regardless of how women actually feed their baby. Thus, some literature considers identity work women do to justify breastfeeding in familial or community context where bottle-feeding is considered normal and less troublesome; where mothers breastfeed for longer than a few months; and where breastfeeding is not going to plan, meaning babies are not gaining weight very fast (Bailey et al. 2004; Murphy 2004; Marshall, Godfrey, & Renfrew 2007). However, given the overarching policy and cultural context of 'breast is best', it is unsurprising to find that moral jeopardy is most pronounced where mothers use formula milk. It is when they formula feed that mothers most often struggle to defend the notion that they are 'good mothers' (Murphy 1999, 2003; Lee 2007a, b; Stapleton et al. 2008; see also Chapter 9 in this volume).

However, variations in maternal experience associated with formula feeding have been noted. Mothers do not simply consider themselves bad mothers when they fail to comply with the advice to breastfeed exclusively. Feelings of guilt have been found to be most apparent among first-time mothers, especially those who held a strong antenatal expectation that they would breastfeed (Lee 2007a). As discussed above, it has also been suggested that it is women from middle-class circles who most clearly experience formula feeding as a moral problem, as it contradicts peer-group expectations (Pain et al. 2001). Other mothers, however, respond with anger, rather than guilt, to the suggestion they are second-rate mothers because they use formula milk, and some treat those who criticise them with contempt and hostility (Lee 2007a, b, 2008). A range of strategies has also been detected, through which mothers defend themselves as good mothers when they formula feed. Important among these is recourse to first-hand and experiential knowledge rather than expert pronouncement; reference is often made to healthy children known to the mother who were formula-fed (Murphy 1999, 2004). Mothers also assert their authority to decide what is best, suggesting this should count for more than expert opinion when it comes to their child (Murphy 1999; Lee 2007a). As noted previously, some also defend formula feeding by emphasising the benefits of paternal bonding.

5.5 Conclusion

The research discussed in this chapter points to an important tension between policy imperatives and the everyday experience of mothers. One conclusion which can be drawn is that the worlds of policy, and of mothers, appear very distant from each other. In policy terms, infant feeding is a practice that needs to be modified in the interests of achieving large policy goals. For mothers, feeding a baby is one part of a relationship, which is surrounded by a complex set of influences and demands. Mothers inevitably respond pragmatically and in ways they have not anticipated to the experience of feeding a baby. This makes their experience often far more ambiguous that the statement 'breast is best' can possibly capture.

The studies considered above also indicate that a policy discourse which more and more attaches only benefits to breastfeeding, and risk to formula feeding, forms part of a context which makes the experience of feeding a baby fraught for many mothers. There is mounting evidence that mothers struggle to maintain positive identity when they formula feed, and also that informal solidarity between mothers as well as relations between mothers and healthcare professionals are negatively influenced by the approach to infant feeding that presently dominates.

An important area for socio-cultural research looking forwards is the potential for the moralisation of parental behaviour to further intensify. As noted in the introduction, the most notable innovation in current policy agendas is the identification of breastfeeding as a practice to be encouraged by programmes to improve 'parenting'. Breastfeeding is in this way now identified as a marker of an approved parenting style, which involves emotional closeness, deemed associated with improved outcomes for children, including in the realms of behaviour and educational success. In this form, the harms threatened by formula feeding expand notably, to include not only harms to physical health but also to the emotional relationship between parent and child. In turn, social problems such as anti-social behaviour and poor attainment at school are reframed as consequences of impaired attachment between parent and child, with infant feeding practices implicated therein. This thinking is articulated this way, by the National Assembly for Wales (2001, p. 10):

> The very intimate relationship that evolves between the mother and suckling baby, the act of nurture, and its reverberations through the family unit may also confer benefit to the cognitive, behavioural and emotional development of the infant and young child....It is therefore sad to find in Wales, along with many other developed countries so many babies not able to receive what amounts to their birthright.

The process through which the incorporation in this way of a particular account of the significance of the mother-child 'bond' into wider social policy is an important area for research, as is how this development shapes and influences parental experience.

References

Bailey, C., & Pain, R. (2001). Geographies of infant feeding and access to primary health-care. *Health and Social Care in the Community, 9*(5), 309–317.

Bailey, C., Pain, R., & Aarvold, J. E. (2004). A 'give it a go' breast-feeding culture and early cessation among low-income mothers. *Midwifery, 20*(2), 240–250.

Blum, L. M. (1999). *At the breast: Ideologies of breastfeeding and motherhood in the contemporary United States*. Boston: Beacon.

Bowes, A., & Domokos, T. M. (1998). Negotiating breastfeeding: Pakistani women, white women and their experiences in hospital and at home. *Sociological Research Online, 3*(3). Retrieved 10 April 2009, from http://www.socresonline.org.uk/socresonline/3/3/5.html

Burrows, R., Nettleton, S., & Bunton, R. (1995) Sociology and health promotion: Health, risk and consumption under late modernism. In R. Bunton, S. Nettleton, & R. Burrows (Eds.), *The sociology of health promotion* (pp. 1–9). London: Routledge.

Cairney, P., & Alder, E. (2001). A survey of information given by health professionals, about bottle-feeding, to first time mothers in a Scottish population. *Health Bulletin, 59*(2), 97–101.

Cairney, P., & Barbour, R. (2007). A research study of sources of support for bottle-feeding in new mothers. *Community Practitioner, 80*(6), 30–34.

Carter, P. (1995). *Feminism, breasts and breast-feeding*. Basingstoke: Macmillan.

Cloherty, M., Alexander, J., & Holloway, I. (2004) Supplementing breast-fed babies in the UK to protect their mothers from tiredness or distress. *Midwifery, 20*(2), 194–204.

Crossley, M. L. (2009). Breastfeeding as a moral imperative: An autoethnographic study. *Feminism and Psychology, 19*, 71–87.

Department for Education and Skills (2003). *Every child matters*. Nottingham: DfES Publications.

Department of Health (2004a). *Good practice and innovation in breastfeeding*. Retrieved 22 April 2009 from http://www.dh.gov.uk/en/Publicationsandstatistics/Publications/PublicationsPolicyAndGuidance/DH_4097202

Department of Health (2004b). *Choosing health*. London: Department of Health.

Department of Health (2007). *Infant feeding survey 2005*. London: The Information Centre.

Earle, S. (2000). 'Why some women do not breast feed: bottle-feeding and fathers' role. *Midwifery, 16*(4), 323–330.

Earle, S. (2002). Factors affecting the initiation of breastfeeding: Implications for breastfeeding promotion. *Health Promotion International, 17*(3), 205–214.

Fitzpatrick, M. (2001). *The tyranny of health*. London: Routledge.

Furber, C. M., & Thomson A. M. (2005). Breaking the rules' in baby-feeding practice in the UK: Deviance and good practice? *Midwifery, 22*, 365–376.

Furedi, F. (2008). *Paranoid parenting*. London: Continuum.

Gillies, V. (2005a). Raising the meritocracy: Parenting and the individualisation of social class. *Sociology, 39*(5), 835–852.

Gillies, V. (2005b) Meeting parents needs? Discourses of 'support' and 'inclusion' in family policy. *Critical Social Policy, 25*(1), 70–90.

Hausman, B. (2003). *Mother's milk: Breastfeeding controversies in American Culture*. London: Routledge.

Hays, S. (1996). *The cultural contradictions of motherhood*. New Haven: Yale University Press.

Knaak, S. (2005). Breast-feeding, bottle-feeding and Dr Spock: The shifting context of choice. *Canadian Review of Sociology and Anthropology, 42*(2), 197–216.

Knaak, S. (2006). The problem with breastfeeding discourse. *Canadian Journal of Public Health, 97*(5), 412–414.

Kukla, R. (2006). Ethics and ideology in breastfeeding advocacy campaigns. *Hypatia, 21*(1), 157–180.

Lee, E. (2007a). Health, morality, and infant feeding: British mother's experiences of formula milk use in the early weeks. *Sociology of Health and Illness, 29*(7), 1075–1090.

Lee, E. (2007b). Infant feeding in risk society. *Health, Risk and Society, 9*(3), 295–309.

Lee, E. (2008). Living with risk in the age of 'intensive motherhood': Maternal identity and infant feeding. *Health, Risk and Society, 10*(5), 467–477.

Lee, E., & Bristow, J. (2009). Rules for infant feeding'. In S. Day Sclater, F. Ebtehaj, E. Jackson, & M. Richards (Eds.), *Regulating autonomy, sex reproduction and the family* (pp. 73–92). Oxford and Portland, Oregon: Hart.

Lee, E., & Furedi, F. (2005). *Mothers' experience of, and attitudes to, using infant formula in the early months*. SSPSSR, University of Kent. Retrieved 20 May 2004 from http://www.kent.ac.uk/sspssr/staff/academic/lee/infant-formula-full.pdf

Maclean, M. (1988). Implications of a health promotion framework for research on breastfeeding. *Health Promotion International, 3*(4), 355–360.

Marshall, J. L., Godfrey, M., & Renfrew, M. J. (2007). 'Being a 'good mother': managing breastfeeding and merging identities. *Social Science and Medicine, 65*(10), 2147–2159.

Miller, T., Bonas, S., & Dixon-Woods, M. (2007). Qualitative research on breastfeeding in the UK: A narrative review and methodological reflection. *Evidence and Policy, 3*(2), 197–230.

Murphy, E. (1999). 'Breast is best': Infant feeding decisions and maternal deviance. *Sociology of Health and Illness, 21*(2), 187–208.

Murphy, E. (2003). Expertise and forms of knowledge in the government of families. *The Sociological Review, 51*(4): 433–462.

Murphy, E. (2004). Risk, maternal ideologies, and infant feeding. In J. Germov & L. Williams (Eds.), *A sociology of food and nutrition* (pp. 200–219). Oxford: Oxford University Press.

Murphy, E., Parker, S., & Phipps, C. (1999) Motherhood, morality and infant feeding. In J. Germov & L. Williams (Eds.), *A sociology of food and nutrition* (pp. 250–266). Oxford: Oxford University Press.

National Assembly for Wales (2001). *Investing in a better start: Promoting breastfeeding in Wales*. Cardiff: National Assembly for Wales.

Nettleton, S. (1995). *The sociology of health and illness*. Cambridge: Polity.

Nettleton, S. (2004). Surveillance and health promotion. In J. Gabe, M. Bury & M. A. Elston (Eds.), *Key concepts in medical sociology* (pp. 155–162). London: Sage.

Pain, R., Bailey, C., & Mowl, G. (2001). Infant feeding in North East England: Contested spaces of reproduction. *Area, 33*(3), 261–272.

Rosin, H. (2009). The case against breastfeeding. *The Atlantic*, April. Retrieved 7 April 2009 from http://www.theatlantic.com/doc/200904/case-against-breastfeeding

Schmidt, J. (2008). Gendering in infant feeding discourses: The good mother and the absent father. *New Zealand Sociology, 23*(2), 61–74.

Shakespeare, J., Blake, F., & Garcia, J. (2003). Breast-feeding difficulties experienced by women taking part in a qualitative interview study of postnatal depression. *Midwifery, 20*(3), 251–260.

Sloan, S., Sneddon, H., Stewart, M., & Iwaniec, D. (2006). 'Breast is best? Reasons why mothers decide to breastfeed or bottlefeed their babies and factors influencing the duration of breastfeeding. *Child Care in Practice, 12*(3), 283–297.

Stapleton, H., Fielder, A., & Kirkham, M. (2008). Breast or bottle? Eating disordered childbearing women and infant-feeding decisions. *Maternal and Child Nutrition, 4*(2), 106–120.

Stewart-Knox, B., Gardiner, K., & Wright, M. (2003). What is the problem with breastfeeding? A qualitative analysis of infant feeding perceptions. *Journal of Human Nutrition and Dietetics, 16*(4), 265–273.

Van Esterick, P. (2002). Contemporary trends in infant feeding research. *Annual Reviews in Anthropology, 31*, 257–278.

Wall, A. (2006). What choice in infant feeding methods? *The Journal of Family Health Care,* 16(1), 13–15.

Wall, G. (2001). Moral constructions of motherhood in breastfeeding discourse. *Gender & Society, 15*(4), 590–608.

Wolf, J. (2007). Is breast really best? Risk and total motherhood in the National Breastfeeding Awareness Campaign. *Journal of Health Politics, Policy and Law, 32*(4), 595–636.

Wray, J. (2005). Choice: Fad or fashion? *The Practising Midwife, 8*(3), 4–5.

Part II
Motherhood, Work, and Infant Feeding Practices

Chapter 6
Shifting Identities: Social and Cultural Factors That Shape Decision-Making Around Sustaining Breastfeeding

Joyce L. Marshall and Mary Godfrey

Contents

6.1 Introduction

Childbirth and breastfeeding are at once both very personal and public, social phenomena. Having a baby impacts upon daily living, social relationships and women's sense of themselves, including their embodied selves. Infant feeding, and in particular the act of breastfeeding, is not just about meeting the nutritional needs of babies, it is imbued with cultural and social meaning with significance for women's successful transition to motherhood. A major life change, motherhood profoundly affects women's assumptive worlds and disrupts the 'normal' pattern of life 'before baby'. Motherhood is a source of joy, of anxiety relating to its successful accomplishment and concerns about loss of freedom and self-identity (Oakley 1979, 1993; Miller 2005).

At the same time, women are located within webs of relationships comprising partners, family members and friends. Focus on women's 'social networks' – the structure and composition of these relational ties (Wellman, Carrington et al. 1988; Wellman, Wong et al. 1997) – directs attention at how women's emotions, attitudes

J.L. Marshall (✉)
Maternal and Child Health, University of Huddersfield, Harold Wilson Building, The University of Huddersfield, Queensgate, Huddersfield, HD1 3DH
e-mail: joyce.marshall@hud.ac.uk

P. Liamputtong (ed.), *Infant Feeding Practices*, DOI 10.1007/978-1-4419-6873-9_6,

© Springer Science+Business Media, LLC 2011

and behaviour relating to motherhood and infant feeding are shaped by the reactions of these 'significant' others (Carter 1995; Blum 1999). Women also draw on support and resources from within their social networks to manage the transition to motherhood. Even so, the weight and intensity of influence of network members will vary with the perceived significance of, and support derived from, particular relationships within the network.

Although generally women subscribe to the dominant scientific and health discourse that 'breast is best', they encounter contradictory views among 'significant others' within their social networks (Blum 1999; Marshall, Godfrey, & Renfrew 2007) and have to make sense of their experience of motherhood and infant feeding in light of the practical realities of their lives. This includes managing an acceptable self/work/family balance. Consequently, it is important in any discussion about breastfeeding to consider influences at a variety of levels – individual, immediate social networks and broader societal and structural factors. In this chapter, our primary focus is on the relational or social network level. We explore how women's sense of themselves as 'good mothers' through their infant feeding practices takes account of the perceptions of significant members of their social networks, including health professionals, and facilitates negotiation through the conflicting expectations of these others with whom they interact.

6.2 Infant Feeding in England: The Social and Political Context

The social and political context within which women make the transition to motherhood at least in part shapes the development of cultural knowledge, beliefs, meanings and practice of infant feeding (Van Esterik 1989; Maher 1992; Palmer 2009). This can be appreciated by the considerable variation in breastfeeding rates evident within Europe (Cattaneo, Yngve, Koletzko, & Guzman 2005). In the United Kingdom, around 70% of women start to breastfeed but only a quarter are doing so 6 weeks later (Bolling, Grant, Hamlyn, & Thornton 2007). These rates are among the lowest in Europe, a stark contrast to Scandinavian countries (Norway, Sweden, Denmark) and Switzerland where initiation rates are over 90% and more than 80% of women are still breastfeeding between three and 4 months later (Cattaneo et al. 2005). See also Chapter 5 in this volume.

In light of expert guidance (World Health Organisation 2003) and to increase UK breastfeeding rates, breastfeeding has become a prominent feature of recent public health policies (see Chapter 5). Thus, Choosing Health (Department of Health 2004a), Every Child Matters (Department for Education and Skills 2004), the National Framework for Children and Maternity Services (Department of Health 2004b) and the High Quality Care for All: Next Stage Review (Darzi 2008) emphasise the health benefits of breastfeeding initiation and continuance. However, the reasons women who start to breastfeed but do not persist are multidimensional and interactive, and such policies to date appear to have had little impact on breastfeeding rates.

At the structural and broader societal level, the changing patterns of women's participation in the labour market and differing maternity leave policies provide some explanation. In a review of the literature, Galtry and Callister (2005) found an association between time off work and duration of breastfeeding, with return to work in the United Kingdom being among the factors predictive of early breastfeeding cessation (see also Chapters 7, 8, and 9 in this volume). In Sweden, which has a high breastfeeding initiation rate and a high maintenance rate at 6 months (97 and 73% respectively), supportive family policies mean that although a large proportion of mothers continue in paid employment, few return to work in the early months of their baby's life taking on average 11 months parental leave and tending to work on a part-time basis (Galtry 2003).

Since 1997, successive Labour governments have introduced policies aimed at reconciling work and family through extended maternity leave, introducing a right to request flexible working and increasing availability of childcare (Lewis & Campbell 2007; see Chapter 5 in this volume). Thus, paid maternity leave was extended to 18 weeks in 1999 and to 26 weeks in 2003, with a commitment to increase it to 40 weeks in 2010. These changes mainly post-date data collection in our study (between 2000 and 2002). Further, the primary focus of policy was on maternal not parental leave with minimal provision for fathers, and protection of women to return to work if they took more than 6 months leave was restricted to the right of return to a similar (and not the same) job (Department of Trade and Industry 2006). This contrasts with more extensive and flexible maternity and paternity leave in Sweden.

In the past, medicalisation has been suggested as an explanation for the decline in duration of breastfeeding. It has been argued that rather than being viewed as a natural event, childbirth and related practices such as infant feeding were seen as pathological (Miller 2005). Increased dependence on technology and professional expertise (Illich 1976; Oakley 1979) was seen as displacing traditional knowledge acquired from family and friends (Arnup, Lévesque, & Pierson 1990). Midwives and health visitors, the main health professionals who support breastfeeding women in England, have often been linked to the medicalisation of breastfeeding (Carter 1995; Murphy 2000, 2003). It is likely that some practices previously encouraged by health professionals have been detrimental to breastfeeding success, for example, separation of mothers and babies, restriction of breastfeeding and supplementation with formula. Yet, this line of argument does not explain the wide variation in breastfeeding rates between high-income countries also subject to medicalisation.

Breastfeeding initiation rates have increased in recent decades, particularly among higher income groups. There is a strong 'natural' discourse around breastfeeding that has been attributed to feminism, linked with the attempt to demedicalise pregnancy and birth and to increase women's empowerment (Oakley 1979; Saha 2002; Crossley 2009). Teaching curricula and professional practice among midwives and health visitors emphasise the health benefits of breastfeeding, and these health professionals generally work with an ideology that places women at the centre of care. Although most women still give birth in hospital, length of in-patient stay is steadily decreasing with more care being provided by community midwives in the woman's home – an environment more likely to be conducive to smoother transition to motherhood and greater maternal control of infant feeding.

Murphy (2003) argues that although mothers are ultimately in control of how babies are fed, expert opinion sets the moral context within which women negotiate their changing identity. One consequence is that women may experience a sense of 'failure' and 'guilt' when they do not continue to breastfeed (Lee 2007; Crossley 2009). Our thesis in this chapter, however, is that the situation is considerably more complex and that the moral context of infant feeding is not only set by the influence of 'experts' but also women encounter considerable dissonance from within their social networks regarding constructions of 'good mothering' and feelings of responsibility (Murphy 1999; Wall 2001). For women, making sense of, and managing, these tensions as they embark on the journey into motherhood, involving their changing self identity, building a relationship with their baby and simultaneously maintaining a positive image of themselves as mothers present a considerable challenge. We now turn to discuss the study that investigated not only how women manage these changes and contradictions but also the part played by midwives and health visitors in supporting them.

6.3 Study Methods and Introducing Women

The qualitative study reported here adds to the small but expanding literature exploring women's baby feeding practices from their perspectives. It is unique in that in addition to in-depth interviews with women, some encounters with midwives and/or health visitors were observed. This enables exploration of women's experiences and practices of breastfeeding including the meanings constructed through interaction with others in their social networks, as well as with health professionals.

Health professionals were accompanied by a researcher (JM) during their daily work. A total of 158 interactions between women who had chosen to breastfeed and midwives or health visitors were observed in the community setting. Interactions with women from a range of socio-economic and ethnic groups were sought, and to achieve this, fieldwork was carried out in a geographical location comprising inner city, suburban and rural areas. Although many women took part in the research and were very willing to invite a researcher into their home, 22 women provided their own detailed breastfeeding stories, including their views and experiences in the early weeks. A full account of the research methodology has previously been reported (Marshall et al. 2007). Here, we introduce these women to provide the reader with some contextual information about their lives.

The study was conducted in the North of England and included women who had chosen to initiate breastfeeding. They ranged in age from 19 to 34 with a mean of 28 years. They were interviewed at different times in the childbirth trajectory: the earliest interview was 10 days after the baby's birth and the latest when the baby was 6 months old, although most women were interviewed between 6 and 16 weeks following the birth. For all but six women, it was their first experience of motherhood. The majority were still breastfeeding when they were interviewed, although many not exclusively. Two women never really established breastfeeding and both had expressed breast milk to feed to their baby.

Sally had given up her job in a newsagent and moved to another town to live with her boyfriend. Before the birth, Sally and her partner returned to stay with Sally's mother in an average-sized semidetached house in an inner city area. Sally wanted to have her baby at home as she hated hospitals but was transferred to hospital during labour. After her baby's birth, Sally was distraught because she was not given the opportunity to breastfeed within the first hour (she had read that this was important), but described the 'special moment' when she finally breastfed. After the first couple of feeds Sally found she was unable to breastfeed and asked for help from the midwives. This resulted in a myriad of suggestions from various midwives that left Sally very confused and upset. She eventually took her own discharge from hospital and at home with help from her mother (who had breastfed her three children). Sally continued to exclusively breastfeed. Sally described her partner as emotionally supportive but said he kept encouraging her to give the baby a bottle. Sally had a good relationship with the community midwife who she trusted implicitly.

Emily was working in a temporary job when she became pregnant. She lived with her partner in a terraced house on the outskirts of the city. Emily did not like hospitals but had given birth there. Although she felt exhausted after the birth she said her baby had fed easily from the first feed and described feeling a 'connection' with him. Although several of her family had breastfed including her mother, Emily said she could not remember seeing anyone except her sister breastfeeding. She said she believed her partner felt 'left out' through not being able to feed the baby but never the less breastfed exclusively for ten weeks, and was feeding alternate breast and formula at twelve weeks. Emily described a wide social network of people close to her who she could talk to and whilst she found this helpful, she also pointed out that 'everyone's opinions are different about everything aren't they, whether it's breast-feeding or changing a nappy?' She 'tried not to take on board everyone's opinions' but to 'figure it out' herself.

Amelia was a solicitor but had changed her job because she did not want to continue working the long hours the job required as she felt this was not compatible with family life. Although planning a family, she was surprised to find she became pregnant very quickly after getting married. She experienced few problems during pregnancy apart from some sickness in the early weeks and continued to work. She did not have strong views about breastfeeding saying:

'if I can do it great, if I can't I'm not too worried'. Amelia described two contrasting embodied experiences of breastfeeding prior to becoming pregnant, the first, on a train journey was a woman breastfeeding an older child that she described as 'revolting'. The second, a very good friend, a glamorous, beautiful girl who breastfed discretely she described as 'really natural'. Her baby breastfed soon after birth and suckled straight away. Amelia said she enjoyed feeling close and that it felt 'natural'. After some initial help to learn the skill of breastfeeding in hospital, she experienced few difficulties. She decided to introduce a formula feed in the evening to involve her husband more as he had made comments like 'It's only your mum can help'. Amelia intended to breastfeed for four months when she planned to return to work.

We now turn to explore how women made sense of and managed complex contradictory notions related to breastfeeding within the broader context of motherhood. Women's experiences are presented chronologically to build up a picture of the way they manage breastfeeding as part of early motherhood.

6.4 Moral Dilemmas in the Decision to Breastfeed

During pregnancy, the moral nature of the infant feeding decision was clearly demonstrated in discourses equating breastfeeding with health of the baby, such as: 'improving the baby's immunity' and 'reducing allergies'; decreasing the chance of the child getting diabetes; 'not having to worry about diarrhoea'; and improving the child's IQ. Although such ideas about infant feeding were garnered from a range of sources including books and magazines, midwives played a significant role in this when delivering parent education classes. Several women spoke of feeling 'pressure' to breastfeed; such messages were not always explicit, but could result from simply more time spent discussing breastfeeding than formula feeding. Health professionals were clear that promoting breastfeeding was part of their role, and Alison (a community midwife) spoke of this during fieldwork:

> She said that during the class one of the mothers had said to her 'you really promote breastfeeding don't you?' and replied 'well I'm a health professional and I have to promote healthy rather than unhealthy things, like I have to discourage people from smoking'. She described how she had said to this woman 'it's a shame it has to be that way because it's a natural thing that should not have to be promoted. It's natural, like getting pregnant, and none of you needed my help for that!' This made them laugh and the woman said 'well when you put it like that...' (Fieldwork with MW4)

Not all health professionals believed in framing breastfeeding as 'best' but rather focussed on the need to convey breastfeeding as normal – perhaps an impossible goal as many women had little or no embodied knowledge of it. Molly, a health visitor, said:

> It needs to be that health professionals as a whole send the message that breastfeeding is the norm, not even the best, it's just the norm. (HV6 interview)

Women generally expected health professionals to promote breastfeeding but some expressed concerns about not feeling free to choose. For example, Deborah, who breastfed for 10 weeks, remarked that:

> . . .it [breastfeeding] is encouraged sometimes I think without, how can I put it? That certain people can't breastfeed, certain people don't want to breastfeed. I think sometimes there's a negative vibe that comes out perhaps from the midwife or perhaps in general that if those people aren't prepared to give it a try. I think that's unfair sometimes. It is not something for everybody. (Deborah aged 29, rural area)

Although these examples concur with the idea of a moral imperative to breastfeed, women's narratives also revealed many conflicting aspects important to their changing identity during pregnancy such as their sexuality. For example, Sally said:

> I just think that breasts kind of aren't viewed, as means of feeding a baby anymore you know what I mean. They are for sex, they're for men, more than anything else. . .and then, it, that all changes when you meet your little baby. (Sally aged 21, inner city)

Women generally involved their partner in the initial decision to breastfeed and most were supportive. For example, Paula said her husband wanted her 'to try breastfeeding'. Unusually, Natasha described how her partner had encouraged her to change her mind when she intended to bottle-feed, she said 'he persuaded me to give it a go'. Some partners were supportive but ambivalent about how to feed the baby. Uniquely, Laura said her partner 'wasn't particularly supportive' and related how she had returned from a 'talk' on breastfeeding given by her midwife and wanted to discuss feeding with him:

> I said, you know 'Do we want to bottle or breastfeed him?' . . . 'Personally', I said 'I'd like to breastfeed him 'cause I think it's natural, it's the best thing' . . . and he kind of said 'Whatever you wanna do, I'll leave it to you because you know'. So fair enough I breastfed him. But then from the word go I think he felt quite pushed out (Laura aged 27, rural area)

So, whilst the moral nature of the breastfeeding enterprise was apparent during pregnancy – the emphasis clearly on 'breast is best', there also existed ambivalence among 'significant others' in women's social networks that they had simultaneously to negotiate. We now consider women's experiences of breastfeeding and the factors that impinge on it as they embraced motherhood.

6.5 Women's Experiences of Breastfeeding

In the early days, acquiring the physical skills of breastfeeding was of paramount importance to women. Accounts of breastfeeding at this time revealed feelings of uncertainty and vulnerability both in their selves as mothers and in their ability to breastfeed. For many, the sense of not knowing what to do was overwhelming in the first days after leaving hospital. A consistent theme within women's narratives during this period was the need to know they were 'doing it right', partly because women recognised breastfeeding as a skill that had to be learnt but also because they felt they were being tested out as 'competent' new mothers.

> It's important for me to have someone to kind of say, you know 'What am I doing? Am I doing this right?' Because you know ... you can read as much as you want but, you know it's nice to know that you're doing the right thing. (Laura)

Partners played a supportive role, albeit as observers, through the sometimes difficult period of acquiring practise skills, primarily through re-inforcing the women's own decision to breastfeed, as exemplified in Holly's account:

> Well he was just really going along with anything that I said, you know, he couldn't really do much. He watched, he knew what the midwives were saying and if I was having trouble on my own then he would say 'Oh have you remembered to do this' and 'are you doing this?'. . .Basically just reminding me what the midwives had said. So he was supportive, but he couldn't really do a lot. (Holly aged 32, rural area)

Some women encountered a degree of ambivalence from partners between wanting to be involved in all aspects of baby work, yet feeling excluded from feeding. Sally, who experienced difficulties in the beginning, described her partner as supportive although:

> I mean, he doesn't really know what to do. . .he has he's been an absolute star as far every thing else, looking after the baby goes. . ., but. . . he sits there and he kind of puts his arms around me: 'there, there, I know your nipples hurt, poor you', you know what I mean. He is kind of emotionally supportive, but he hasn't got the foggiest idea . . .where to begin helping somebody to breastfeed. . . He was . . . a lot more keen than me to just give her a bottle, I think. . . it was really upsetting him that she was crying and hungry and I was crying and in pain,. . . and as far as he could see the easiest solution was to give her a bottle and then we both shut up. So I mean he was sort of like 'are you sure you don't want to give her a bottle why don't we just like feed her with a bottle it'll be fine'. And it was me who was just like she can't have a bottle it's not fair she needs breast milk.

Confronted with difficulties in breastfeeding and ambivalence from partners, women actively sought and relied upon help to continue from 'knowledgeable and reinforcing' others within their social networks (as well as from health professionals). Holly maintained telephone contact with a friend experiencing similar problems and Emily received support from her friends with babies. Lisa regularly attended social and breastfeeding support groups with the mothers she had met at the child health clinic. Sally turned to her mother who had breastfed.

Whilst women's mothers were often a source of support and advice, they could also be seen as unhelpful in the practice of breastfeeding. Thus, Jenny kept her mother at a distance when the baby was feeding frequently but not gaining weight and turned to the midwife for help:

> Because she never breastfeed, cause I was a month early, in an incubator, so she never breastfed me and then when my sister came along she just didn't think about it. So I think because she hasn't breastfed she can't understand. There's like, they need to feed more regularly don't they than bottle fed babies . . .and she was thinking 'I'm not giving him enough milk'. (Jenny aged 30, rural area)

Over time, having mastered the technique of breastfeeding, women's priorities shifted to focus on the need to know the baby was receiving adequate nutrition – the underlying problem being their inability to directly observe the quantity of breast milk the baby was taking. In the absence of unequivocal observable evidence, women drew upon indirect cues such as the way their breasts felt in relation to feeds and the baby having wet and dirty nappies. These ways of making the invisible visible worked to increase women's confidence in their ability to provide sufficient milk for their baby and to counter criticisms that they were not performing adequately. Paula, who was happily breastfeeding her second baby, described what happened at a family gathering when her baby became unsettled, cried and needed feeding more frequently than usual:

> They were saying: 'oh you need to talk to your health visitor or your midwife, because it doesn't look as if you have got enough milk there or it might not be strong enough'. So I was tired anyway so I was getting really upset. But I knew he was putting weight on, so I thought well there is nothing wrong with him. (Paula, aged 22, second baby, rural area)

Paula was able to draw on her previous experience and the empirical knowledge that her baby was gaining weight to reassure herself.

Such cues were not foolproof as an unsettled baby could easily undermine women's confidence in their milk supply. Deborah was confronted with multiple and conflicting expectations that affected her perception of breastfeeding as equating to good mothering:

> The hardest thing for me was the fact that when Abigail was awake she was never content and that I found really, really difficult... used to tear me up inside really, because I couldn't understand why when she was awake she was always crying... And that towards the end was one of the major factors in coming off and going on to the bottle ...And it was difficult because on the one hand my mum was really trying to encourage me to keep going. [Partner's] mum was the opposite; her answer to everything was the bottle...And it nearly came to the stage where we had words...In the end I had to say 'Look I'll make the decision as to when and where and how this baby is fed'.

Sarah also was a first-time mother and felt upset that her mother-in-law judged that she was not 'coming up to scratch' as a mother:

> I think she [mother-in-law] was horrified to see Simon didn't sleep (pause) at all... and she was you know, 'ooh he's not very settled...I felt pretty bad...he was at his worst really...and they also made a big deal every time he was grouchy like: 'ooh babies don't cry for no reason there must be something wrong with him'. And passing him round saying to me: 'have you fed him...he's hungry; have you fed him. (Sarah aged 31, suburban area).

For Sarah, the fact that she viewed her baby's behaviour as atypical and that her relationship with her mother-in-law was not very close meant that she could put aside her mother-in-law's negativity, albeit taking an immediate knock in confidence. Women's status as 'good mothers' then was not universally equated with breastfeeding by key members of their social networks. Where women attributed high value to breastfeeding, they actively sought out positive reinforcers from within their networks. Negativity – either in the context of periods of particular vulnerability or from network members whose influence was particularly salient – could threaten continuance.

6.6 Pressure or Support? Interactions with Health Professionals

Commentaries in the literature suggest that medicalised discourses around motherhood and breastfeeding simultaneously position mothers as responsible for the well-being of their children and reliant upon experts (Arnup et al. 1990; Apple 1995, 2006; Murphy 2000, 2003). Here, as discussed earlier, the discourse of 'breast is best' was pre-eminent in the antenatal period, and this was clearly reflected in women's accounts linking breastfeeding with improved health of their babies. However, although it could be argued this may set a moral imperative for breastfeeding (Murphy 2000), our findings suggest that in the postnatal period a much more complex picture emerged. Whilst for women breastfeeding was generally equated with good mothering to the extent that the baby was seen as healthy, happy and thriving, where observable indicators did not support this (the baby was feeding often but unsettled and not gaining weight), the link between breastfeeding and good mothering was open to doubt. Within this context health professionals did not simply continue to promote infant feeding and help women with the technical aspects of infant feeding but also carried out extensive emotional work (Nettleton 2006) supporting women in their struggle to see themselves and be seen as 'good mothers' (cf. Chapter 9 in this volume).

Women referred to different elements of support from health professionals that they found helpful and this varied over time. In the early days, practical help with the physical aspects of breastfeeding was paramount. As feeding became established, suggestions about how to manage the life-baby balance became more important as was the knowledge that the baby was growing and developing well. Support at this stage was usually offered with attention to how women felt – their emotional well-being. Women spoke of being encouraged by health professionals telling them they were 'doing well' and being reassured that their baby's behaviour was 'normal'. Even women who knew their baby was healthy and happy liked this to be reiterated by health professionals, as illustrated by Amelia:

> I could feel her feeding quite regularly and getting quite a lot and then going to sleep. So I thought it, but you still want somebody to tell you it's all right . . . even thought you feel its right, it's still nice to have that reassurance...

Most women believed there was a 'right way' to do things and that health professionals would be able to give them this information. For example, Sally said '. . .you just need someone who knows'. Women valued timely and relevant information from health professionals not simply to ensure continued breastfeeding but also to help them to maintain their identity as 'good mothers', ensure a happy healthy baby and manage the life/baby balance.

Women frequently talked about the need for input from health professionals to resolve a particular issue of relevance to them – general or abstract advice or help was rarely perceived to be useful. Observational data revealed that health professionals made considerable efforts to encourage women to express their concerns. This was done in a variety of ways, such as asking open questions: 'how is the feeding going? or 'how are you getting on?' Their body language often conveyed interest (e.g. sitting close to women on the same level and maintaining good eye contact) and they listening attentively to women's stories and offered suggestions that specifically responded to these. Women usually described their concerns as a series of events that had occurred – as a narrative of the baby's feeding pattern. Such stories did not merely recount events but also conveyed messages to health professionals about the way the woman *felt* about those events, enabling them to provide relevant and useful information and/or emotional support in response to the uniqueness of their individual situations. The following excerpts from field work with one health professional (Beverley) illustrate this variation:

(Khalda – an Asian woman, a paediatrician, having her second baby. Her first child had lost a large amount of weight after birth)

Beverley:	How's the feeding going?
Khalda:	She's going 4 hours... [More talk about times of feeds]... I got [another midwife] to watch me feed her because she was making gulping noises.
Weighed baby	– baby had lost weight. Further discussion about feeding pattern in more detail...
Khalda:	I don't know if she is using me as a dummy...
Beverley:	Just go with that...'

(Lisa's baby was 14 days old and her first baby)

Beverley:	I presume she's been doing fine since I saw you last?
Lisa:	Yes she fed ever so often yesterday. (Further discussion)
Beverley:	Are you drinking?
Lisa:	Yes I'm drinking loads.
Beverley:	She's putting on weight?
Lisa:	Yes she is. The health visitor popped in this morning. (talks to the baby)
Beverley:	They do this at times when they are feeding all the time to boost the milk supply; you have to go with the flow. It's about 6 weeks when they have a big growth spurt.

These data illustrate that whilst dialogue was specifically relevant to each woman, there was a common theme of encouraging women to breastfeed more – 'to go with the flow'.

Health professionals said they tried to present information in a meaningful way and this sometimes meant altering the language they used to explain things taking account of what they knew about women:

> I thought this was basic simple communication skills? (Laughs} If I said to you that I had, I don't know, a 16 or 17 year old here, who may not have attended school very much, if I said 'research has shown', I sound like a sales person off the telly, selling bras or something. But you've got to make it meaningful for them. (Lindsey, health visitor)

Health professionals assessed many factors with potential to impact women's ability to breastfeed their baby and modified what they said in the light of these. For example, some health professionals suggested middle-class women should view breastfeeding like a job to encourage full commitment to it.

The relationship with health professionals was also important. Women in this study described health professionals using words such as 'nice and supportive', 'interested', 'patient with me', identified openness and honesty as important characteristics and needed to feel that health professionals listened to and had time for them but at the same time wanted to remain in control, as the following quote illustrates:

> I mean Beverley [MW5] was brilliant because she was really open about everything . . ..with the pregnancy and the birth and everything . . .. Really sort of laid back and doesn't push things on you and make you feel she's taken charge of your life or anything. (Emily)

Health professionals also recognised the need not to attempt to direct women's lives, for example:

> I am not here to shape anybody's culture yes, . . .I'm not about to tell them they mustn't do this, I will say 'well try this' or 'I don't think it is a good idea to that', or 'see what you think about it', 'if you try it the first time and it doesn't work then you will know', you know. That way you gain their confidence of the women you don't go in and try to direct people's lives. . .. (Olivia, midwife)

Interactions between breastfeeding women and health professionals after the birth of their baby were more of a negotiated encounter than has been previously suggested. It was apparent that health professionals generally encouraged women to breastfeed. However, they did this in a way that was sensitive to the context within which women were operating – both with an understanding of the multiple pressures affecting women as they breastfed and their need to maintain a view of themselves as 'good mothers'.

6.7 Conclusion

Women aspired to become and be 'good mothers' and although all of them in this study had made the decision to start breastfeeding, continuing with it and for how long was contingent upon a range of factors. Not only was there the challenge of 'doing it right' but also of balancing the growth and health of their babies with the demands of their daily lives. Within their social networks women's status as 'good mothers' was not universally equated with breastfeeding. Where women attributed high value to breastfeeding, they actively drew on salient sources of support from their social networks and sought to minimise their exposure to challenges to their identity as 'good mothers'. Whilst health professionals encouraged women to sustain breastfeeding, they also recognised their struggle to maintain a positive self-identity in the face of varying conceptions of 'good', 'bad' and 'adequate' mothering.

References

Apple, R. (2006). *Perfect motherhood: Science and childrearing in America.* New Brunswick: Rutgers University Press.

Apple, R. D. (1995). Constructing mothers: Scientific motherhood in the nineteenth and twentieth centuries. *Social History of Medicine, 8*(2), 161–178.

Arnup, K., Lévesque, A., & Pierson, R. R. (1990). Delivering *motherhood: Maternal ideologies and practices in the 19th and 20th centuries.* London: Routledge.

Blum, L. M. (1999). *At the breast: Ideologies of breastfeeding and motherhood in the contemporary United States.* Boston: Beacon.

Bolling, K., Grant, C., Hamlyn, B., & Thornton, A. (2007). Infant Feeding Survey 2005. London: The Information Centre for Health and Social Care.

Carter, P. (1995). *Feminism, breasts and breastfeeding.* New York: St Martins Press.

Cattaneo, A., Yngve, A., Koletzko, B., & Guzman, L. R. (2005). Protection, promotion and support of breast-feeding in Europe: Current situation. *Public Health Nutrition, 8*(01), 39–46.

Crossley, M. L. (2009), Breastfeeding as a moral imperative: An autoethnographic study. *Feminism and Psychology, 19*, 71–87.

Darzi, A. (2008). *High quality care for all: NHS next stage review final report.* London: Department of Health.

Department for Education and Skills. (2004). *Every child matters: Change for children.* London: The Stationary Office.

Department of Health. (2004a). *Choosing health: Making healthier choices easier.* London: The Stationary Office.

Department of Health. (2004b). *National service framework for young people and maternity services.* London: The Stationary Office.

Department of Trade and Industry (2006). *Work and families. Choice and flexibility. Additional paternity leave and pay. Government response to consultation.* London: Department of Trade and Industry.

Galtry, J. (2003). The impact on breastfeeding of labour market policy and practice in Ireland, Sweden and the USA. *Social Science and Medicine, 57*, 167–177.

Galtry, J., & Callister, P. (2005). Assessing the optimal length of parental Leave for child and parental well-being: How can research inform policy? *Journal of Family Issues, 26*(2), 219.

Illich, I. (1976). *Limits to medicine.* London: Marion Boyers.

Lee, E. (2007). Health, morality, and infant feeding: British mother's experiences of formula milk use in the early weeks. *Sociology of Health and Illness, 29*(7), 1075–1090.

Lewis, J., & Campbell, M. (2007). UK work/family balance: Policies and gender equality, 1997–2005. *Social Politics: International Studies in Gender, State and Society, 14*(1), 4–30.

Maher, V. (1992). *Anthropology of breastfeeding.* Oxford: Berg.

Marshall, J. L., Godfrey, M., & Renfrew, M. J. (2007). Being a 'good mother': Managing breastfeeding and merging identities. *Social Science & Medicine, 65*(10), 2147–2159.

Miller, T. (2005). *Making sense of motherhood: A narrative approach.* Cambridge: Cambridge University Press.

Murphy, E. (1999). 'Breast is best': Infant feeding decisions and maternal deviance. *Sociology of Health and Illness, 21*, 187–208.

Murphy, E. (2000). Risk, responsibility, and rhetoric in infant feeding. *Journal of Contemporary Ethnography, 29*(3), 291–325.

Murphy, E. (2003). Expertise and forms of knowledge in the government of families. *Sociological Review, 51*(4), 433–462.

Nettleton, S. (2006). *The sociology of health and illness.* Cambridge: Polity.

Oakley, A. (1979). *From here to maternity: Becoming a mother.* Oxford: Martin Robinson.

Oakley, A. (1993). *Essays on women, medicine and health.* Edinburgh: Edinburgh University Press.

Palmer, G. (2009). *The politics of breastfeeding: When breasts are bad for business.* London: Pinter and Martin.

Saha, P. (2002). Breastfeeding and sexuality: Professional advice literature from the 1970s to the present. *Health Education and Behaviour, 29*(1), 61–72.

Van Esterik, P. (1989). *Motherpower and infant feeding.* London: Zed Books.

Wall, G. (2001). Moral constructions of motherhood in breastfeeding discourse. *Gender and Society, 15*(4), 592–610.

Wellman, B., Carrington, P., & Hall, A. (1988). Networks as personal communities. In B. Wellman & S. D. Berkowitz (Eds.), *Social structures: A network approach* (pp.130–184). Cambridge: Cambridge University Press.

Wellman, B., Wong, R. Y., Tindall, D., & Nazer, N. (1997). A decade of network change: Turnover, persistence and stability in personal communities. *Social Networks, 19*, 27–50.

World Health Organization (2003). *Global strategy for infant and young child feeding.* Geneva: World Health Organization.

Chapter 7
Breastfeeding Under the Blanket: Exploring the Tensions Between Health and Social Attitudes to Breastfeeding in the United States, Ireland and the United Kingdom

Caroline Jane Gatrell

Contents

7.1 Breastfeeding and Health in the United Kingdom and the United States

In this chapter, I seek to position breastfeeding as a form of women's work which, in the United Kingdom, Ireland and the United States, is often unrecognised due to assumptions that breastfeeding is a 'natural' attribute of motherhood. I further seek to highlight the difficulties of trying to combine breastfeeding with employment.

For new mothers within the United Kingdom and the United States, the issue of whether, and how, breastfeeding and employment may be combined is a pressing

C.J. Gatrell (✉)
Department of Management Learning and Leadership, Lancaster University Management School, Lancaster University, Lancaster, LA1 4YX, UK
e-mail: c.gatrell@lancaster.ac.uk

P. Liamputtong (ed.), *Infant Feeding Practices*, DOI 10.1007/978-1-4419-6873-9_7,
© Springer Science+Business Media, LLC 2011

one. This is because, over the past three decades, there has been a significant and sharp growth in the numbers of women who maintain continuous employment after childbirth (Padavic & Reskin 2002; Gatrell 2008). At the same time, the pressure exerted on mothers by health professionals to breastfeed beyond the first year of babies' lives has become intense. This pressure has arisen because Health Agencies in Britain, Ireland, and America prioritise breastfeeding as an important public health, and health promotion, issue. Thus, the American Academy of Pediatricians (2009, p. 1) states on its website that:

> Advocating for children through the protection, promotion, and support of breastfeeding is a high priority for the AAP.

The designation of breastfeeding as a health priority has occurred because breast milk is believed, within UK/Irish-American medical contexts, to provide the best available source of infant nourishment (Department for Health and Children 2005). Current health research within the United Kingdom and the United States argues that the health benefits of breastfeeding are conclusive for both infants and their mothers (Galtry 1997; Witters-Green 2003; Wolf 2006). Breastfeeding is said to build infant immunities and enhance good health through childhood and beyond, protecting the wider population from infectious disease and chronic health problems such as asthma, diabetes and some psychological syndromes (Jackson 2004; Raymond 2005; Berger, Hill, & Waldfogel 2005). Breastfeeding (especially if continued over a 2 year period) is also seen to benefit maternal health by significantly reducing the risks of breast cancer and osteoporosis (Wolf 2006). See also Chapter 20 in this volume.

Thus, health agencies invest time and resource measuring and collating breastfeeding rates, and the promotion of breastfeeding is foregrounded as a priority within health campaigns. Over the past decade, the emphasis on increasing breastfeeding rates has shifted to include not only improved *initiation* rates but also emphasises the importance of increasing *duration* rates of breastfeeding. This is partly because, although campaigns to promote breastfeeding appear to have contributed to enhanced rates of breastfeeding initiation (Bailey & Pain 2001; Earle 2002), breastfeeding duration rates in the United Kingdom and the United States show that many mothers switch to formula when children are between 3 and 9 months of age. Bailey and Pain (2001) observe that while 66% of new mothers in the United Kingdom initiate breastfeeding, only 27% are still breastfeeding when babies are 4-months-old and only 14% of mothers still breastfeed when babies are 9 months. In the United States, while 69.5% of mothers initiate breastfeeding, only 10% of mothers who work full-time are still breastfeeding babies at 6 months (though this figure rises to just below 30% for 'stay-at-home mothers' (Boswell-Penc & Boyer 2007).

Thus, as well as seeking to persuade mothers to initiate breastfeeding, health agencies are now focusing on encouraging them to *continue* breastfeeding as an exclusive mode of infant feeding well beyond the first few weeks after birth. The introduction of formula milk, and/or solid foods, before 6 months is discouraged. As explained on the American health advice web site Web MD (2009):

> Experts recommend breastfeeding exclusively (no formula, juice, or water) for six months. If you supplement with formula, your milk production may go down.

Web MD goes on to advise that, while solid foods may be introduced at 6 months of age, breastfeeding should nevertheless be continued, with babies being fed on a combination of breast milk and solid foods until they are at least 1 year old, and preferably into the second year.

Health promotion campaigns in the United Kingdom, Ireland and the United States are thus aimed at increasing not only the numbers of women who breastfeed but also at extending the period during which breastfeeding is encouraged. Within breastfeeding promotion campaigns, the weight of responsibility for infant nutrition through breastfeeding is allocated to individual mothers, rather than social institutions more generally (Murphy 2003; Gatrell 2008). Thus, for example, in the 'Infant Feeding Recommendations' produced by the British NHS to facilitate hospital and community midwives in encouraging breastfeeding (Department of Health 2004), it is explained to health workers that individual mothers are the main 'target audience' for the promotion of breastfeeding as the optimum mode of infant nutrition. Similarly, in the advice offered via Web MD (2009) much of the guidance offered is aimed at persuading individual mothers, rather than organisations or social institutions, of the importance of breastfeeding.

7.2 Convenience Food? Breast Milk and Discourses of 'Natural' Motherhood

Social and health research has indicated that health promotion campaigns have been effective at raising awareness, among mothers, of the notion that 'breast is best' (Murphy 2003; Boswell-Penc & Boyer 2007). However, although mothers are now aware of the benefits of breastfeeding for child health, it could be argued that health agencies fail to acknowledge sufficiently the challenges involved in breastfeeding an infant up to and beyond the first year. As Bailey and Pain (2001), Miller (2005) and Gatrell (2007) have pointed out, breastfeeding may be difficult to establish, and problematic to maintain. Discourses about the benefits of breastfeeding often appear to gloss over the hard work entailed, focusing instead on the idea of breastfeeding as a 'natural' activity. For example, La Leche League describes breastfeeding as a 'natural', 'normal' activity. The La Leche League guidance on 'Beginning Breastfeeding' (2005) could be seen to minimise the notion of breastfeeding as challenging work, framing it instead as a 'womanly art' which the womanly body is programmed to perform, albeit with practice. La Leche League (2005, p. 5) advises mothers that once

> [you]overcome difficulties, remember that the time will come when you'll think of breast milk as the perfect convenience food.

Discourses such as this, which emphasise the 'natural' and 'womanly' qualities of breastfeeding, could be seen to obfuscate the probability that breastfeeding may be both physically painful and emotionally draining, especially for women who believed it would come 'naturally' to them, but in the event found it a gruelling challenge (Bailey & Pain 2001; Kitzinger 2003; Gatrell 2007). Discourses of 'natural' motherhood further tend to play down the time and energy consumed by breastfeeding. Kitzinger (2003, p. 401) points out that babies who are fed 'on demand' need to be fed every 2–4 hours, and each feed may take minimally thirty minutes. Mothers may feel 'very drained when nursing is long and drawn out [especially] if [mothers] are tired and the baby is constantly demanding to be fed'. Breastfeeding, then, may be difficult to establish and hard work to maintain, despite social expectations that 'normal', 'womanly' mothers should manage to breastfeed 'naturally'. The notion of breastfeeding as 'natural' and 'normal' fails to recognise the physical, emotional and temporal labour that women must invest in order to initiate and maintain breastfeeding. For women with more than one child to look after, especially if they are responsible for household domestic labour, the notion of breastfeeding for over a year may appear impractical and, indeed, 'inconvenient'. For some mothers who are feeling exhausted and trying to cope either with first babies, or with new babies and other siblings, formula milk might thus appear to be a more 'convenient' form of infant feeding than breast milk.

7.3 Discretionary Breastfeeding: Social and Cultural Attitudes Towards Breastfeeding

Furthermore, although breastfeeding up to and beyond the first year is promoted to mothers as the 'best' form of infant nutrition, the notion that breastfeeding is 'normal' and 'natural' does not appear to extend to the public setting, especially if babies are over 3 months old. As Kitzinger (2005) points out, breastfeeding might be presented to mothers by health agencies and pro-breastfeeding campaigners as a 'normal' maternal activity, but in the United States, the United Kingdom and Ireland, it is an activity which women are usually expected to conduct at home. Kitzinger (2005) thus observes a sense of social antipathy towards women who breastfeed their infants in public settings. In contrast to the idea of breastfeeding as a 'normal' activity, women who breastfeed outside the home are generally required to manage this with the utmost discretion as if breastfeeding is 'shameful' when performed in public. Breast might be 'best', but mothers are nevertheless expected to conceal breastfeeding babies under blankets or clothing – a social requirement which becomes increasingly difficult to fulfil as babies grow older (and more wriggly!). Kitzinger (2005, pp. 40–41) thus argues that women who breastfeed all but the tiniest of infants within public spaces may be criticised for failing to 'conform to normal standards of decency,' and may be accused of 'exhibitionism', 'immodesty' and 'distasteful' behaviour. Gatrell (2008) observes how even women breastfeeding infants under 1 month old may be singled out and excluded from public spaces such as restaurants (see Chapter 3 about an incident in Australia). Even within their own homes, as Bailey and Pain (2001) observe breastfeeding mothers may experience criticism from other family members who disagree either with breastfeeding per se, or who feel uncomfortable when mothers breastfeed within shared space, in the company of other household members or guests. See also Chapter 20 in this volume.

Kitzinger (2005) and Gatrell (2008) suggest that, for many women, fear (or personal experience) of such social disapproval is often a key factor in the decision to move from breast milk to formula. In the same vein as cultural feminist writers such as Martin (1989), Shildrick (1997) and Grosz (1994) have suggested, Kitzinger (2005, p. 39) attributes antipathy towards breastfeeding to a social fear of the fluidity of the 'leaky' maternal body. She argues that although breastfeeding might be considered the best form of infant nutrition, breast milk is concurrently (at least if feeding is performed in any 'public' setting) 'perceived as an unclean secretion', which is both unpredictable and 'revolting'. Kitzinger (2005, p. 39) likens breast milk to other fluids that are 'specifically female [such as] menstrual blood and amniotic fluid, [which are treated by others as if] offensive, too....they are not only polluting but dangerous ...From puberty onwards, girls are educated to be secretive and ashamed about [female bodily fluids]. All women's body products are to be hidden'.

7.4 Breastfeeding and Employment

Given the potential or actual social reaction to breastfeeding as a public activity, it seems unsurprising that women are reluctant to combine breastfeeding with employment. McKinlay and Hyde (2004), Bailey and Pain (2001), Ortiz, McGilligan, & Kelly (2004), Hausman (2004) and Gatrell (2007, 2005, 2007) all consider that a proportion of women give up breastfeeding because they cannot envisage combining breastfeeding with paid work (see also Chapters 8 and 9 in this volume). McKinlay and Hyde (2004) have argued that mothers who do seek to breastfeed infants, or to express milk, within the workplace face hostility and discouragement. Witters-Green (2003) explains that this occurs partly because employers fear that breastfeeding might cause other employees to feel 'discomfitted' and because it might induce lapses of concentration among employed mothers (Witters-Green 2003, p. 424). Like Kitzinger (2005), Hopfl (2000) suggests that organisational antipathy towards breastfeeding stems from employers' fears about women's 'leaky' bodies which are regarded, by employers, as unreliable and unpredictable, in a way which does not apply to the bodies of male employees. Hopfl (2000, p. 101) highlights the problems of trying to integrate the post-childbirth body into the workplace, and asserts that breastfeeding is treated as an undesirable symbol of motherhood: 'the organization [is] not a place for women with physical bodies which produce... breast milk and maternal smells'.

The theoretical hypothesis that the pregnant body may be a source of social abjection and disgust (Grosz 1994; Kitzinger 2005; Gatrell 2007) suggests that, for women who do seek to breastfeed at work, the experience of infant feeding might be challenging. This points to the need for further research on how mothers experience trying to combine breastfeeding and employment. Drawing upon data gathered from Internet discussion sites (described as 'netnographic' data),

I demonstrate below how, despite policies supposedly offering protection and support to new mothers, employed breastfeeding women face a contradiction in terms. On one hand, mothers are exhorted by health agencies to continue breastfeeding as the optimum form of infant feeding, while on the other hand, employed women feel pressured to switch to formula milk, due to workplace expectations that breastfeeding should be ceased unless mothers can manage it without disrupting employers' routines. See also Chapters 8 and 9 in this volume.

7.5 The Study

Following a study in which I explored women's experiences of pregnancy and work (Gatrell forthcoming) through netnographic research, I extended this study to examine how breastfeeding mothers managed to feed their infants at home and in the workplace rather than my usual method of qualitative interviews. Increasingly, women choose the Internet as a source of collective support and information. Lagan, Sinclair, and Kernohan (2006, p. 20) state that, 'for many women, the internet provides a new kind of safe haven. Often anonymous, it offers a never-ending source of information and reassurance . . . and can link individuals who . . . share common issues.' Netnography seemed appropriate as a research method to understand how breastfeeding women establish and maintain breastfeeding, including on their return to paid work.

While anonymity and ethics are paramount in research on a sensitive topic such as breastfeeding and employment, traditional rules on research ethics are not easy to apply to 'netnography'. This is because, although the world-wide-web is an 'open space', meaning that message board conversations are available to anyone with internet access, the researcher has no personal contact with those who correspond in cyber space. Thus, researchers have no means of knowing whether (or not) Internet users would 'choose' for their cyber conversations to be researched. Because Internet space is open to all, most Internet users choose pseudonyms to protect their identities (Lagan et al. 2006). Nevertheless, additional steps to safeguard the identity of research subjects have been taken for the purpose of this chapter. I have thus anonymised all texts cited, replacing chosen Internet identifiers with pseudonyms. I have also excluded personal details and have avoided detailed reference to geographical locations.

Having selected my data, I interpreted this thematically, classifying electronically, via cut and paste, in relation to breastfeeding at home and in the workplace. This was time-consuming, but facilitated a 'closeness' with the data.

7.6 Getting Established: Breastfeeding as 'Work'

Most mothers who discussed breastfeeding on Internet sites were aware that breast milk was considered the 'best' form of infant nutrition. While some mothers (like those in Murphy's 2003 study) resisted the obligation placed upon them to breastfeed, Internet correspondence indicated that most women did attempt to initiate breastfeeding. It is important to recognise that some mothers were keen to point out to others the positive aspects of breastfeeding, especially given the 'close bond' it enabled them to form with their new babies.

However, it is also imperative to acknowledge that most correspondents who had initiated breastfeeding indicated that this was a 'skill' which did not come 'naturally', but which required hard work, practice and training by 'experts'. Many women observed how individual health professionals and the 'how to breastfeed' texts emphasised the burden of maternal responsibilities to feed infants exclusively with breast milk, but 'glossed over' the difficulties of breastfeeding. In contrast to the idea of breastfeeding as a 'normal', 'natural' process, breastfeeding is described by some mothers, especially in the early stages, as 'toe curlingly painful'; a 'nightmare'.

The notion of breastfeeding as a painful 'struggle' (as opposed to a 'natural' 'womanly' process) is summed up neatly by Linda, who writes in response to an anxious message from pregnant correspondent Jo, who is 'scared' of failing to establish breastfeeding. Linda stated:

> Many pro breastfeeders are so keen to promote that breast is best [that] they tend to gloss over the fact that many women DO struggle, and ... . Like every new skill, it takes a while to perfect, and yup, it can be uncomfortable, sore, exhausting and so on!! ... But I think many people who are struggling give it up because they think they cant do it. There is help available though, to be honest I struggled at first, but once I'd got it, it was easy peasy.

For Linda, who felt she had 'got it', it seemed that the pain associated with breastfeeding was temporary. For others, however, pain was an everyday factor in breastfeeding, and this pain did not reduce as mothers become more skilled. June warned:

> ayowtch at that first drag!!! Don't think, however long one breastfeeds, that that sensation ever becomes ignorable.

For women such as Linda who eventually succeeded in establishing breastfeeding, even if they 'struggled' to do this, a sense of pride was apparent. However, for women who tried but failed to establish breastfeeding, or who gave up after a short time, the guilt and anxiety experienced was acute, as were their fears that they would be evaluated as 'failing' in their duties as mothers. Linda referred to the pressure exerted on mothers by 'pro-breastfeeders'; and among web-site correspondents, it appeared that women experienced intense pressure from health professionals to establish infant feeding from the breast.

7.7 Pressure to Breastfeed

While it was acknowledged that hospital midwives were 'doing their job', and that this was understandable, the pressure to breastfeed and the sense that mothers were being judged on their decision and/or ability to breastfeed were resented by some women. For example, Amie reported:

> My experience... is that a 'breastfeeding police force' exists in many maternity hospitals. Not only are women put under pressure to breast feed, but those who run into trouble are made to feel guilty.

Some women felt pressured to the point where they felt obliged to exercise deceptive tactics to escape what they saw as the opprobrium of health staff, when they switched to formula milk. Guilt and anxiety at giving up breastfeeding appeared to be especially severe among new mothers who failed to keep going with breastfeeding following ill health and/or a traumatic birth experience. Poor maternal or infant health did not appear to 'excuse' mothers from the requirement to breastfeed, with health professionals expecting mothers to 'work through the pain' and continue, even in circumstances where, it could be argued, formula feeding might have provided a more realistic option.

For example, Mel, who is quoted below, struggled to breastfeed following a birth which she describes as 'traumatic'. As in the case of many women who found breastfeeding difficult, Mel appeared to feel under scrutiny by health staff, and she associated successful breastfeeding with being assessed as a 'good' mother. Her failure to manage breastfeeding was linked in her mind to being evaluated as, in her words, a 'horrible' mother. Like the women in Murphy's (2003) study, Mel's worries about being rated as a bad mother, and her reaction to being pressured to breastfeed, led Mel to lie to health professionals that she intended to continue breastfeeding, rather than admit her plans to switch to formula. Over 3 years later, Mel (similarly to some of the women in Gatrell's 2007 study) still expressed a strong sense of guilt about giving up:

> I felt pressured to breastfeed while still in the hospital after a traumatic birth experience of my premmie (who is a healthy 3 year old today). In fact, I came back to my hospital bed with a breast pump machine already parked beside it! I ended up just lying to the hospital staff that I was planning to continue breast feeding just to get them off my case, but then I would go home and cry, being made to feel like a horrible mom for not breastfeeding. I wonder if maybe this pressure has any link to the increasing rate of moms going into postpartum depression? It just seems like yet another thing to make moms feel horrible.

Similarly, Joanne found breastfeeding painful and problematic following a difficult birth. No attempt appears to have been made, on the part of hospital staff, to relieve Joanne's worries about failing to breastfeed. Rather, it appears she was encouraged to continue, despite heavy bleeding from her nipples (one of which developed a blood clot). After struggling for 4 weeks, Joanne finally gave up breastfeeding in a state of acute distress. Despite support from her husband and her own mother, Joanne appeared to feel profoundly guilty at switching to formula, as well as deeply fearful that others would measure her performance as a mother negatively, assessing her as failing the 'good mother' test, due to her inability to breastfeed her daughter:

> I was a firm believer in breastfeeding being the best option ...I read the books [and] took a pre-natal breastfeeding class. My daughter fed almost constantly for the first three days [following a traumatic birth]. Even though she was latched on properly I was in agony...At 3am on the third night I felt a searing pain in my right breast and my nipple was bleeding badly. I broke down exhausted and terrified while a midwife took my baby away to give

> her some formula. I spent the rest of the night and most of the next day crying with guilt at 'letting my baby down' so badly... I was told not to put her to the breast for 24 hours and ...I had to spend 5 days in hospital in total because of this feeding problem and I got no sleep there so was exhausted. ...Finally after 4 weeks I stopped trying to breastfeed. I felt like such a failure and cried many times over this. I was ashamed to feed my baby ... in public because I thought people would judge me for not breastfeeding'.

The guilt experienced by women like Jo, who initiate breastfeeding but give up, is an important topic of discussion on web boards. Like Jo and Mel, many correspondents express feelings of guilt if they switch to formula milk having 'struggled' to breastfeed – this despite reassurance from other women on message boards that: 'You shouldn't let others make you feel guilty – just do what is best for you'.

7.8 'Normal', 'Natural' or 'Immodest'? Breastfeeding at Home

For women who do succeed in establishing breastfeeding, maintaining this within UK/Irish-American cultural settings may not be easy. It is important to acknowledge here that some women report their partners and relatives – often especially their own mothers – as very supportive of their breastfeeding activities. Some mothers recount how expressing milk may enable partners to feed and feel close to new babies. However, breastfeeding, even in their own homes, was not straightforward for all mothers. For example, some women found they were expected to breastfeed alone and in private space, rather than in front of family members or guests. Some mothers who did persist in breastfeeding in front of others within their own households found that family attitudes towards breastfeeding differed from the views espoused by health staff and breastfeeding 'experts'. For example, some women's mothers and mothers-in-law heralded from generations where breastfeeding was regarded as appropriate only in the first few weeks of life. Family members were sometimes critical of the contemporary guidance that babies should be breastfed up to and beyond the first year of life and questioned whether this was 'normal', one woman being told by her own mother that her decision to continue breastfeeding after her baby was 4 months old was 'ridiculous'.

Breastfeeding mothers were also, in some cases, subject to opprobrium because the feeding of infant children in front of other adults within the home was seen as neither 'natural' or 'normal', but rather as 'immodest' and inappropriate. For example, Jen wrote about her husband's preference that she should shut herself away to breastfeed on occasions when male guests were invited to her home:

> Even if I go into the other room to get my daughter latched and all set up, then come back out holding her and covered with a blanket my husband gets upset if his guy friends are over. I don't get it ... how is breastfeeding UNDER A BLANKET immodest? ... I hate having to go and sit in a room by myself for a half hour. It sucks. How can I help my husband to understand that it's OK for me to breastfeed in front of other men ESPECIALLY if I'm covered up and everything – plus, since I get her latched on in another room, ... you don't even see or hear ANYTHING. Or do you agree with him that its 'weird' and 'immodest' for me to breastfeed in front of other men?

In keeping with Kitzinger's (2005) assertions that breastfeeding is treated as a 'shameful activity', Jen's own husband positions breastfeeding as an activity which Jen should perform in privacy. Significantly, in contrast to the description of breastfeeding by La Leche League as 'normal' and 'natural', Jen's desire to breastfeed in the company of others, rather than in isolation, is regarded by her husband as 'immodest'. Later in Jen's message, she mentioned that her husband is afraid that breastfeeding their infant might make his male friends 'uncomfortable'. This may be partly due to the kind of social discomfiture around women's unpredictably 'leaky' maternal bodies as described by Martin (1989), Grosz (1994), Longhurst (2001), Kitzinger (2005) and Gatrell (2008). In addition, male discomfiture regarding breastfeeding may relate to tensions between the notion of breasts and both maternal and sexual. Both Young (2005) and Giles (2004) have psychologised men's uneasiness about breastfeeding, suggesting that some men regard maternal satisfaction in breastfeeding as likely to reduce or displace women's heterosexual relationship with men. Thus, some men may resent breastfeeding mothers (even those women who are not their own partners).

7.9 Breastfeeding and the Workplace

The experiences of the women quoted above indicate firstly that breastfeeding may not come 'naturally' to women, but may be a 'struggle', and secondly that breastfeeding may not be treated as 'normal' within social spaces, even those which are familiar, such as the home. In this context, it may come as no surprise that many women who seek to combine breastfeeding with employment may find this challenging. As McKinlay and Hyde (2004) observe, many mothers wishing to breastfeed their infants, or to express breast milk in organisational spaces, face antipathy and discouragement. This situation may be problematic for some UK mothers, but is likely to be especially problematic in the United States, where maternity leave is short and is often unpaid (Calnen 2007). Although there are occasional examples of good organizational practice (Ortiz et al. 2004; Groskop 2006), most workplaces do little to support breastfeeding mothers (Witters-Green 2003; cf. Chapter 8 in this volume). On returning to work, previous studies have suggested that mothers who do attempt to continue breastfeeding at work are likely to find that health guidance about breastfeeding infants for minimally 1 year is ignored by employers (if they are aware of it at all). Most organisations have no policy relating to breastfeeding, and no room set aside for feeding or expressing. The only refrigerators available are those provided for general use, and these are often dirty and/or full of packed lunches and cows' milk for coffee. It is left to mothers (rather than employers) to procure requisite space and time: 'It is up to you to work out where to pump, where to chill and store your milk and how to schedule work breaks that coincide with let-down times' (Boswell-Penc & Boyer 2007, p. 561). Often, women wishing to express breast milk are left with no option other than to do this in the lavatory, especially if they are in junior and/or lower paid roles and without access to private office space (Boswell-Penc & Boyer 2007; Gatrell 2007; see also Chapter 8).

Internet correspondence between mothers who are attempting to continue breastfeeding on returning to work suggests little improvement on these experiences. Occasionally, instances of kindness and support are reported, and these usually relate to the actions of individual line-managers who are sympathetic to mothers' plight. For example, Barbara, having confessed to her line-manager how unhappy she was at the prospect of giving up breastfeeding, found that:

> [The next day] my boss came into my office with a huge surprise. He had bought me a double electric pump, complete with breastmilk storage bags, a cooler, bottles, you name it! And ... he gave me 2-20 minute breaks (paid) everyday, and a private room to pump. He also gave me [exclusive] space in the refrigerator to store my breast milk. I was able to enjoy my job even [and] continue feeding my daughter only breast milk while working full time, thanks to [his] support.

Most women, however, tell a different story from Barbara's. As Belle described:

> Let me tell you all – it's not easy being a fulltime working mom and breastfeeding. Between office politics of women who know what you are doing and being not so supportive scheduling breaks if your boss is a jerk, staying healthy and not runned down – [continuing to breastfeed can be challenging].

While individual managers may be helpful, organisations continue to offer minimal 'official' support to breastfeeding mothers. Ironically, Betty's experiences below suggest that even healthcare providers (some of whom, at least in theory, have policies in place to support breastfeeding mothers) may be discouraging in practice. Betty explained how, because she worked in a hospital, she had anticipated that:

> ...there would be no problem with me pumping. Well for some reason [my boss] said that she wasn't willing to change any of my breaks around or give me a few extra minutes [needed] from the time I start pumping until the end...My boss said if I can't do it during my breaks that I can't do it! ... So I don't know if I should go to Human Resources ... I don't want my boss to get mad at me, I have to work with her everyday!... I am now thinking that maybe I should just quit pumping. . . .I know that if I quit I will feel really guilty that I am not giving my daughter my milk anymore . . . I hate that there is no turning back if I quit pumping, I am going to feel so guilty.

Office worker Jodie did manage to continue breastfeeding after returning to work, but recounted this as a difficult and unpleasant experience. Because she sensed that breastfeeding was a 'taboo' subject at work, it prevented her from asking for private space to pump and suitable storage for her milk, and this meant that she had to express her milk in the lavatory. Jodie had the impression that her workplace must have known that she was expressing milk in the bathroom, but nobody appeared to offer her any alternative. Once back at work, it seemed she was expected to conceal her maternity and her maternal body, and to present herself within the workplace as if the birth of her daughter had never occurred.

> I wanted to do my best for [daughter] and to nurse her right through but there were no policies that I know of and I did not dare ask about nursing so I used the restrooms on my break to pump. I brought cold storage to work and kept the milk under my desk. I guess they must have knew, but no one mentioned it. I don't know how I did this, its hardly nice

> pumping in a stall, but I wanted to feed her with my milk and they don't talk about this kind of thing at work so what else to do? Its like, they want me to carry on as before, as if i never had a child.

7.10 Understanding Social Antipathy to Breastfeeding

Breastfeeding, the challenges of initiation and duration and the problem of social antipathy to breastfeeding attract much discussion among new mothers on message boards. Some women attempt to analyse why breastfeeding invokes negative reactions when performed in any kind of public setting. Like Young (2005) and Kitzinger (2005), Tilly, considering American attitudes towards breastfeeding, related antipathy towards breastfeeding to the tensions between the notions of the sexual and the maternal breast.

> Why is it that America is the only culture that looks down on breastfeeding? I'm not saying all Americans but the majority, even those that breastfeed aren't comfortable with it when around others. As a society we've gotten it ingrained in our heads that breasts equal sex rather than the food source they are intended to be.

Similarly to Hopfl (2000), Kitzinger (2005) and Gatrell (2007, 2008), Marie-Therese related antipathy towards breastfeeding to the notion of disgust. In Marie-Therese's interpretation, the pressure on women to breastfeed their infants is totally at odds with the sense that the maternal body is a source of social disgust; this making the idea of breastfeeding within any social space other than the home highly problematic:

> In the wider society I think pregnancy, childbirth and breastfeeding is regarded if not quite with 'utter disgust', then at least with something heading in that direction.

7.11 Conclusion

The views of both Tilly and Anne-Marie support the findings of this study to the effect that, while breastfeeding may be promoted within health policy as the ideal form of infant nutrition, such policies fail to take into account a range of obstacles faced by new mothers who are attempting to breastfeed. Given the extent of these obstacles, it seems unsurprising that breastfeeding duration rates decline sharply when babies are a few weeks old, with relatively small numbers of children being fed exclusively on breast milk for 6 months, and few babies being breastfed beyond the first year.

Specifically, the study indicates that one reason for the drop in breastfeeding duration rates is because, while health agencies are focused almost exclusively on the need for mothers to breastfeed in order to maximise infant health, little attention is given to the intensive physical and emotional labour required of breastfeeding mothers. The hard work required to initiate and to maintain breastfeeding appears often to be unrecorded, and/or discounted by health agencies. Arguably, the discounting of breastfeeding work occurs because breastfeeding is presented to mothers and wider society as a 'normal', 'natural' 'womanly' activity. This view of breastfeeding as 'natural' obfuscates the difficulties of establishing and continuing breastfeeding, especially in circumstances where mothers have experienced a traumatic birth and are feeling exhausted and/or ill.

The second reason why breastfeeding duration rates are lower than health agencies would wish is because breastfeeding promotion policies, which are aimed principally at mothers, do not sufficiently account for negative social attitudes towards breastfeeding (cf. Chapters 3, 4 and 5 in this volume). Mothers may be encouraged by health professionals to initiate and maintain breastfeeding in preference to formula milk, but are likely to face discouragement and antipathy if they perform the work of breastfeeding anywhere other than within the home. Even then, women might be seen as 'immodest' if they attempt to breastfeed at home but in the company of others.

To add to the obstacles facing breastfeeding mothers, breastfeeding is difficult to combine with employment as it is rarely accommodated within the workplace. The latter part of this chapter has highlighted the tensions between health professionals' expectations of the 'good' mother who breastfeeds her child and social imperatives about how employed mothers should comport themselves at work. Employed women such as Jodie are expected to hide breastfeeding practices, appearing in the workplace as if the birth of their babies had not occurred. For Jodie, the maternal work of breastfeeding thus became 'hidden' in the most literal sense. Women like Barbara, who seek workplace support to facilitate the expressing of milk, may be refused permission on the basis that breastfeeding must not disrupt workplace routines. In the light of these difficulties, it is unsurprising that so many women switch from breastfeeding to formula milk on returning to employment (see also Chapter 8 and 9 in this volume).

Finally, perhaps the most disturbing result of this study relates to the feelings of guilt and anxiety expressed by so many of the women who fail to establish breastfeeding, or who switch to formula milk because they are 'struggling' to breastfeed. Mothers are keenly aware of the health message that breastfeeding is best for babies. Most acquiesce with the idea that mothers must bear responsibility for enhancing infant health (or otherwise), depending on whether they feed their infants with breast milk or formula (Murphy 2003; Gatrell 2007, 2008; see Chapter 9 in this volume). In this context, the notion that breastfeeding is a 'natural' element of good mothering means that mothers who switch to formula feel they are measured against, and are failing the criteria of, 'good' motherhood. Breastfeeding is presented to mothers as a task at which they 'ought' to succeed if they are 'natural' mothers (La Leche League 2005). Thus, while breastfeeding might enhance both infant and maternal health when all goes to plan, the distress caused to mothers who are unable to breastfeed is palpable. Some mothers are so oppressed by the pressure to breastfeed successfully that they lie to health professionals, pretending that they are still breastfeeding when this is no longer the case. The possibility that some women feel pressured into telling lies could cast doubt on present estimates of breastfeeding duration rates, which (if mothers feel obliged to lie) may in practice be lower than statistics indicate.

Perhaps it is time to recognise that the notion of 'breast is best' needs to encompass the needs of mothers as well as their infants. Health promotion initiatives could be targeted more broadly, towards achieving a social situation whereby mothers are better supported than at present, and are no longer pressured into breastfeeding (or into concealing breastfeeding problems), 'under a blanket'.

References

American Academy of Pediatricians (2009). Breastfeeding initiatives. Retrieved 12 August 2010, from http://www.aap.org/breastfeeding/index.html

Bailey, C., & Pain, R. (2001). Geographies of feeding and access to primary health care. *Health and Social Care in the Community, 9*(5), 309–317.

Berger, L. M., Hill, J., & Waldfogel, J. (2005). Maternity leave, early maternal employment and child health and development in the US. *The Economic Journal, 115*, F29–F47.

Boswell-Penc, M., & Boyer, K. (2007). Expressing anxiety? Breastpump use in American wage workplaces. *Gender, Place and Culture, 14*(5), 151–167.

Calnen, G. (2007). Paid maternity leave and its impact of breastfeeding in the United States: Historic, economic, political and social perspectives, *Breastfeeding Medicine, 1*(2), 34–44.

Department of Health (2004). *Good practice and innovation in breastfeeding.* London: Crown Copyright.

Department of Health and Children (2005). *Breastfeeding in Ireland: A five year Strategic Action Plan.* Galway: Department of Health and Children.

Earle, S. (2002). Factors affecting the initiation of breastfeeding: Implications for breastfeeding promotion. *Health Promotion International, 17*(3), 205–214.

Galtry, J. (1997). Suckling and silence in the USA: The costs and benefits of breastfeeding. *Feminist Economics, 3*, 1–24.

Gatrell, C. (2005). *Hard labour: The sociology of parenthood.* Maidenhead: Open University Press.

Gatrell, C. (2007). Secrets and lies: Breastfeeding and professional paid work. *Social Science and Medicine, 65*, 393–404.

Gatrell, C. (2008). *Embodying women's work.* Maidenhead: Open University Press.

Gatrell, C. (2009). Policy and the pregnant body at work: Strategies of secrecy, silence and supra-performance, *Gender, Work and Organization.* DOI 10.1111/j.1468-0432.2009.00485.

Giles, F. (2004). 'Relational and strange': A preliminary foray into a project to queer breastfeeding. *Australian Feminist Studies, 19*, 301–314.

Groskop, V. (2006). Boardroom babies. *Sunday Times 'Style'*, February 26, p. 22.

Grosz, E. (1994). *Volatile bodies: Toward a corporeal feminism.* Bloomington: Indiana University Press.

Hausman, B. L. (2004). The feminist politics of breastfeeding. *Australian Feminist Studies, 19*, 273–285.

Hopfl, H. (2000). The suffering mother and the miserable son: Organizing women and organizing women's writing. *Gender, Work and Organization, l7*(2), 98–105.

Jackson, W. (2004). Breastfeeding and type 1 diabetes mellitus. *British Journal of Midwifery, 12*(3), 158–165.

Kitzinger, S. (2003). *The new pregnancy and childbirth: Choices and challenges.* London: Dorling Kindersley.

Kitzinger, S. (2005). *The politics of birth.* Edinburgh: Elsevier Butterworth Heinemann.

La Leche League Great Britain (2005). *Beginning breastfeeding.* Nottingham: La Leche League Great Britain.

Lagan, B., Sinclair, M., & Kernohan, W. G. (2006). Pregnant women's use of the internet: A review of published and unpublished evidence. *Evidence Based Midwifery, 4*(1), 17–23.

Longhurst, R. (2001). *Bodies: Exploring fluid boundaries.* London: Routledge.

Martin, E. (1989). *The woman in the body: A cultural analysis of reproduction.* Boston: Beacon.

McKinlay, N. M., & Hyde, J. S. (2004). Personal attitudes or structural factors? A contextual analysis of breastfeeding duration. *Psychology of Women Quarterly, 28*, 388–400.

Miller, T. (2005). *Making sense of motherhood: A narrative approach.* Cambridge: Cambridge University Press.

Murphy, E. (2003). Expertise and forms of knowledge in the government of families. *The Sociological Review, 51*, 433–462.

Ortiz, J., McGilligan, K., & Kelly, P. (2004). Duration of breast milk/expression among working mothers enrolled in an employer-sponsored lactation program. *Pediatric Nursing, 30*(2), 111–119.

Padavic, I., & Reskin, B. (2002). *Women and men at work.* Thousand Oaks, CA: Sage.

Raymond, J. (2005). Another reason for you to breastfeed. *Working Mother, 28*(4), 70–74.

Shildrick, M. (1997). *Leaky bodies and boundaries: Feminism, postmodernism and (bio) ethics.* London: Routledge.

Web MD (2009). Your guide to breastfeeding. Retrieved 20 June 2009 from http://www.webmd.com/parenting/baby/breastfeeding-9/nursing-basics

Witters-Green, R. (2003). Increasing breastfeeding rates in working mothers. *Families, Systems and Health, 21*, 415–434.

Wolf, J. (2006). What feminists can do for breastfeeding and what breastfeeding can do for feminists. *Signs: Journal of Women in Culture and Society,* 31, 397–424.

Young, I. M. (2005). *On female body experience: 'Throwing like a girl and other essays'*. Oxford: Oxford University Press.

Chapter 8
Breastfeeding Beliefs and Practices Among Employed Women: A Thai Cultural Perspective

Susanha Yimyam

Contents

8.1 Introduction

Breastfeeding has long been recognised as superior to artificial feeding in a variety of aspects. The evidence of the nutritional, immunological, behavioral, economic, and environmental benefits of breastfeeding for both developed and developing countries is overwhelming and indisputable (WHO 2001; American Academy of Pediatrics [AAP] 2005). Scientific studies show it has significant benefits to infants, mothers, and societies (Villalpando & Lopez-Alarcon 2000; Singhal, Cole, & Lucus 2001; American Academy of Pediatrics 2005; Yimyam 2005; UNICEF 2006).

The twentieth century has seen large variations and swings in breastfeeding practices. There was a rapid decline in the prevalence of breastfeeding in Western countries between the 1940s and early 1970s. This period coincided with economic changes that encouraged major migrations from rural to urban areas, both in developed and in developing countries (Menon & Amin 2006; UNICEF 2006). In the

S. Yimyam (✉)
OB-GYN Nursing Department, Faculty of Nursing, Chiang Mai University, Chiang Mai 50200, Thailand
e-mail: syimyam@mail.nurse.cmu.ac.th

P. Liamputtong (ed.), *Infant Feeding Practices*, DOI 10.1007/978-1-4419-6873-9_8,
© Springer Science+Business Media, LLC 2011

developing world, rates of initiation and duration have periodically risen and fallen over the past several decades, with large variations within and between countries and regions. Generally, breastfeeding duration has fallen as urbanisation has increased, and optimal breastfeeding practices are rare (WHO 2001; Yimyam & Morrow 2003). However, an improvement in infant feeding practices after the adoption of the Innocenti Declaration are indication to work of policy makers, health promoters, health care providers, child advocates, communicators, and donors who made infant and young child feeding a priority (UNICEF 2006). The past 15 years have witnessed much success in improvement in terms of the rate of exclusive breastfeeding and timely complementary feeding increase between 1990 and 2004. Overall, the global prevalence of exclusive breastfeeding both in developed and in developing countries for the first 6 months increased from 34 percent to 39 percent. Increases in exclusive breastfeeding rates tended to be much greater in developing countries, from 34 percent to 41 percent. Rates in some countries doubled, tripled, and even quadrupled, particularly where health and community workers had been trained to give mothers appropriate breastfeeding counseling and support (UNICEF 2006).

Surveys have consistently shown that breastfeeding prevalence and duration are higher among educated, more affluent mothers in industrialised countries, but higher among rural, poorer and less educated women in developing countries (Donath & Amir 2000). Rural occupations are usually more compatible with child care, including breastfeeding (Wongboonsin & Ruffolo 1993; Yimyam 1998; Holla-Bhar 2006). Some experts (Wilmoth & Elder 1995; Narasimhan 2006) suggest the urban reduction in breastfeeding stems from media portrayal of bottle-feeding as modern and convenient, and declines in extended family households able to care for the growing number of women in paid employment. Lack of family assistance with household tasks, which makes mothers busier and hence cause reduction in frequency of suckling, were cited to explain early weaning (Yimyam 1998). Other variables often associated with infant feeding are ethnicity, marital status, age, parity, and employment status, but the direction of association is inconsistent within and between countries and regions (Scott & Binns 1999; Yimyam & Morrow 1999; Menon & Amin 2006).

Although breastfeeding has long been recognised and advocated by the government, there have only been modest efforts to promote breastfeeding in Thailand. The government put the campaign in the National Food and Nutritional Policy (NFNP) under the Fourth National Economic and Social Development Plan (NESDP) for 1977–1981 (Chatranon 1988). Since then, breastfeeding has been included in every NESDP and promoted continuously in Thailand (Chatranon 1988; Chayovan, Knodel, & Wongboonsin 1990). Early activities included policy meetings, seminars and training with various professionals, the adoption of the Marketing Code of Infant Food Products in 1981, and public campaigns promoting breastfeeding. Further steps were needed within the health care system (Winichagoon, Viriyapanich, & Dhamamitta 1992) for improving the health care services. These have involved education and training of health professionals. Sminars, workshops, and training programs for health professionals have been held in Thailand to promote breastfeeding since 1977. Hospital policy and environment, which allows early contact between infants and mothers, reduces the period of mother–infant separation, as well as increases rooming-in and discourages the use of medications during delivery, has been modified (Chayovan et al. 1990; Durongdej & Mangklasiri 1993). In 1992, Thailand was one of twelve countries launching the 'Baby Friendly Hospital Initiative'. The Ministry of Public Health (MOPH) has formally adopted the 'Ten Steps to Successful Breastfeeding' for improving the hospital environment to accommodate and promote breastfeeding (Winichagoon et al. 1992; Family Health Division 1994). By July 1996, 99.5 percent of public hospitals under the MOPH (760 of 763 hospitals) have become 'Baby Friendly Hospital Initiative'. However, only one private hospital has received this certificate (Taintavorn 1996). See also Chapters 4 and 19 in this volume.

The revised 'Thailand Code for Advertisement and Sale of Breast-milk Substitutes and Related Products 1995' provided guidelines for business sectors, medical and health personnel, and other concerned parties (Taintavorn 1996). Thailand was chosen as the site for the WABA Global Forum on 'Children's Health, Children's Rights: Action for the 21st Century', held in Sukothai Thammathirat Open University, Bangkok, in 1996. This brought participants from 86 countries who signed for 'Ten Links for Nurturing the Future'. With cooperation between the government and the non-governmental organisations, 'Breastfeeding Month' campaigns are organised in each August. This involve activities at national, provincial, district, and village levels by providing information through every type of mass media (radio, newspapers, magazines, television, and public address systems), distributing leaflets, posters, and flip charts as well as organising annual health competitions among breastfed children (Yimyam 2005). Although the public campaigns have increased awareness, they have been less successful at increasing the rates of breastfeeding.

Breastfeeding is imbued with positive cultural values in terms of nurturing. Many Thai mothers contend that the breastfed infant is often easy to raise (Van-Esterik 1988; Vong-Ek 1993; Yimyam 1998). Studies have reported that, in general, Thai mothers have positive attitudes toward breastfeeding and most knew about the nutritious and immunological qualities of breast milk. They believe that breastfed babies are healthier than bottle-fed babies, that breast milk is safe and clean, and promotes child growth and development (Vong-Ek 1993; Family Health Division 1994; see also Chapter 9 in this volume). A combination of socio-economic and demographic change together with certain misunderstandings about lactation pose threats to this heritage (Vong-Ek 1993; Yimyam & Morrow 2003). Breastfeeding in Thailand is a nearly nationwide practice; initiation rates (one day of birth) in the large survey were 84.8 percent (National Statistical Office 2007). However, the national surveys have shown a decline in duration, and extremely low rates of exclusive breastfeeding; only 5.4 percent of Thai children are exclusively breastfed for the first 6 months after birth, one of the lowest exclusive breastfeeding rates in the world. Rural infants were breastfed more than urban infants. Moreover, infants from the Northern region were exclusively breastfed more than infants from other regions. Meanwhile, the Central region (including Bangkok) had the lowest number of infants who were breastfed (National Statistical Office 2007).

Furthermore, some cultural beliefs and practices are obstacles to successful breastfeeding. We know relatively little about the process of infant feeding decision-making in relation to these beliefs and practices. In particular, the cultural change and socio-economic circumstances that affect living and environments and patterns of time allocation, which in turn affect health and health behaviors such as breast-feeding, need fuller explication if we are to design the most optimal public health policies. Investigating the interaction between national policies, social and cultural changes, socio-economic circumstances, and breastfeeding requires exploration of several dimensions of women's traditional beliefs and practices.

In this chapter, I will provide discussions on a study that delved into the experiences of employed women as mothers in northern Thailand. The focus is on breastfeeding culture in Thai society. Particular issues included are the recognition of the benefits of breastfeeding, breastfeeding preference, influence of confinement on breastfeeding, misunderstanding of breastfeeding, and perception of breastfeeding and breast milk. The chapter concludes with comments on the implications of the findings of my study in terms of the current international discourse on health promotion, particularly in the context of basic human rights.

8.2 The Study of Thai Women in Chiang Mai

As the social changes of modernisation and urbanisation proceed rapidly around the world, creating new dynamics for women, it is increasingly important to understand the public health ramifications of changing lifestyles and the potential need for new policies and interventions. Women in this study were recruited from Chiang Mai (estimated population 1.6 million in 2008) for this study for two reasons. First, Chiang Mai represents a society with rapid growth, which has brought about far-reaching cultural, social, and economic change. Second, it was due to a familiarity with the political, cultural, and social circumstances of the author, who lives and works there.

Data gathering was undertaken in three stages. Stage 1 used multiple qualitative approaches: interviews with key informants, observation of health facilities and references to breastfeeding in the media, interpretation of policy documents, and in-depth interviews with 10 employed mothers. Findings from Stage 1 were used to develop the research instrument for Stage 2 and as a context for interpreting final results. Stage 2 consisted of interviews with 300 employed mothers using a semi-structured questionnaire based on a literature review and findings from Stage 1. In the third stage, 30 mothers were interviewed in-depth to clarify and illustrate important findings from *Stage 2*. Findings from Stage 3 were used as a context for interpreting final results.

The main participants were employed mothers of babies between 4 months and 3 years of age who had initiated breastfeeding and were completely weaned at the time of interviewing. They were asked for information about their infant feeding and employment experiences. For Stage 1, convenience and purposive sampling was used to select 10 women from varied employment sectors. For Stage 2, the mothers were recruited using quota sampling from the record of University Hospital based on the occupational profile of women delivery in that year. Therefore, 300 mothers were chosen including 66 (22 percent) government or state enterprise employees and 156 (52 percent) private employees in the formal sector, and 25 (8 percent) pieceworkers and 53 (18 percent) self/family employees in the informal sector. The interviews were conducted at a time and place convenient to the mothers. The mothers in Stage 3 were selected from interesting participants in *Stage 2* to clarify and illustrate important findings.

This combined qualitative and quantitative study was reviewed and approved by the Human Research Ethics Committees of Chiang Mai University. It also received permission from an appropriate person in authority at the provincial level and hospital level (the Chiang Mai Provincial Chief Medical Officer and directors of hospitals) to carry out this project among health facilities in Chiang Mai.

8.3 Breastfeeding Culture in Thai Society

The benefits of breastfeeding in contemporary Thai society are widely recognised and valued. The findings and discussions draw on observations of the way breastfeeding is presented in the media, as well as interviews through all stages of data collection.

8.3.1 Recognition of the Benefits of Breastfeeding in Contemporary Society

As women in many societies (see Liamputtong Rice 2000; Holla-Bhar 2006; Tsianakas & Liamputtong 2007), Thai women view breastfeeding as best for infants. '*Ka nam nom*' (the value of breast milk) is not only a term to describe the benefits of breastfeeding but also has taken on a wider cultural meaning used commonly in Thailand. It says much about the significance of this term that it is also used more generally to describe the concept of obligation to one's mother. It has connotations of acknowledging the sacrifice mothers make for their infants, and the expectation that when infants grow up and can earn income, they will pay back this debt by financial, practical, and emotional support for their parents when they are old. If the daughter marries, the groom gives property to the bride's parents as a repayment for '*ka nam nom*'.

In Thai society, it is believed that the components of breast milk are derived from blood flowing through mammary glands. As in the other study (Vong-Ek 1993), many women in my study said they accepted this concept. The Thai popular folk song entitled '*ka nam nom*' refers to the view that breast milk is best because 'breast milk was squeezed from maternal blood circulation', and blood is necessary to human life. Therefore, if a mother gives breast milk to her baby, it means she gives a great deal of her life to her infant. Marisa (pseudonym) stated:

> I gave breast milk to my baby because breast milk comes from mother's blood.

Most mothers mentioned that it is better to give breast milk than formula or cow's milk because it is a human product. They explained that all valuable foods taken by the mother yield good milk for the infant. According to Somchit,

> Breast milk is higher nutritional value than formula because a breastfed baby can receive all of the food a mother eats through breast milk. Compared to breast milk, formula may not be good because it comes from cattle, and cattle always eat grass.

Many women spontaneously asserted that a proper diet is essential for milk production and quality.

> I must be careful about the food that I eat . . . . If I eat a nutritious diet, my breast milk will be of good quality. (Marisa)

Moreover, some believed that breast milk can transfer the characteristics of mother to baby. Many mothers in this study expressed views similar to those of Wilawan:

> Human babies should have human breast milk, not cow's milk. Cow's milk is for calves. If infants are fed cow's milk, they will be naughty like cattle.

8.3.2 Breastfeeding Preference

Data among the 300 employed women reveal that all women in this study preferred and planned to breastfeed (either with or without formula). When women were asked to cite their main reason for preferring breastfeeding, they responded as follows: breastfeeding's nutritional value (23 percent), protection against infection and immunity content (21 percent), cost consideration (19 percent), mother/infant bonding (13 percent), healthy and good development for the infant (13 percent), and convenience (11 percent).

8.3.2.1 Breastfeeding's Nutritional Value

The women in this study believed in the nutritional value of breastfeeding. Comments made by women support the questionnaire responses. Marisa explained:

> I love my baby, and I want to give the best to my infant. I know breast milk has a suitable nutritional value. It is my responsibility to ensure that I give my infant a healthy start.

Wantanee stated:

> Nothing is better than breast milk. I intend to breastfeed as long as I can.

8.3.2.2 Protection Against Infection and Immunity Content

Although some women gave similar credit in terms of 'nutritional value' to breast milk and formula, others drew a distinction about immunological components. Pimporn said:

> I think both breast milk and formula have the same nutritional value . . . . but I think breast milk has substances which can prevent my baby from getting sick.

8.3.2.3 Cost Consideration

Cost was considered as one main aspect of breastfeeding preference among the women. Many reported that they preferred breastfeeding because it was cheaper. Sunee, a pieceworker working from home, told me that:

> If you breastfeed you save on expenditure. Formula is expensive, if I can breastfeed I will save money.

Julai, who was working in the family business outside the home, said:

> It doesn't cost anything if I breastfeed my baby. I planned to bring the baby to work and continue breastfeeding.

8.3.2.4 Healthy and Good Development for the Infant

Some mothers gave 'healthy and good development of the infant' as the first reason for breastfeeding. Somjai stated:

> My mum said that breast milk is best for every infant. I was also breastfed when I was young. I agree with her. I saw my neighbor's infants, who were breastfed, are healthy. I want my infant to be like them.

And Wandee said:

> I think breastfed babies won't have as many problems with constipation or diarrhea as bottle-fed babies. They won't get too fat. Breastfed babies may develop better, and are smarter than bottle-fed babies.

8.3.2.5 Mother/Infant Bonding

'Maternal and infant bonding' is another reason that mothers in this study mentioned for breastfeeding. Vimon expressed it that:

> I believe that my baby felt warm and safe. Whenever I breastfed him I also felt very happy. I can't explain how wonderful it is. I will never forget that period of my life.

Many women mentioned that a breastfed infant always has a closer relationship with the mother than a bottle-fed infant. Sudthida stated:

> If you breastfed your babies, they will love you more than bottle-fed infants.

Some mothers cited the benefits of maternal and infant bonding during breastfeeding for good emotional development of the infant. Wantanee mentioned:

> The best way for the baby to feel warm and secure is to breastfeed. They feel secure, and they are the happiest babies because they're comfortable. They won't have a cold heart.

8.3.2.6 Convenience

Convenience was another reason for mothers working in the informal sector to prefer to breastfeed. Umpai, a pieceworker, explained:

> Breastfeeding is more convenient for me. I won't waste my time preparing and cleaning bottles. Also, when I go out I don't need to carry a big load of things.

These findings suggest that the circumstances of women's lives influence their views and practices. As Marchand and Morrow (1994) have argued, the maternal decision for breastfeeding results from the complex interaction of societal, cultural, economic, family dynamic, and personal considerations. Most women (56 percent) said they hoped to breastfeed for a year or more since they thought that weaning before this time was too soon. As Pikul told me:

> It is too early to wean a baby less than one year. The baby is not strong enough and should still be breastfed.

And Ladda stated:

> It was ashamed to wean my baby before one year. I think that a baby within this age always needs breast milk as an important source of food. . . . An infant over one year of age can eat by himself. If he is weaned, he can eat more rice and other foods.

8.3.3 Influence of Confinement on Breastfeeding

The study found that the rates of breastfeeding at discharge and at 1 month postpartum were 90 percent and 94 percent, respectively. The higher rate at 1 month suggests that it is discouraging circumstances in hospital which interfere with successful initiation such as separate from the infant and early supplementation. The peak rate at 1 month also coincided with the period of *'yu daun'*, a traditional confinement practice in the northern region (see Liamputtong 2004). Although most Thai women today have given up the complicated restriction practices of the traditional confinement period, they still follow some of these customs. After discharge, almost all women in this study practiced '*yu duan*' for about 1 month. Within this practice, most felt themselves to be very weak after delivery. Certain food prohibitions and curtailed activities were deemed necessary to recover. In general, these traditional beliefs and practices provide an opportunity for the women to adjust to a new role of mother. Since both the mother and the baby are kept together, they are able to learn from one another. Moreover, strong social endorsement of the value of breastfeeding (and the obligation it places on the next generation) reinforces the benefits of breastfeeding during confinement. For the new mother, often her mother and mother- in-law come to stay with her in order to support and advise her how to take care of herself and her infant, especially, breastfeeding.

However, some traditional notions may be barriers to successful breastfeeding. For example, the belief that mothers should not go outside for a period after birth (or during a confinement period) poses difficulties for women whose babies are in special care units at the hospital, as the mother may be reluctant to leave home to breastfeed. In my study, some mothers who were discharged before their babies did not come to the hospital because they felt they should stay inside during this period. Thongdee, who had a premature baby, gave her view about this matter.

> Because my baby was too small [birth weight = 2,000 grams], he had to be in hospital for a week whilst I was discharged the morning of the second day. My husband came to visit him every day but I didn't because I had to observe '*yu duan*'.

Fortunately, with support from her mother, Thongdee could successfully establish breastfeeding.

> When I first started breastfeeding at home, he refused to suck but my mum suggested I should keep trying. Finally he began to latch on, and was breastfed until he was 15 months.

Similarly, concern about food prohibitions can act as an impediment if women feel they are unable to eat as lactating women 'should' once they return to work. For example, Pattama explained:

> I couldn't be as careful with my diet as before. At '*yu duan*' my husband and my mother took care of my baby and me. . . . They prepared and served me appropriate food every meal, especially '*hua pli*' (banana tree flower). Once I returned to work, I had to do both my work and housework. I'd never pack my lunch to work. It is easy to buy food in the workplace. So, I didn't restrict my diet. Sometime I had pickled bamboo shoots. I think some kinds of foods that I ate may not produce good milk and even make my baby sick. So, I weaned him when I went back to work.

Other cultural beliefs and practices can act as barriers to breastfeeding. These include perceptions that 'there is no breast milk in the first few days', 'breastfeeding can cause infant illness', 'breast milk later in lactation is inadequate in nutritional value', and the practice of giving a bottle of water or formula at an early age. Together with a lack of knowledge about the mechanics of breastfeeding, or how to solve breastfeeding problems, these notions may diminish confidence and lead to early weaning.

8.3.4 Misunderstanding of Breastfeeding in Contemporary Thai Society

8.3.4.1 Confusion with Breastfeeding on Demand and Night Feeding

Breastfeeding on demand is used in common practice for Thai mothers as mothers in other countries such as in Hungary (Ungvary 2006) and in Malta (Brog 2006). However, it can be confusing as some mothers cannot understand the baby's cues. They are likely to put baby on the breast continuously, therefore starting a vicious circle of frustration as feeding becomes a hard work instead of a pleasure. Perceptions of timing are influenced by the myth that healthy happy babies would systematically feed quickly and sleep for a few hours. Most mothers will try to manage things to work out this way.

In Thailand, it is traditionally common for the Thai mother to sleep in the same bed with their baby for a total period of postpartum and some of the lactation period. Thus, they could easily breastfeed through the night. However, some breastfeeding mothers in my study were advised to give a bottle to baby before night time so that baby would sleep longer and that the mothers' sleep would not be disturbed as they had to work the next day. A major maternal milestone as perceived by 'baby sleeping through the night' in this study corresponded with the study in New Zealand (James 2006).

8.3.4.2 Breastfeeding in Public

As other studies have shown (see Borg 2006; Carmen Sortino 2006; James 2006; Ungvary 2006), while there are no laws prohibiting breastfeeding in public in Thailand, it does not receive much support. Most public institutions still have no location reserved for breastfeeding, though this situation seems to be changing slowly. Thus, most women seem not to breastfeed in public, since people often find it inappropriate and unsuitable. Breastfeeding in public might receive diverse reactions, from total support to total disapproval. Anuree said that:

> I often prepare a bottle of formula when I have to bring baby outside. It is very hard to find suitable place for hiding during breastfeeding.

Women experience different reactions to breastfeeding in different settings, from warmth and acceptance to being asked to leave or stop breastfeeding. This situation seldom occurs in contemporary Thai society. However, breastfeeding in public does not find too much support. There is a greater tolerance for breastfeeding young babies in public places than for breastfeeding toddlers in some countries such as New Zealand (James 2006) and Argentina (Carmen Sortino 2006). See also Chapter 7 in this volume.

8.3.5 Mistaken Perception of Breastfeeding and Breast Milk

8.3.5.1 Perceptions of Breast Milk Insufficiency

There were deficiencies in the knowledge of mothers in my study. Other studies (Quarles, William, Hoyle, Brimeyer, & William 1994; Yusof, Mazlan, Ibrahim, & Jusoh 1995) have found that insufficient breast milk syndrome was the most common reason given by mothers for early supplementation, as in this study (see also Chapter 20 in this volume). Similar to Asian women in other studies (Morrow, 1996; Fok, 1997; Liamputtong Rice 2000; Holla-Bhar, 2006; Menon & Amin, 2006; Narasimhan, 2006), many mothers in my study believed that during the first few days their milk had not arrived or they did not have enough milk to nourish their babies. Therefore, some of them bottle-fed and waited passively for breast engorgement to occur in order to feel assured that their milk had come in. This misperception about the need to suckle from birth, unawareness of the existence of sufficient colostrum for a new baby's needs, and lack of knowledge of the benefits of early frequent suckling, reflect some weaknesses in knowledge about the process and mechanics of breastfeeding. It also indicated inappropriate advice and inadequate support from health professionals. Maliwan explained her experience:

> My milk hadn't come yet for the first few days after delivery. So I gave formula to my baby. After I was discharged from hospital, I felt my breasts full and knew I had milk. Then I started breastfeeding.

As in many countries (WHO 1993; Castiglia 1999; Holla-Bhar 2006; Janssens 2002), the increasing prevalence of the nuclear family which accompanies rapid industrialisation and urbanisation means many mothers have little contact with breastfeeding role models within their extended family. This is a real deficiency, especially because older female relatives were credited with saving the breastfeeding relationship for several mothers in this study. Moreover, the ready availability of bottles and formula may act on a subconscious level as a backstop for those with problems.

Experts (Hill 1991; WHO 1996; Holla-Bhar 2006; Mojab 2009) report that a mother's lack of confidence about the adequacy (in quality or quantity) of her breast milk to satisfy her infant's needs is an underlying cause of the insufficient breast milk syndrome. The other determinant is infrequent feeding, which can result in decreased milk production. In this study, at some time many women wondered whether they had enough milk for their babies because their babies cried a lot. As Suchada stated:

> I gave formula to him because he always cried and I felt that I had not enough milk since giving birth. I had fed him with breast milk and formula for a month. I really realized that I had not enough milk for him. So, I weaned him.

However, in a similar situation, but with her mother's support, Somchit overcame her problem and breastfed for 18 months:

> At a few days after delivery, my milk didn't come out well. I felt that I didn't have enough milk for my baby. She always cried. I gave formula every feed after breastfeeding until I was discharged from hospital. At home, my mother helped me to put my baby on the breast. She encouraged me to massage my breasts and to breastfeed frequently. I followed her advice. After that, everything was okay. I could breastfeed her until she was one and a half years old. She was not given formula any more.

Some mothers clearly had inadequate support and sympathy from health professionals in this matter. Seepan told me about her unhappy maternity experience:

> I didn't have enough milk for a few days after birth . . . . Whenever I complained about my breastfeeding difficulty, they [health professionals] didn't take it seriously. They always blamed me because I didn't put my baby to the breast frequently. I said that I followed their advice, but it was not successful. It seemed that they didn't believe me at all. They didn't understand me. Perhaps it was because they didn't have any experience of their own. Most of them were young and single.

Some health professionals themselves accepted the belief that 'insufficient milk' might occur during the first few days. Therefore, they might suggest formula to the mother. Saisunee stated:

> During my first few days in hospital after giving birth, I had no milk, so the nurse suggested I give her formula.

The negative impact of not being a *Baby Friendly Hospital* is apparent in this example. The findings related to early breastfeeding management by hospital staff, as other studies have shown (Losch, Dungy, Russell, & Dusdieker 1995; Wilmoth & Elder 1995; Amir & Ingram 2008; Mulford 2008), indicate that health professionals may be knowledgeable about the benefits of breast milk, yet not be supportive of the act of breastfeeding. This may manifest in the lack of verbal and practical support for women who intend to or are in the process of breastfeeding, and in the provision of infant formula for all infants who had complications or whose mothers had complications. These reflections by mothers bring to life the delicate nature of the breastfeeding relationship and the need for correct management by health staff.

Moreover, the plain water is almost universally provided to breastfed children in Thailand regardless of how young the child (Kanchana 2003; cf. Chapter 19 in this volume). The major reason of some mothers for providing plain water in this study was the fear that their infants were thirsty. In addition, some mothers believed that: 'It is necessary to give water to baby after breastfeeding as adult drinks water after meal to clean its tongue'. This may have an impact on breastfeeding, as less suckling results in reduced breast milk production (Menon & Amin 2006).

8.3.5.2 Perceptions of Breastfeeding Can Cause Infant illness

As in other studies (Vong-Ek 1993; Marchand & Morrow 1994; Morrow 1996), some mothers in this study thought breast milk itself caused illness, and therefore they should take their baby off the breast. They blamed themselves for 'spoiling' their breast milk, either by eating foods which did not agree with their babies or by emotional upsets such as anxiety or fright. Vipa stated:

> I ate a lot of spicy foods, I love '*Nam Plick*' (chilli dip), but it can pass through my milk and give my baby diarrhea.

Pranom, who had marital troubles when her baby was 5 months old, explained:

> I breastfed her for a few months only. I weaned her because I often had problems with my husband. Sometimes we had fights. Maybe this would make my milk deteriorate and make my baby sick. I thought it was better to stop breastfeeding.

Moreover, some health professionals may have given confusing suggestions. Puangthong, a pieceworker at home, told me:

> After being breastfed for one and a half months, my daughter got diarrhoea. I took her to a private clinic in the city. The doctor said that she might be allergic to breast milk and suggested I stop breastfeeding for a while and use a special formula from the clinic. One week later, she was better and I took her to follow up at the clinic. The doctor advised me to continue to feed her with that formula until it was finished, then she could have a normal formula.

It is of great concern that misperceptions and lack of knowledge among mothers are not always corrected by health professionals. Indeed, some health workers actively contributed to misperceptions which resulted in weaning.

8.3.5.3 Perception of 'Breast Milk Later in Lactation Is Inadequate in Nutritional Value'

Some women worried about the quality of their breast milk. They believed that good breast milk should be 'thick', 'sweet' and 'white color', thus, they would stop breastfeeding if breast milk became 'clear' and 'tasteless'. Although Chompunuch had a lot of breast milk, she did not continue breastfeeding after she found that her breast milk became 'clear' and 'tasteless' when she tried it at 4 months. She explained:

> My milk became clear, not white and '*khoon*' (opaque). It was tasteless. I had heard from older people that if this happens the milk doesn't have much benefit to the baby any more. Perhaps, I thought, this was the time that I should give supplementary foods. I started giving formula and 'Cerelac' at four months.

Such mistaken beliefs attributed to others in the community are very unfortunate. They also demonstrate that some women are not knowledgeable about the changing appearance and taste of breast milk.

8.4 Conclusion

It appears that cultural beliefs and practices, combined with support from family members, may be the most important factors influencing initiate breastfeeding practices in the first month. The benefits of breastfeeding in contemporary Thai society are widely recognised and valued. The findings suggest that the circumstances of women's lives influence their views and practices. The preference for breastfeeding derives from a variety of nutritional, health/medical, social, economic, cultural, and psychological reasons, sometimes related to a level of knowledge about psychology, immunology, correct weight gain, or cost consideration. The peak rate at 1 month also coincided with the period of '*yu duan*,' which promotes a close contact between the mother and her newborn infant. However, some beliefs, for example, perceptions of breast milk insufficiency, use of water at an early age, postpartum food restrictions and practices, and misconceptions about breast milk and breastfeeding, can present barriers for successful breastfeeding.

The findings from this study recommend several strategies to promote breastfeeding concerning on cultural beliefs and practices. As shown in Table 8.1, the study findings, in terms of whether they are likely to facilitate or threaten successful breastfeeding, were grouped under the headings 'positive' (= facilitating) and 'negative' (= threatening). According to the Ottawa Charter for Health promotion, the five key areas for action to promote good health are public policy, creating a supportive environment, strengthening community action, developing personal skills and re-orienting health services. Strategies include modifying hospital policies and practices; improving attitudes and knowledge of health personnel; using public and social support; educating employed women; providing support and encouragement; and initiating legislation and political action to create policies aimed toward healthier infant feeding practices.

It is essential that breastfeeding promotion campaign should integrate cultural beliefs and practices, and programs should modify negative beliefs and practices. Additionally, Thai health authorities must move to re-orient health services, improve attitudes and knowledge of health personnel, and use public and social support for supporting and empowering all women to establish and continue breastfeeding.

Table 8.1 Finding and recommendations

Study findings	Recommendations
***Positive:* cultural belief and practices** – Recognition of *'breast is best'* – Highest breastfeeding rate is during *'yu duan'*, the traditional 1 month confinement period ***Negative:* cultural beliefs and practices** – The use of bottle of water and/or formula at an early age – Postpartum food restrictions and practices – Misconceptions about breast milk and breastfeeding (1) Belief that there is no breast milk in the first few days (2) Perception of breast milk insufficiency (3) Belief that breastfeeding causes infant illness (4) Belief that breast milk given to older infants is nutritionally inadequate	**Breastfeeding promotion campaign should integrate cultural beliefs**: – Support and strengthen positive cultural beliefs and practices related to breastfeeding via mass media such as television, radio, magazines, and newspapers – Public endorsement of mother staying together with the infant **Modifying hospital policies and practices** – In cases of child illness, facilitate the stay in hospital of the mother if the child is admitted – Stop the routine provision of bottles of infant formula and/or water to mother – Encourage and help mother to breastfeed immediately after delivery **Improve attitudes, knowledge, and practices of health care personnel** – Train all staff, give specialized training for lactation consultant and continue to educate (1) Integrate breastfeeding issues into curriculum for medical and nursing students (2) Improve the availability of books and other printed matter, so new information can be rapidly disseminated **Programs to modify negative beliefs and practices** – Health personnel should discuss with mothers non-scientific practices which are potentially harmful, while ignoring others – Public discussion of misconceptions about breast milk and breastfeeding via mass media such as television, radio, magazines, and newspapers

Acknowledgments I am grateful to the Thai government who provided me with the financial support. I thank the Faculty of Nursing of Chiang Mai University for giving me the material and professional support during my field work. I am also indebted to the employed mothers who participated in this study for their willingness to take time from their busy lives to talk with me at length about themselves and the issue. I thank Professor Wichit Srisuphan for her encouragement and Dr. Martha Morrow for her support and valuable comments in the preparation of this chapter.

References

American Academy of Pediatrics [AAP]. (2005). Breastfeeding and the use of human milk. *Pediatrics, 100*, 1035–1039.

Amir, L. H., & Ingram, J. (2008). Health professionals' advice for breastfeeding problems: Not good enough! *International Breastfeeding Journal, 3*(22). Retrieved 20 May 2009, from http://www.internationalbreastfeedingjournal.com/content/3/1/22

Brog, C. (2006). Nursing triplets – Malta. In R. Holla-Bhar (Ed.), *Against all odds: Gendered challenges to breastfeeding* (pp. 87–97). Penang, Malasia: Juta.

Carmen Sortino, M. (2006). Taking breastfeeding to the community – Argentina. In R. Holla-Bhar (Ed.), *Against all odds: Gendered challenges to breastfeeding* (pp. 22–39). Penang, Malasia: Juta.

Castiglia, P. T. (1999). Extended families: Social support systems for children. *Journal of Pediatric Health Care, 13*(3), 139–141.

Chatranon, W. (1988). *Thailand's national breastfeeding promotion programs.* Paper presented at the International Asian Regional Lactation Management Workshop and Related Events, Bali, Indonesia, 29 June–9 July 1988.

Chayovan, N., Knodel, J., & Wongboonsin, K. (1990). Infant feeding practices in Thailand: An update from the 1987 Demographic and Health Survey. *Studies in Family Planning, 21*(1): 40–50.

Donath, S., & Amir, L. H. (2000). Rates of breastfeeding in Australia by state and socioeconomic status: Evidence from the 1995 National Health Survey. *Breastfeeding Review, 8*(3), 23–27.

Durongdej, S., & Mangklasiri, R. (1993). *The impact of hospital policy and performance on the initiation and maintenance of breastfeeding*. Unpublished document.

Family Health Division. (1994). *A study of breastfeeding situation.* Bangkok: Family Health Division, Ministry of Public Health, Thailand.

Fok, D. (1997). Breastfeeding in Singapore. *Breastfeeding Review, 5*(2), 25–28.

Hill, P. D. (1991). The enigma of insufficient milk supply. *American Journal of Maternal and Child Nursing, 16*(6), 312–316.

Holla-Bhar, R. (2006). *Against all odds: Gendered challenges to breastfeeding.* Penang, Malasia: Juta.

James, L. (2006). Bridgeing cultures in support of breastfeeding – New Zealand. In R. Holla-Bhar (Ed.), *Against all odds: Gendered challenges to breastfeeding* (pp. 98–114). Penang, Malasia: Juta.

Janssens, A. (2002). *Family and social change: The household as a process in an industrializing community.* Cambridge: Cambridge University Press.

Kanchana, S. (2003). Breastfeeding promotion policy. In S. Jittinun, V. Chattranon, S. Swadivorn (Eds.), *Breastfeeding: Theory to practice* (pp. 331–337). Bangkok: Bangkokwetsasarn.

Liamputtong, P. (2004). *Yu duan* practices as embodying tradition, modernity and social change in Chiang Mai, Northern Thailand. *Women & Health, 40*(1), 79–99.

Liamputtong Rice, P. (2000). *Hmong women and reproduction*. Westport: Bergin & Garvey.

Losch, M., Dungy, C. I., Russell, D., & Dusdieker, L. B. (1995). Impact of attitudes on maternal decisions regarding infant feeding. *Journal of Pediatrics, 126*(4), 507–514.

Marchand, L., & Morrow, M. H. (1994). Infant feeding practices: Understanding the decision-making process. *Family Medicine, 26*(5), 319–324.

Menon, L., & Amin, S. (2006). *Breastfeeding: A Reproductive health and rights issue.* Penang, Malasia: Juta.

Mojab, C. G. (2009). The cultural art of breastfeeding. Retrieved 8 January 2009, from http://www.llli.org/llleaderweb/LV/LVOctNov00p87.html

Morrow, M. (1996). Breastfeeding in Vietnam: Poverty, tradition, and economic transition. *Journal of Human Lactation, 12*(2), 97–103.

Mulford, C. (2008). Is breastfeeding invisible, or did the health care system just choose not to notice it? *International Breastfeeding Journal, 3*(13). Retrieved 8 January 2009, from http://www.internationalbreastfeedingjournal.com/content/3/1/13

Narasimhan, S. (2006). Obstacle to exclusive breastfeeding – India. In R. Holla-Bhar (Ed.), *Against all odds: Gendered challenges to breastfeeding* (pp. 73–86). Penang, Malasia: Juta.

National Statistical Office (2007). *The Multiple Indicator Cluster Survey (MICS) December 2005–February 2006.* National Statistical Office, Ministry of Information and Communication Technology. Denmark: Gerbeer Creative.

Quarles, A., William, P. D., Hoyle, D. A., Brimeyer, M., & William, A. R. (1994). Mother's intention, age, education and duration and management of breastfeeding. *Maternal–Child Nursing Journal, 22*(3), 102–107.

Scott, J. A., & Binns, C. W. (1999). Factors associated with the initiation and duration of breastfeeding: A review of the literature. *Breastfeeding Review, 7*(1), 5–16.

Singhal, A., Cole, T. J., & Lucus, A. (2001). Early nutrition in preterm infants and later blood pressure: Two cohorts after randomized trials. *Lancet, 357*, 413–419.

Taintavorn, W. (1996). *Report of Thai children health development program for the mid-decade goals.* Paper presented at the WABA Global Forum on Children's Rights: Action for the 21st Century, Sukothai Thammathirat Open University, Bangkok, 2–6 December 1996.

Tsianakas, V., & Liamputtong, P. (2007). Infant feeding practices and Afghan immigrant women in Australia. In P. Liamputtong (Ed.), *Childrearing and infant care issues: A cross-cultural perspective* (pp. 249–273). New York: Nova Science.

Ungvary, R. W. (2006). Institutional challenges to breastfeeding – Hungary. In R. Holla-Bhar (Ed.), *Against all odds: Gendered challenges to breastfeeding* (pp. 61–72). Penang, Malasia: Juta.

UNICEF–United Nations Children's Fund (2006). *1990–2005 Celebrating The Innocenti Declaration on the protection, promotion and support of breastfeeding.* Florence, Italy: UNICEF Innocenti Research Centre.

Van-Esterik P. (1988). The cultural context of infant feeding. In B. Winikoff, M. A. Castle, & V. H. Laukaran (Eds.), *Feeding infants in four societies: Cause and consequences of mothers' choices* (pp. 187–202). New York: Greenwood.

Villalpando, S., & Lopez-Alarcon, M. (2000). Growth faltering is prevented by breast-feeding in underprivileged infants from Mexico City. *The Journal of Nutrition, 130*(3), 546–552.

Vong-Ek, P. (1993). Socio-cultural factors influencing breastfeeding duration in Thailand. In B. Yoddumnern-Attig, G. A. Attig, W. Boonchalaksi, K. Richter, & A. Soonthorndhada (Eds.), *Qualitative methods for population and health research* (pp. 401–410). Nakhonpathom: the Institute for Population and Social Research, Mahidol University.

Wilmoth, T. A., & Elder, J. P. (1995). An assessment of research on breastfeeding promotion strategies in developing countries. *Social Science and Medicine, 41*(4), 579–594.

Winichagoon, P., Viriyapanich, T., & Dhamamitta, S. (1992). Breastfeeding in Thailand: Trends and promotion efforts. In P. Winichagoon, Y. Kachondham, G. A. Attig, & K. Tontisirin (Eds.), *Integrating food and nutrition into development: Thailand's experiences and future visions* (pp. 124–132). Thonburi: P.I. Printing.

Wongboonsin, K., & Ruffolo, V. P. (1993). The future of Thailand's population policy: Potential directions. *Asia-Pacific Population Journal, 8*(3), 3–18.

World Health Organization (1993). *Breastfeeding: The technical basis and recommendations for action.* Geneva: World Health Organization.

World Health Organization (1996). *Not enough milk.* Geneva: Division of Diarrhoeal and Acute Respiratory Disease Control, World Health Organization.

World Health Organization (2001). *The optimal duration of exclusive breastfeeding: Results of a WHO systematic review.* Geneva: World Health Organization.

Yimyam, S. (1998). Breastfeeding work and women's health among Thai women in Chiang Mai. *Breastfeeding Review, 6*(1), 17–22.

Yimyam, S. (2005). Breastfeeding promotion for healthy mothers and healthy babies. In W. Kunaviktikul (Ed.), *Towards the success of health promotion* (pp. 155–171). Chiang Mai, Thailand: Chotana.

Yimyam, S., & Morrow, M. (1999). Breastfeeding practices among employed Thai women. *Journal of Human Lactation, 15*(3), 225–232.

Yimyam, S., & Morrow, M. (2003). Maternal labor, breast-feeding, and infant health. In J. Heymann (Ed.), *Global inequity at work* (pp. 105–135). New York: Oxford University Press.

Yusof, Y. A., Mazlan, M., Ibrahim, N., & Jusoh, N. M. (1995). Infant feeding practices and attitudes of mothers in Kelantan towards breastfeeding. *Medical Journal of Malaysia, 50*(2), 150–155.

Chapter 9
Good Mothers and Infant Feeding Practices Amongst Women in Northern Thailand

Pranee Liamputtong and Somsri Kitisriworapan

Contents

9.1 Introduction

Breastfeeding is profoundly supported by both professionals and lay individuals (Schmied & Lupton 2001; Cricco-Lizza 2005; see Chapters 2–5 in this volume). It is claimed that breastfeeding is beneficial for both a newborn infant and a mother (Witters-Green 2003; Wolf 2006). For the infant, breast milk is the ideal food in both quantity and quality. With its anti-infective properties, breast milk provides protection against infection and health problems (Marild, Hansson, & Jodal 2004; Jackson 2004; Berger, Hill, & Waldfogel 2005; Raymond 2005; Quigley, Kelly, & Sacker 2007; WHO 2007). Breastfeeding also provides bonding between mother and her infant (Jelliffe & Jelliffe 1978; Dettwyler, 1995). Hence, breastfeeding is seen as promoting not only the health of the infant but also its development and psychological well-being (Abel, Julie, Tippene-Leach, Finau, & Lennan 2001; Riordan 2005). For the mother, breastfeeding soon after birth reduces the risk of postpartum

P. Liamputtong (✉)
School of Public Health, La Trobe University, Bundoora, Victoria, Australia 3086
e-mail: pranee@latrobe.edu.au

P. Liamputtong (ed.), *Infant Feeding Practices*, DOI 10.1007/978-1-4419-6873-9_9,
© Springer Science+Business Media, LLC 2011

haemorrhage (Gonzalez 1990; Coutsoudis 2005), breast cancer and osteoporosis (Coutsoudis 2005; Wolf 2006), and provides a natural form of birth spacing (Gray et al. 1990; Coutsoudis 2005). Economically, breastfeeding saves money which the family has to spend on expensive formula if bottle-feeding is adopted (Abel et al. 2001; Oddy 2001; Gartner et al. 2005).

However, not all women and their families necessarily perceive it as such. Infant feeding practices occur within the social and cultural context of the society in which women live (Dykes 2005). Although women understand the value of breast milk, many women choose not to breastfeed their infants or may try to combine breastfeeding with bottle-feeding (Earle 2000; Dykes 2005; Scavenius, van Hulsel, Meijer, Wendte, & Gurgel 2007). Previous studies have identified the many reasons women cite as the choice of infant feeding, for example, work (Yimyam & Morrow 2003; Oritz, McGilligan, & Kelly 2004; Duong, Lee, & Binns 2005; Calnen 2007; Gatrell 2007; Scavenius et al. 2007), insufficient milk (Hillervik-Lindquist 1991; Moffat 2002; Sacco, Caulfield, Gittelsohn, & Martínez 2006; Tsianakas & Liamputtong 2007; Scavenius et al. 2007), infant and maternal health (Rossiter 1992, 1999; Craig & Scambler 2006), lack of social support (Schmidt 2008; Barona-Vilar, Escribá-Agüira, & Ferrero-Gandıa 2009), availability of infant formulae (Riordan & Gill-Hopple 2001; Liubai, Doan Thi Phuong, Nguyen-Thi, & Hiroshi 2002; Mistry, Freedman, Sweeney, & Hollenbeck 2008) and women's perceptions of breastfeeding (Rossiter 1992, 1999; Rodriguez-Garcia & Frazier 1995). As Bailey and Pain (2001), Miller (2005) and Gatrell (2007) point out, breastfeeding can be difficult to establish and problematic to maintain. If women do not breastfeed, we need to understand why. This necessitates a research project which will take into account the socio-cultural influences on infant feeding decisions among women. Our project attempts to fill this gap in literature in Thai society.

In the several past decades, rapid social and economic transformations have changed women's lives in many parts of the world (Duncan, Edwards, & Reynolds 2003; Ehrenreich & Hochschild 2003; Vincent, Ball, & Pietikainen 2004). Thai women have also been caught in this change. Women in Thailand have entered the labour force as a way to increase their family income since the 1960s when the country's economy has become increasingly dependent on the global market economy (Tantiwiramanond & Pandey 1991; Lim 1993; Yimyam 1997; Liamputtong 2007). Many women in the North, as Yimyam (1997) points out, work outside the home as well as perform housework. These changes have profoundly affected women, motherhood and infant feeding practices (see also Chapter 8 in this volume).

Similar to many other developing countries, the duration of breastfeeding declined in Thailand during the 1970s (Knodel, Chayovan, & Wongboonsin 1990; Yimyam 1997; Chapter 8). Although the decline was moderate, it was pervasive enough to affect women from rural and urban settings as well as women from different educational attainments. How would mothers in Thailand see themselves as mothers and practise infant feeding in a changing social and economic environment? If women have to work outside their homes and try to breastfeed at the same time, will this impact on their perceptions and practices of infant feeding? In this chapter, we discuss infant feeding practices in Northern Thai society. In particular, we focus on how mothers perceive and experience breastfeeding and how they in fact feed their infants.

9.2 Breast and Bottle-Feeding: Moral and Deviant Mothers

The dominant idea that 'breast is best' (Stanway & Stanway 1978) is pervasive in literature on infant feeding patterns and in policy and health promotion attempting to educate women about their infant feeding practices (Nadesan & Sotirin 1998; Murphy 1999; Guttman & Zimmerman 2000; see also other chapters in this volume). Within the lay population, this idea is also promulgated. Due to the societal perception of the superiority of breastfeeding, as Murphy (1999, p. 187) contends, mothers' intention not to breastfeed their babies may tarnish the 'moral status' of motherhood. By choosing to bottle-feed their infants, a mother is subjected to the accusation that she is a 'bad' mother, who 'places her own needs, preferences or conveniences above her baby's welfare' (Murphy 1999, p. 187). On the contrary, the 'good mother' is 'deemed to be one who prioritises her child's needs, even (or perhaps especially) where this entails personal inconvenience or distress' (Murphy 1999, pp. 187–188), such as trying to breastfeed against many obstacles (see also Chapter 12 in this volume).

Motherhood, Nadesan and Sotirin (1998, p. 221) contend, is 'often represented as the ultimate expression of womanhood while breast-feeding is represented as the ultimate experience of motherhood'. Because of this, as Murphy (1999, p. 188) suggests, the decision to bottle-feed is likely to be considered as 'questionable' (McHugh 1970).

> It leaves women open to the charge of being a poor mother, in short, of maternal deviance. The intention to formula feed threatens women's claims to qualities such as selflessness, wisdom, responsibility and far-sightedness all of which are widely seen as evidence of being a 'good mother' (Murphy 1999, p. 188).

Guttman and Zimmerman (2000, p. 1458) argue that 'the discourses on motherhood, nurture, naturalness and modernity' has created the moral image of breastfeeding. As Earle (2000, p. 327) points out in her study with women in Coventry, England, women perceived breastfeeding as natural. A woman who did not breastfeed was perceived as 'a horrible mother'. As such, women who intend to bottle-feed their infants open themselves to a charge of deviance (Goffman 1963) or 'immoral mothers' (Liamputtong 2006).

Deviance, according to Murphy (1999, p.189), 'involves a charge that public morality is being violated' and in the case of infant feeding, mothers break the rules of infant feeding. But more than that, as Murphy (1999, p. 188) theorises, 'the moral mother is not simply one who follows the rules. Rather, she is one who follows the rules *knowingly*'. Hence, simply breaking the rules does not make the mother deviant. Rather, as McHugh (1970, p. 188, original emphasis) suggests, 'her deviance rests upon a judgement that she has broken the rules *knowingly*'. In the case of infant feeding, mothers who choose not to breastfeed their infants and know very well about the likely impacts of the practice on infant's health are potentially subject to the charge of deviance as 'immoral mothers'.

Social rules, Sykes and Matza (1957, p. 666, original emphasis) argue, are '*qualified* guides to action'. The charge of being immoral or deviant mothers, Murphy contends 'is always defeasible in the sense that it is open to the possibility of refutation'. Dingwall (1976) suggests this possibility is dependent on the ability of the individual to appeal to some 'possible grounds for refuting the accusation'. Therefore, Murphy (1999, pp. 189–190) suggests, despite the fact that breastfeeding is socially constructed as 'the optimal method of infant feeding', which has ramifications for the judgement of moral motherhood, 'the rule that "good mothers breastfeed" is not so rigid as to be binding under all circumstance'. There appears to be some possibilities for women who intend to bottle-feed to 'challenge or resist the interpretation of their behaviour as morally sanctionable'. To do so, Sykes and Matza (1957) and Scott and Lyman (1963) suggest the use of 'techniques of neutralisation', particularly 'justification'. According to Scott and Lyman (1963) and Murphy (1999, p. 190), justification involves 'an acceptance that the act is deviant, while seeking to rebut any suggestion that it is therefore morally or socially sanctionable'.

In relation to infant feeding, however, Murphy (1999, p. 190) contends, women who intend to bottle-feed must prove that, while it breaks the rule, it is nonetheless justified. When the decision to formula feed her baby is questioned, a mother must justify that her intention is 'non-conventional'; that is 'she could not have done otherwise'. She has no other choices and hence her intention should not be sanctioned since it can be justified. Therefore, the charge of deviance should be abolished. As Wright, Clark, and Bauer (1993, p. 262) contend, when breastfeeding is socially valued in societies, women choosing not to breastfeed may use socially and culturally acceptable grounds for their actions, such as the need to work in a paid employment and having insufficient milk to justify their actions. This will help them to escape being seen as 'bad mothers'.

In this chapter, we will show that the morality of breastfeeding is also pervasive among Thai women in Northern Thailand. We will also examine the ways in which women talk about their accounts/stories which are used to deny the charge that their choices are deemed deviant even though they might bottle-feed their infants.

9.3 The Study

This chapter is based on in-depth interviews with 30 Thai women who are living in Chiang Mai, Northern Thailand. Fifteen women were recruited from Chiang Mai City and fifteen from Mae Chantra sub-district (fictitious name), 49 km from the municipality of Chiang Mai. This was to ensure that women from different social class backgrounds would be selected. Women from Chiang Mai City were mainly from urban and middle-class backgrounds with a higher educational level, while women from Mae Chantra sub-district were from a peasant background and had lesser educational attainment and income. The majority of the women in this study had recently given birth, but only few were pregnant at the time of this study being conducted.

Women were firstly recruited through a personal network of the researcher as well as through a 'snowball' sampling technique (Liamputtong 2009); that is, women were asked to nominate or contact their friends or relatives who would be interested in participating in the study. Each woman was informed about the nature of the research and her participation. An informed consent form (in Thai) was signed once the women agreed to participate in the study. Ethical approval was sought and granted by the Ethics Committees of La Trobe University.

An in-depth interviewing technique was employed to elicit information (Liamputtong 2009). The women were individually interviewed about traditional beliefs and practices regarding infant feeding practices and motherhood as well as background information on socio-demographic characteristics. The interviews were held in the women's homes. All interviews were conducted in Thai. Each woman was interviewed once, with the interview lasting between one to two hours, depending on the participant. All interviews were tape-recorded for later transcription and analysis. All interviews were transcribed in the Thai language to maintain the subtlety and meaning of the women's voices as accurately as possible. The analysis was also done from the Thai transcripts, and only those quotations that are presented in the chapter were translated into English (Liamputtong 2010). The translation retains, verbatim, what the women said, with some syntactical corrections.

The data concerning were analysed using a thematic analysis method guided by phenomenology (Liamputtong 2009). The interview transcripts were used to interpret how women described their meanings and experiences of traditional beliefs and practices regarding infant feeding and motherhood in their everyday lives. Their responses were then organised into coherent themes (Liamputtong 2009), as presented in the following sections. Women's names have been changed for confidentiality.

9.4 'Breast Is Best' Notion: Women's Accounts

There is no doubt that the women in this study perceived breast milk as the best food for their newborn and young infants (cf. van Esterik 1988; Vong-Ek 1993; Yimyam 1997; Liamputtong Rice 2000; Liamputtong Rice & Naksook 2001; Scavenius et al. 2007; see also Chapters 2, 4, 5, 6, 7, 8 in this volume). It is said that breast milk contains antibiotics and all nutrients that could not be equalled by consuming all the five food groups. Women remarked that only breast milk contains all the goodness that newborn and young infants need. Pimpilai, an urban educated woman, provided the following explanation when asked about breast milk:

> Mother's milk is best as it provides good immunity to the baby, so that the baby will have a high resistance to ill health and diseases. People say that breastfed babies will have a good resistance and immunity and these children will not get sick or catch a cold easily.

Saijai, an urban middle-class woman, similarly remarked:

> I have been breastfeeding for 10 months. I have read many books and they all say that breast milk is best for the baby. I wanted my baby to get all the best things in her life and so I breastfeed her.

Not only breast milk provides the best sort of nutrients to an infant, the act of breastfeeding also provides warmth and psychological well-being to their newborn as well. Wilai, an urban educated woman, had some interesting remarks about breastfeeding. She suggested that the nutrients in infant formula nowadays is more or less similar to breast milk, but the act of feeding is in fact provides more closeness, warmth and emotional well-being to both the mother and her newborn. Similarly, Sumalee, a rural woman, reflected on her belief about breast milk that:

> I think the best food for my baby is mother's milk. It is the purest form of food that screens from our own body. The baby will receive warmth and love from a mother. Mother's goodness will then be passed onto the baby through breast milk. And this is the best way for the baby to be passed on good stuff from us as mothers.

When prompted about bottle-feeding, Sumalee remarked that:

> With bottle-feeding, even though we feed the baby ourself, it is not the same as feeding the baby from our body. It is like putting cow's milk into the baby's body. When we breastfeed, we can cuddle the baby, we can hold the baby close to our body. But, it is not the same when we use the bottle. We might cuddle the baby, but it does not give me the same sort of feelings like breastfeeding. So, feeding the baby by a bottle is not the same as feeding from our breasts because it is not coming out from our own bodies.

Of interest is the perception among rural or poor women who contended that breast milk not only makes the infant strong and healthy but was also financially sound. Mothers did not have to spend money on buying infant formula. This is clearly seen in the account given by Isara, a rural poor woman who breastfed her infant for 3 months. The infant became very ill and had to be hospitalised. While in hospital, the nursing staff bottle-fed him, and as a result her breast milk dried up. In Isara's mind, this was unfortunate for not only her infant but also for her financial situation, as now she had to find money to purchase infant formula for her baby, rather than being able to save money for other necessities needed in the family.

Orachorn, also a rural poor woman, contended that breast milk was not only best for her babies, but also because of her financial circumstances, she had no other option. This was her explanation:

> I breastfed my babies, all of them, because what else I could feed them apart from breast milk. I am not in a position to buy any infant food to give them. Breastfeeding was the only option I had.

Of note is the fact that more rural poor women initiated and continued breastfeeding for a long period of time. This was partly due to their financial constraints as well as their understanding of the goodness of breast milk.

Others talked about the hygienic aspect of breastfeeding. They would compare this with that of bottle-feeding. Sirin, an urban educated woman, remarked:

> I believe breast milk is best because if we bottle-feed, we have to make up the bottles and they may not be clean enough and this will create the likelihood of the baby getting germs

more than from mother's milk. This is why people say mother's milk is the best for her baby.

Women made sense of the benefit of breast milk from their lived experiences with breastfeeding and other feeding methods. Sinjai, an urban educated woman, compared the health of her two children, one was bottle-fed and another breastfed:

As far as I can see is that a breastfed baby is much healthier and stronger than a formula-fed baby. [...] is not that strong, when he was a little baby, he was very thin and always had some sort of ill health like it was very easy for him to get a cold or diarrhoea. He was formula fed. But [...] who was breastfed is always healthy; never got sick. I can easily see the differences between them.

9.5 Breast Milk: *Luad Nai Ok* – Mother's Blood and Mother/Child Connection

Breastfeeding, van Esterik (1988, 1989) suggests, is perceived as 'a holistic and integrated activity' within a more traditional society like Thailand. Indeed, as Dykes (2005, p. 2287) points out, within traditional communities, breastfeeding is illustrated 'as entirely relationally orientated with absence of any dichotomy between the baby's nutritional and emotional needs'. The women in Dykes's study (2005, p. 2286) made reference to 'intimacy, closeness and nurture, seeing breastfeeding as much more than providing breast milk to the baby'. Zeitlyn and Rowshan (1997) theorise that through breastfeeding, women and their breastfed children are 'interconnected and indivisible'. This is clearly reflected in the Thai women's discourses regarding the origin of breast milk. The notion that breast milk is best stems largely from a traditional belief among Thai people that it is produced from the blood of the mother. Often, breast milk is referred to as *luad nai ok*, literally means 'blood from mother's chest'. It symbolises sacrifice and maternal love of a mother toward her infant. Zeitlyn and Rowshan (1997) point out that Bangladeshi women also see the connection between a mother and a child through breastfeeding. In a similar manner, Sumalee, a rural woman, contended that:

Breast milk comes from our own blood; it is filtered from our blood – mother's blood. This is why there is always a strong connection between a mother and her child.

Suriya, a rural poor woman, remarked that:

The best milk for a baby is mother's milk. It is much better than anything else because it provides warmth and closeness to the baby, much more than bottle-feeding, because mother's milk is made from the mother's blood.

The interconnectedness between mothers and infants can be seen from an interesting account given by Saijai, an urban middle-class woman. In this case, it deserves our attention. Saijai has been breastfeeding her baby for 10 months. When she had to return to work, she twice tried to wean the baby form breastfeeding. Both attempts failed, according to her. She elaborated on these attempted that:

> I tried to wean him twice. When he was about 7 months old, I stopped him from my breast but he would cry until he vomited. Once he cried to the point that he was in shock. It was like his cry was frozen. I was so sorry for the baby and said to myself I would not wean him. So, I continued breastfeeding. You should see his face when I put him back on my breast. Even it was just a short suck, he was smiling and I was feeling so sorry for him. I was in tears. How could I as a mother wean my baby when he is like this?

Our interpretation is that breastfed mothers, as Murphy (1999, p. 200) suggests, 'simultaneously display adequate maternal knowledge (that 'breast is best') and appropriate maternal morality (that they would prioritise the baby's welfare)'. Women knew very well what was best for their babies, and they intended to do so. As such, as Murphy (1999, p. 201) suggests, 'breastfeeding was treated not only compatible with, but indeed, indicative of, maternal morality'.

Some women would suggest that breast milk is made from food a mother consumes during the *yu duan* (confinement) period (see also Chapter 8 in this volume). The consumed food is made into the mother's blood and then turned into breast milk (cf. Zeitlyn & Rowshan 1997). Hence, women would be particularly cautious about food consumption during the first month after birth, as it could affect the health of their infants. Clearly, this is a reflection of the mother–baby connection through breastfeeding. Isara, a rural poor woman, told us that:

> Breast milk is from our own blood; our blood is filtered and made into breast milk. So, whatever we eat during lactation will get into the baby's body too; like if we eat hot food, the baby might have a stomach ache. So, we have to be careful with what we eat during the first month. I would *kam kin* – restrict myself with diet during this time; things like hot food or pickles I would not eat during *yu duan* at all.

But, for some well-off women, the consumption of good food must start early. Sinjai volunteered that:

> Breast milk is from the food we eat. We have to nourish our bodies; make our bodies healthy and strong. It will help us to produce good blood and then this blood will turn into breast milk for the baby. This is why we have to make sure that we eat good food from when we become pregnant.

On the contrary, many poor women would feel that due to their poverty, their food intake was not sufficient and nutritious enough for them to produce good breast milk for their babies. As such, their babies might not receive good milk and hence this might affect their connection with their babies. Malai, a rural poor woman, remarked on this:

> The mother [she] did not have good food to eat during pregnancy; only rice and sweet potatoes. How could the baby get good breast milk then? When I was pregnant, I only had rice noodle curry [cheap dish to prepare], so my baby did not get good nutritious food either. I was not in good health, and so the baby would not be born healthy. I did not have the chance to drink milk or any other nutritious food and this is because I am poor. I live in poverty, hence I could not live and eat well and this affected the quality of breast milk.

9.6 Mothers' Decision to Bottle-Feed

Despite their knowledge about the goodness of breast milk, several mothers in our study decided to bottle-feed their infants. Araya, an urban educated woman, when asked what she believed to be the best food for a new born infant, expressed her idea that: 'Of course, mother's milk because breast milk is beneficial as mothers will eat all the good things in order to produce beast milk for our babies'. But, when asked if she breastfed her newborn, she said 'No, my baby is having a bottle'. Her main reason was 'I did not have enough milk. At first, I did have some as I stimulated my breasts but because I had a problem with my cut from my caesarean birth, I could not feed the baby. I then started feeding him with infant formula'.

For some women, a mixed feeding method was adopted for practical reasons such as the need to leave the baby with others due to commitments that they needed to attend to as part of their living reality. Pimpan, a rural woman, told us that she has breastfed the second baby for 11 months now, but she also gave the baby infant formula as a supplement. She had to attend to many tasks and if she only breastfed the baby, the baby would be clingy and it would not be practical for her to do her work properly. If the baby was accustomed to taking infant formula as well, she could leave the baby with a family member while she was doing something else.

There were two major reasons that the women in this study used to justify their decisions to bottle-feed their infants.

9.6.1 The 'Not Enough Milk' Syndrome

Breastfeeding is full of contradictions. As Zeitlyn and Rowshan (1997, p. 57) point out, despite the fact that breast milk is important for child survival, 'insufficient milk' is a commonly reported phenomenon, particularly among urban middle-class and educated women in many parts of the world (see Tully & Dewey 1985; Hill 1991; Hillervik-Lindquist 1991; Marchand & Morrow 1994; WHO 1996; Beasley, Chick, Pybus, Weber, MacKenzie, & Dignam 1998; Dykes & Williams 1999; Murphy 2000; Abel et al. 2001; Dykes 2002, 2005; Hamlyn, Brooker, Oleinikova, & Wands 2002; Sacco et al. 2006; see also Chapters 8, 18 and 20 in this volume). Often, insufficient milk is used as a justification for many women to progress to bottle-feeding (Murphy 2000; Dykes 2005).

In Dykes's study (2005, p. 2287), the most striking and consistent theme that she found was that women lacked confidence and trust in their bodies. Women did not feel confident in their abilities to produce enough milk, or the right-quality milk. This lack of confidence was expressed not only by the women themselves but was also obvious amongst the midwives. This is in a similar vein to the findings of Zeitlyn and Rowshan (1997, p. 58), in their research on insufficient milk in Bangladesh, who found that breast milk is perceived 'with ambivalence'. Both mothers and health professionals often gave 'insufficient milk' as a reason for not breastfeeding.

As Zeitlyn and Rowshan (1997, p. 63) point out in their study, women believed that their babies did not have enough breast milk and often the women would remark that 'their milk "dried up" or that the baby cried and was believed to be hungry'. Some women remarked that breast milk did not 'satisfy' their babies or 'fill' their stomachs. That unsettled behaviours of their infants were associated with the women's perceptions of insufficient milk are also evident in other studies (see Hillervick-Linquist 1991; Beasley et al. 1998; Dykes & Williams 1999; Hamlyn et al. 2002; Dykes 2005; Sacco et al. 2006). Yimyam (1997; see Chapter 8) also suggests that the most common breastfeeding problems given by Thai women in her study was due to insufficient milk. In our study, despite women's intention to breastfeed and for most, they attempted to do so for a long period of time, in reality, many could not do this. Sumalee, a rural woman, provided a clear account about the goodness of breastfeeding (see earlier section), but she was only able to breastfeed for 2 months, and it was not exclusive either. She adopted a mixed method. She defended herself as not only due to having 'insufficient milk' but also the physiology of her nipples and the consequences of taking contraceptive pills.

> I managed to breastfeed my baby for 2 months because I used a mixed method. The baby was always hungry; I could tell because she always curled her lips and sucked the air, and this indicated that she was hungry. I did not have enough milk to feed her; it did not really come out even she was sucking. My nipples were very short too so it was hard for her to grasp. When she could not suck she would cry and I felt sorry for her. So, I gave her some formula after breastfeeding. By the end of the second month, my milk was totally dried up.

All too often, as Dykes (2005, p. 2287) points out, women's bodies have been seen as 'weak, defective and deeply untrustworthy' and hence 'denigrated'. This has led women to think that their bodies are not suited to breastfeeding (see also Martin 1992; Davis-Floyd 1992, 1994; Blum 1993; Duden 1993; Shildrick 1997; Dykes 2002, 2005). Due to this, breastfeeding may be seen 'as something which will be difficult (or impossible) to achieve successfully' (Earle 2000, p. 326) by women. Vong-Ek (1993) and Dykes (2002, 2005) argue that beliefs in insufficient milk may lead women to adopt formula feeding or weaning of breast milk. This has been demonstrated by some of the women in this study.

9.6.2 Paid Work and Breastfeeding

Maternity leave entitlement in Thailand is not very generous, nor uniform across the work forces. As Yimyam, Morrow, and Srisuphan (1999, p. 958) contend, 'there is no comprehensive, universal legislation protecting the breastfeeding rights of employed women and few private companies or government agencies provide regular support in this sphere'. It has been observed that only women who work in the government sector or some privileged business sectors may receive a better deal of maternity leave than those working in the private sector or factories. The current legislation regarding maternity leave in Thailand was enacted in May 1993 (Yimyam 1997; Yimyam & Morrow 2003). For those who are Thai government and state enterprises employees, they are entitled to 90 days maternity leave with full pay.

However, women may request a further 180 days unpaid personal leave for childrearing. For those in the private sector, if they are permanent employees, they will be given 90 days maternity leave with pay. According to the Labour Protection Law, employers are to be paid up to 45 days from their own funds and the other 45 days can be claimed from the national Social Security Fund, to which the employees have also contributed. For many women, who work as casual, part-time, and subcontract workers, or those who work on a daily basis and for small businesses, do not have access to maternity leave at all (van Esterik 1988; Richter & Yoddumnern-Attig. 1992; Yimyam 1997; Yimyam & Morrow 2003). As such, it is clear that the ability of mothers to breastfeed their babies is dependent upon 'regulations on maternity leave time'. Boonwanich (1993) examined the impact of the duration of postnatal leave and other factors on the pattern of breastfeeding amongst 790 public employees in Bangkok and found that about fifty percent of the babies were weaned by the completion of maternity leave of the mothers. Those who took leave of less than 90 days weaned their babies at the period between 1 and 2 months. These mothers, as Boonwanich suggested, initiated early weaning as a way to prepare their babies to take infant formula from a child care provider. In Yimyam et al.'s work (1999), they discovered that most women in their study clearly wanted to combine work and breastfeeding. However, many found the demands of these simultaneous roles problematic. Because of the need to combine work and breastfeeding, many mothers weaned their children prematurely. See also Chapters 7 and 8 in this volume.

Returning to work, Yimyam (1997, p. 50) contends, is given by many women as their reason for weaning, including Northern Thai mothers (see also Jackson et al. 1992; Richter & Yoddumnern-Attig 1992; Yimyam & Morrow 2003; Dykes 2005). In our study, women who returned to work early could not continue their breastfeeding. This was problematic for some poor women who needed to return to work soon after their maternity leave entitlement ceased. Naree, an urban poor woman, had to leave her youngest infant with her oldest daughter who was to feed the baby with infant formula. The baby refused the bottle and did not thrive. Naree remarked:

> I had to go to work but the baby would refuse the bottle. I tried infant formula but he would not take it. We had to leave him to cry and he cried until he eventually had to start taking the bottle. So, he was so thin, even now he is still thin. This is the problem for me with feeding because I had to return to work.

But, this was also problematic for some urban women. Manee breastfed her first child for only 1 month, but could do so for 3 months with her second child. Both short periods of breastfeeding were results of her limited maternity leave. She remarked:

> My first baby was breastfed for only one month, as that was all the leave I could get. My second baby was able to take breast milk for three months as I was able to take three months leave. After that they both had to take the bottle.

Due to financial needs, women returned to work, and hence these women made their decisions to bottle-feed. Women's decisions to bottle-feed, Murphy (1999, p. 194) suggests, is a clear indication of their justification that they are indeed good mothers, mothers who would do anything to ensure 'a reliable supply of food' for their infants. This is further evidenced by the way the women managed their two roles. They attempted to do the best for their infants, as Manee told us:

> But, I tried to breastfeed them at night, so that I could continue breastfeeding until they were six or seven months old.

But, for some mothers, returning to work might not extensively interfere with their breastfeeding. It seems, as Yimyam (1997) points out, the type and location of work and the opportunity for mothers to make contact with infants during working hours determined infant feeding behaviour amongst mothers in my study. Clearly, mothers' access to their infants during working hours assisted them to continue breastfeeding (WHO 1993; Yimyam & Morrow 2003). Wilai, an urban educated woman, was able to continue breastfeeding for 6 months. The baby was placed in a child care centre belonged to her work place. She would go to feed the baby three times a day during her working hours. Wilai was fortunate in the sense that she was working at a place where child care was provided for staff and it was in a close proximity. But, even in Wilai's case, she had to gradually introduce the bottle to her child and by 6 months the child was ready to abandon breast milk. Wilai remarked:

> With my second baby, I continued to breastfeed her until 6 months. Even when she attended a child care, I continued to feed her. But, after three months of doing this, I started to give her infant formula. By 6 months, she did not want my breasts anymore; may be the milk did not flow as well as the bottle milk. So, she refused to take my breasts and that was the end of my breastfeeding career.

Warunee and Patanee, who both are urban educated women, continued to breastfeed their babies long after they returned to work. Similar to Wilai, they were able to access the child care organised within their work places and this enabled them to breastfeed their babies during working hours.

Others would find their own practical solutions to enable them to combine breastfeeding and work. Most often, women use a mixed method of feeding; they would breastfeed their infants at night while during the day the infant was given a bottle at a child care centre, or if at home, by family members like a grandmother. Siriporn, an urban educated woman, returned to her work when both of her babies were 3 months old. In the first 3 months, she adopted an exclusive breastfeeding regime. She continued to breastfeed them at night for 9 months with the first child and more than 10 months for the second. At the time of our interview, she was still breastfeeding her second baby. It seems that some women would continue to do what they could despite the need to resume work.

9.7 Not Breastfeeding? Justification of Maternal Morality

As Murphy (2000, p. 309) contends, bottle-feeing is 'presented as compatible with the morality of motherhood', women who intended to bottle-feed their babies in our study knew very well that their intention would be likely to be seen as being 'bad mothers'. Their narratives, however, indicated the trend to defend themselves that bottle-feeding is 'wrong, bad, or irresponsible'. As such, by implication, they are not 'bad mothers' (Murphy 1999, p. 193). Bottle-feeding was used as an 'accountable decision' (Scott & Lyman, 1963) by the women in our study.

Murphy (1999, p. 194), in her study, found that women who decided to bottle-feed attempted to show that 'they cared too much to expose their babies to any risk that food would not be available when required'. These women claimed that mothers who formula feed their babies should be seen as 'good mothers'. By contrast, those who breastfeed 'risk a culpable maternal behaviour', as they made their babies go hungry while they could prevent this by giving them formula substance. Good mothers, according to the women in Murphy's study, should 'ensure that their babies had a dependable, scientifically formulated source of food'. To these women, a good mother can achieve in a different way (Murphy 1999, p. 197).

Likewise, the women in our study who bottle-fed or adopted a mixed method of feeding would defend themselves that they did so because of their love and concern about the health and well-being of their babies. If they were unable to produce enough breast milk, and if they did not initiate bottle-feeding, the infant might not survive or thrive well. With the formula, many women perceived that it contained similar good nutrients to breast milk. It was better to have milk to feed their babies, whatever the milk might be. These women would see that their intention to bottle feed was beneficial to their infants and this was the reflection of maternal love. Hence, they would still be seen as being good mothers despite bottle-feeding their infants. Prapaporn, an urban educated woman, asserted that:

> I used a mixed feeding pattern. I fed the baby with infant formula after breast milk because I did not have enough milk. The baby was frustrated and cried so I had to use the bottle to supplement breastfeeding. My nipples were small and this made it difficult for my baby to suck and I think this is why my milk did not really flow well. I could not leave the baby cry with hunger and hence I used both milks. It is better this way if we can't produce enough milk for the baby... If I had enough breast milk I would not give her the bottle.

As suggested above, many women in our study perceived that infant formula contained similar good nutrients to breast milk. This is the way women justified their intentions and practices. As Murphy (1999, p. 196) points out in her study too that the women used this justification to challenge the fundamental belief that 'breast is best'. These women argued that 'formula feeding was not harmful'. This is what Sykes and Matza (1957) and Scott and Lyman (1963) define as 'denials of injury'. As one woman in Murphy's study (cited in Murphy, 1999, p. 196) remarked, 'there's the same nutrients in both...they say breast milk is better because it's your's and its' nature...there's definitely the same nutrients in both'. To this mother, 'the nutrient values of breast and formula milk are identical and equally suitable for the baby', and this was in contradiction to the option of health professionals.

Women who adopted a mixed method would justify their practices and defend their good mother identity by insisting on giving breast milk to their infant prior to the bottle. This was the way to ensure that their infants would receive good food as much as possible. Darunee, an urban educated woman, contended that:

> I would make sure that the baby took breast milk before the bottle. I would breastfeed until I felt that I would not have milk in my breasts then I would give the baby infant formula. The baby became used to bottle milk and would not want to take my breast, but I would insist on this. He did not like it but I would persevere with it.

Pimpilai, an urban educated woman, justified her mixed method by saying that:

> I believe that mother's milk is best, but if we can't produce enough milk for our babies, we then need to also give infant formula too. The baby should receive a well-balanced of quantity of milk. My milk was little; the baby only sucked a few times I would not have any more milk to feed him. No matter how hard I tried to produce a lot of milk, I did not succeed. So, I felt sorry for my baby as I could see that he was hungry.

9.8 Conclusion

Breastfeeding has become an international agenda. Dykes (2005, p. 2283) contends that the pressure on women to breastfeed has become increasingly pervasive. Internationally prescribed guidelines on breastfeeding proliferate. The World Health Organization (2002) now sets out its recommendation that women should exclusively breastfeed their newborn infants for a minimum of 6 months. This recommendation has gained credence and health professionals in particular insist on this on new mothers.

Infant feeding practices, however, continue to relate to the local moral world. In modernising societies, as Barlow (1985, p. 137) contends, infant feeding practices 'do not exist in isolation from the cultural and socio-economic environments in which they occur. They result from beliefs and values which operate within particular ecological environments and socio-economic situations'. Breastfeeding in any society, as such, is not problem-free either. Each society perceives and deals with problems in culturally specific ways (Millard 1990). The mothers' choice to breastfeed or not, as Nadesan and Sotirin (1998) content, 'encompasses subtle, but compelling conflicting demands, reflecting some of the tensions and contradictions women face in contemporary society'.

Infant feeding practices are indeed contentious issues. As Murphy (1999, p. 205) writes, mothers' decision to feed their babies 'carries considerable moral baggage'. Indeed, the findings of our study suggest that 'infant feeding is a moral minefield'. The ways that women can be judged or judge themselves is clearly articulated in this study. This is an indication that, as Murphy (1999, p. 206) contends, 'mothers are all caught in the cross-currents of complex and sometimes contradictory obligations'. Clearly then, infant feeding decisions are not only about nutrition, but more importantly are about morality.

Whether the women intend to breast or formula feed, they attempt to construct 'an image of themselves as moral members of society' (Murphy 1999, p. 191). Mothers' intention to breastfeed is culturally constructed as an act of a good mother. These women follow the rules knowingly and hence were not questioned about their maternal morality or felt the need to justify their intentions. Breastfeeding, Murphy

(1999, p. 204) contends, could be perceived as 'evidence of being a good mother who is not only knowledgeable but who is also prepared to act on that knowledge'. But, this also holds true for mothers who intend to bottle-feed despite some societal ambivalence about their infant feeding intentions. When a feeding decision is made, a mother knows very well that 'her decision is vulnerable to the charge of sanctionable deviance'. Hence, she must construct an invention in order to defeat such a charge. As such, women must rely on providing a range of justification for their intentions (Murphy 1999, p. 200), as the attempts employed by the women in this study.

It seems clear that the discourse on breastfeeding amongst the Thai women in this study relates to ideals of motherhood. Most often, women refer breast milk to 'mother's milk' (*nom mae*). This emphasises the mother and child relationship ideal. The belief that it is a mothers' blood that creates her breast milk and the characteristics of a mother is transferred to her child through breast milk reinforces the interconnection between a mother and her child.

It is clear in this study that both breast and bottle-feeding mothers see themselves as 'knowledgeable rather than ignorant'. As Earle's study (2000, p. 327) indicates, both breast and bottle-feeding mothers definitely know that breastfeeding is best for their infants. Guttman and Zimmerman (2000, p. 1468) too suggest in their findings that regardless of the infant feeding method they adopted, the women rated highly the health benefits of breastfeeding. Most also believed that breastfeeding is something a 'good mother' should do. However, the actual practice of breastfeeding amongst these women was socially constrained, regardless of their feeding choices. Mothers who bottle-feed attempt to show that their decisions to bottle-feed, which 'superficially, seems irreconcilable with responsible motherhood, is perfectly justified' (Murphy 1999, p. 205). Clearly, as Guttman and Zimmerman (2000, p. 1468) contend, this does not mean that mothers who bottle-feed do not care about the health of their baby. Rather, 'formula may simply be accepted as a "good enough" substitute'.

The campaign 'Breast is best', Nadesan and Sotirin (1998, p. 230) suggest, 'casts the decision to breast-feed as a dualistic choice between "good" and "bad" bodies, images, performances, and policies'. 'Breast is best' is not only a choice over whether women should breastfeed or not, but also 'an injunction to perform culturally authorized gender identities'. In the case of this study, it is the gender identity of women as mothers. In addition, we must be mindful that, as Earle (2000, p. 328) suggests, women do not necessarily lack knowledge to make decisions about infant feeding, but that 'there are other significant factors at play'. And in this chapter, we have shown that there are other significant factors including work and insufficient milk dictate whether women choose to breast or bottle-feed their infants.

Acknowledgements We wish to thank all the Thai women who provided valuable insights for us to construct this chapter and the Faculty of Health Sciences, La Trobe University who provided research grant which made this research possible. We also thank Rosemary Oakes for her valuable comments in the preparation of this chapter. The chapter is an abridged version of a chapter in the first author's book *'The Journey of Becoming a Mother among Northern Thai Women'*, published by Lexington Books, 2007

References

Abel, S., Julie, P., Tippene-Leach, D., Finau, D., & Lennan, M. (2001). Infant care practices in New Zealand: A cross-cultural qualitative study. *Social Science and Medicine, 53*, 1135–1148.

Bailey, C., & Pain, R. (2001). Geographies of feeding and access to primary health care. *Health and Social Care in the Community, 9*(5), 309–317.

Barlow, K. (1985). The social context of infant feeding in the Murik Lakes of Papus New Guinea. In L. B. Marshall (Ed.), *Infant care and feeding in the South Pacific* (pp. 137–154). New York: Gordon and Breach Science.

Barona-Vilar, C., Escribá-Agüira, V., & Ferrero-Gandıa, R. (2009). A qualitative approach to social support and breast-feeding decisions. *Midwifery, 25*, 187–194.

Beasley, A., Chick, N., Pybus, M., Weber, J., MacKenzie, D., & Dignam, D. (1998). 'I was scared I had run out of milk!': Breastfeeding and perceptions of insufficient milk among Manawatu mothers. In A. Beasley, & A. Trlin (Eds.), *Breastfeeding in New Zealand: Practice, problems and policy* (pp. 57–74). Palmerston North: Dunmore.

Berger, L. M., Hill, J., & Waldfogel, J. (2005). Maternity leave, early maternal employment and child health and development in the US. *The Economic Journal, 115*, F29–F47.

Blum, L. M. (1993), Mothers, babies and breastfeeding in late capitalist America: The shifting contexts of feminist theory. *Feminist Studies, 19*, 291–311.

Boonwanich, P. (1993). The study of the effect of the duration of the postnatal maternal leave and other factors to the pattern of breast feeding among the civil servants. *Journal of Provincial Hospital, 12*(5), 9–17 (in Thai).

Calnen, G. (2007). Paid maternity leave and its impact of breastfeeding in the United States: Historic, economic, political and social perspectives. *Breastfeeding Medicine, 1*(2), 34–44.

Coutsoudis, A. (2005). Breastfeeding and the HIV positive mothers: The debate continues. *Early Human Development, 81*, 87–93.

Craig, G. M., & Scambler, G. (2006). Negotiating mothering against the odds: Gastrostomy tube feeding, stigma, governmentality and disabled children. *Social Science and Medicine, 62*, 1115–1125.

Cricco-Lizza, R. (2005). The milk of human kindness: Environmental and human interactions in a WIC clinic that influence infant-feeding decisions of black women. *Qualitative Health Research, 15*(4), 525–538.

Davis-Floyd, R. E. (1992). *Birth as an American rite of passage*. Berkeley: University of California Press.

Dettwyler, K. A. (1995). A time to wean: The hominid blueprint for the natural age of weaning in modern human population. In P. Stuart-Macadam, & K. A. Dettwyler (Eds.), *Breastfeeding: Biocultural perspectives* (pp. 39–72). New York: Aldine De Gruyter.

Dingwall, R. (1976). *Aspects of illness*. London: Martin Robertson.

Duden, B. (1993). *Disembodying women: Perspectives on pregnancy and the unborn*. London: Harvard University Press.

Duncan, S., Edwards, R., & Reynolds, T. (2003). Motherhood, paid work and partnering: Values and theories. *Work, Employment & Society, 17*(2), 309–330.

Duong, D., Lee, A., & Binns, C. (2005). Determinants of breastfeeding within the first 6 months post-partum in rural Vietnam. *Journal of Paediatrics & Child Health, 41*, 338–343.

Dykes, F. (2002). Western marketing and medicine-construction of an insufficient milk syndrome. *Health Care for Women International, 23*(5), 492–502.

Dykes, F. (2005). 'Supply' and 'demand': Breastfeeding as labour. *Social Science & Medicine, 60*, 2283–2293.

Dykes, F., & Williams, C. (1999). "Falling by the wayside": A phenomological exploration of perceived breast milk inadequacy in lactating women. *Midwifery, 15*(4), 232–246.

Earle, S. (2000). Why some women do not breast feed: Bottle feeding and father's role. *Midwifery, 16*, 323–330.

Ehrenreich, B., & Hochschild, A. R. (2003). *Global women*. London: Granta.
Gartner, L., Morton, J., & Lawrence, R. A. (2005). Breastfeeding and the use of human milk. *Pediatrics, 115*(20), 496–506.
Gatrell, C. (2007). Secrets and lies: Breastfeeding and professional paid work. *Social Science and Medicine, 65*, 393–404.
Goffman, E. (1963). *Stigma: Notes on the management of spoiled identity*. Englewood Cliffs: Prentice Hall.
Gonzalez, R. (1990). A large scale rooming-in program in a developing country. Proceeding of the Interagency Workshop on Health Care Practices Related to Breast-feeding. *International Journal of Gynaecology and Obstetrics, 31*, 1–5.
Gray, R., Campbell, O. M., Apelo, R., Eslami, S. S., Ramos, R. M., Gehert, J. C., et al. (1990). The risk of ovulation during lactation. *Lancet, 335*, 25–27.
Guttman, N., & Zimmerman, D. R. (2000). Low-income mothers' views on breastfeeding. *Social Science & Medicine, 50*, 1457–1473.
Hamlyn, B., Brooker, S., Oleinikova, K., & Wands, S. (2002). *Infant feeding 2000*. London: The Stationary Office (TSO).
Hill, P. D. (1991). The enigma of insufficient milk supply. *American Journal of Maternal and Child Nursing, 16*(6), 312–316.
Hillervik-Lindquist, C. (1991). Studies on perceived milk insufficiency. A prospective study in a group of Swedish women. *Acta Pediatrica Scandinavica, 376*, 6–25.
Jackson, D. A., Imong, S. M., Wongsawasdi, L., Silprasert, A., Preunglampoo, S., Leelapat, P., et al. (1992). Weaning practices and breast-feeding duration in Northern Thailand. *British Journal of Nutrition, 67*(2), 149–164.
Jackson, W. (2004) Breastfeeding and type 1 diabetes mellitus. *British Journal of Midwifery, 12*(3), 158–165
Jelliffe, D. B., & Jelliffe, E. E. P. (1978). *Human milk in the modern world*. Oxford: Oxford University Press.
Knodel, J., Chayovan, N., & Wongboonsin, K. (1990). Breast-feeding trends, patterns and policies in Thailand. *Asia-Pacific Population Journal, 5*(1), 135–150.
Liamputtong, P. (2006). Motherhood and "moral career": Discourses of good motherhood among Southeast Asian immigrant women in Australia. *Qualitative Sociology, 29*(1), 25–53.
Liamputtong, P. (2007). *The journey of becoming a mother amongst women in northern Thailand*. Lanham: Lexington Books.
Liamputtong, P. (2009). *Qualitative research methods* (3rd edn). Melbourne: Oxford University Press.
Liamputtong, P. (2010). *Performing qualitative cross-cultural research*. Cambridge: Cambridge University Press.
Liamputtong Rice, P. (2000). *Hmong woman and reproduction*. Westport: Bergin & Garvey.
Liamputtong Rice, P., & Naksook, C. (2001). Breastfeeding practices among Thai mothers in Melbourne. *Midwifery, 17*(1), 11–23.
Lim, L. L. (1993) 'The feminization of labour in the Asia-Pacific rim countries: From contributing to economic dynamism to bearing the brunt of structural adjustment'. In N. Ogawa, & G. Jones (Eds.), *Human resource in development along the Asia-Pacific rim* (pp. 176–209). Singapore: Oxford University Press.
Liubai, L., Doan Thi Phuong, L., Nguyen-Thi, H., & Hiroshi, U. (2002). Prevalence of breast-feeding and its correlates in Ho Chi Minh City, Vietnam. *Pediatrics International, 44*(1), 47–54.
Marchand, L., & Morrow, M. H. (1994). Infant feeding practices: Understanding the decision-making process. *Family Medicine, 26*(5), 319–324.
Marild, S., Hansson, S., & Jodal, U. (2004). Protective effect of breastfeeding against urinary tract infection. *Acta Paediatrica, 93*(2), 164–168.
Martin, E. (1992). *The woman in the body: A cultural analysis of reproduction*. Boston: Beacon.

McHugh, P. (1970). A commonsense conception of deviance. In J. D. Douglas (Ed.), *Deviance and responsibility: The social construction of moral meanings* (pp. 61–88). New York: Basic Books.

Millard, A. V. (1990). The place of the clock in pediatric advice: Rationales, cultural themes, and impediments to breastfeeding. *Social Science and Medicine, 31*, 211–221.

Miller, T. (2005) *Making sense of motherhood: A narrative approach*. Cambridge: Cambridge University Press.

Mistry, Y., Freedman, M., Sweeney, K., & Hollenbeck, C. (2008). Infant-feeding practices of low-income Vietnamese American women. *Journal of Human Lactation, 24*(4), 406–414.

Moffat, T. (2002). Breastfeeding, wage labour, and insufficient milk in peri-urban Kathmandu, Nepal. *Medical Anthropology, 21*(2), 207–230.

Murphy, E. (1999). 'Breast is best': Infant feeding decisions and maternal deviance. *Sociology of Health & Illness, 21*, 187–208.

Murphy, E. (2000). Risk, responsibility, and rhetoric in infant feeding. *Journal of Contemporary Ethnography, 29*(3), 291–325.

Nadesan, M. H., & Sotirin, P. (1998). The romance and science of 'breast is best': Discursive contradictions and contexts of breast-feeding choices. *Text and Performance Quarterly, 18*, 217–232.

Oddy, W. H. (2001). Breastfeeding protects against illness and infection in infants and children: A review of literature. *Breastfeeding Review, 9*(2), 11–18.

Oritz, J., McGilligan, K., & Kelly, P. (2004) Duration of breast milk: Expression among working mothers enrolled in an employer-sponsored lactation program. *Pediatric Nursing, 3*(2), 111–119.

Quigley, M., Kelly, Y., & Sacker, A. (2007). Breastfeeding and hospitalization for diarrheal and respiratory infection in the United Kingdom Millennium Cohort Study. *Pediatrics, 110*(4), e837–e842.

Raymond, J, (2005) Another reason for you to breastfeed. *Working Mother, 28*(4), 70–74.

Richter, K., & Yoddumnern-Attig, B. (1992). Framing a study of Thai women's changing roles and statuses. In B. Yoddumnern-Attig, K. Richter, A. Soonthorndhada, C. Sethaput, & A. Pramualratana (Eds.), *Changing roles and statuses of women in Thailand: A documentary assessment* (pp. 1–7). Salaya: The Institute for Population and Social Research, Mahidol University.

Riordan, J. (2005). *Breastfeeding and human lactation* (3rd edn). Sudbury: Jones and Bartlett.

Riordan, J., & Gill-Hopple, K. (2001). Breastfeeding care in multicultural populations. *JOGN Nursing, 30*, 216–223.

Rodriguez-Garcia, R., & Frazier, L. (1995). Cultural paradoxes relating to sexuality and breastfeeding. *Journal of Human Lactation, 11*, 111–115.

Rossiter, J. C. (1992). Attitudes of Vietnamese women to baby feeding practices before and after immigration to Sydney. *Midwifery, 8*, 103–112.

Rossiter, J. C. (1999). Maternal-infant health beliefs and infant feeding practices: The perception and experience of immigrant Vietnamese women. In P. Liamputtog Rice (Ed.), *Asian mothers, western birth* (pp. 161–174). Melbourne: Ausmed.

Sacco, L. M., Caulfield, L. E., Gittelsohn, J., & Martínez, H. (2006). The conceptualization of perceived insufficient milk among Mexican mothers. *Journal of Human Lactation, 22*(3), 277–286.

Scavenius, M., van Hulsel, L., Meijer, J., Wendte, H., & Gurgel, R. (2007). In practice, the theory is different: A processual analysis of breastfeeding in northeast Brazil. *Social Science and Medicine, 64*, 676–688.

Schmidt, J. (2008). Gendering in infant discourses: The good mother and the absent father. *New Zealand Sociology, 23*(2), 61–74.

Schmied, V., & Lupton, D. (2001). Blurring the boundaries: Breastfeeding and maternal subjectivity. *Sociology of Health & Illness, 23*(2), 234–250.

Scott, M. B., & Lyman, S. M. (1963). Accounts. *American Sociological Review, 33*, 46–62.

Shildrick, M. (1997). *Leaky bodies and boundaries, feminism, postmodernism and (bio) ethics*. London: Routledge.

Stanway, P., & Stanway, A. (1978). *Breast is best: A commonsense approach to breast feeding*. London: Pan Books.

Sykes, D. M., & Matza, D. (1957). Techniques of neutralization: A theory of delinquency. *American Sociological Review, 22*(6), 664–670.

Tantiwiramanond, D., & Pandey, S. R. (1991). *By women, for women: A study of women's organizations in Thailand*. Pasir Panjang Singapore: Institute of Southeast Asian Studies.

Tsianakas, V., & Liamputtong, P. (2007). Infant feeding practices and Afghan immigrant women in Australia. In P. Liamputtong (Ed.), *Childrearing and infant care issues: A cross-cultural perspective* (pp. 249–273). New York: Nova Science.

Tully, J., & Dewey, K. G. (1985). Private fears, global loss: A cross-cultural study of the insufficient syndrome. *Medical Anthropology, 9*, 225–243.

Van Esterik, P. (1988). The cultural context of infant feeding. In B. Winikoff, M. A. Castle, & V. H. Laukaran (Eds.), *Feeding infants in four societies: Causes and consequences of mothers' choices* (pp. 187–202). New York: Greenwood.

Van Esterik, P. (1989) *Beyond the breast-bottle controversy*. New Jersey: Rutger University Press.

Vincent, C., Ball, S. J., & Pietikainen, S. (2004). Metropolitan mothers: Mothers, mothering and paid work. *Women's Studies International Forum, 27*, 571–587.

Vong-Ek, P. (1993). How popular beliefs influence breastfeeding practices in Northeast and Central Thailand. *Journal of Primary Health Care and Development, 6*: 61–76.

Witters-Green, R. (2003). Increasing breastfeeding rates in working mothers. *Families, Systems and Health, 21*, 415–434.

Wolf, J. (2006). What feminists can do for breastfeeding and what breastfeeding can do for feminists. *Signs: Journal of Women in Culture and Society, 31*, 397–424.

World Health Organization. (1993). *Breastfeeding: The technical basis and recommendations for action*. Geneva: World Health Organization.

World Health Organization. (1996). *Not enough milk*. Geneva: Division of Diarrhoeal and Acute Respiratory Disease Control, World Health Organization.

World Health Organization (2002). *Infant and young child nutrition. Global strategy on infant and young child feeding. Fifty-fifth World Health Assembly*. Geneva: World Health Organization.

World Health Organization (2007). *Evidence on the long-term effects of breastfeeding: Systematic reviews and meta-analysis*. Geneva: World Health Organization.

Wright, A. L., Clark, C., & Bauer, M. (1993). Maternal employment and infant feeding practices among the Navajo. *Medical Anthropology Quarterly, 7*, 260–280.

Yimyam, S. (1997). *Breastfeeding experiences among employed Thai women in Chiang Mai*. Unpublished doctoral thesis, Key Centre for Women's Health in Society, The University of Melbourne, Melbourne.

Yimyam, S., & Morrow, M. (2003). Maternal labor, breast-feeding, and infant health. In Heymann, J. (Ed.), *Global inequalities at work: Work's impact on the health of individuals, families, and societies* (pp. 105–135). New York: Oxford University Press.

Yimyam, S., Morrow, M., & Srisuphan, W. (1999). Role conflict and rapid socio-economic change: Breastfeeding among employed women in Thailand. *Social Science and Medicine, 49*, 957–965.

Zeitlyn, S., & Rowshan, R. (1997). Privileged knowledge and mother's "perceptions": The case of breast-feeding and insufficient milk in Bangladesh. *Medical Anthropology Quarterly, 11*(1), 56–68.

Part III
Infant Feeding Practices and HIV/AIDS

Chapter 10
Breastfeeding in Sub-Saharan Africa: Still the Best Despite the Risk of HIV

Lucy Thairu

Contents

10.1 Introduction

Breast milk has long been recognised as the optimal source of nutrition for young infants, preventing unnecessary child deaths. For example, a study conducted in 1912 in the United States (Davis 1912) suggested that infant mortality was highest in bottle-fed infants who were under 3 months of age, and that, compared to breastfed infants, mortality could be up to six times more in bottle-fed infants. By the early 1970s, factors such as urbanisation, participation in paid employment and aggressive marketing by infant formula companies were shown to impact the initiation and duration of breastfeeding in the developing world (Brown 1973). The potential dangers of bottle-feeding for infant health and survival were highlighted, most notably the lack of hygiene in preparing artificial feeds and 'stretching' infant formula to make it last longer when resources were scarce (Brown 1973). Recognising the importance of breastfeeding, policies such as the 1981 International Code of Marketing of Breast-milk Substitutes (World Health Organization 1981)

L. Thairu (✉)
Division of Infectious Diseases, Stanford University School of Medicine, Stanford, CA, USA
e-mail: thairu@stanford.edu

P. Liamputtong (ed.), *Infant Feeding Practices*, DOI 10.1007/978-1-4419-6873-9_10,
© Springer Science+Business Media, LLC 2011

were enacted to ensure the 'provision of safe and adequate nutrition for infants, by the protection and promotion of breast-feeding, and by ensuring the proper use of breast-milk substitutes, when these are necessary, on the basis of adequate information and through appropriate marketing and distribution'. The code was important in that it provided guidelines for the advertisement or promotion of breast milk substitutes, bottles and teats to the general public and forbade the promotion of these products through the health care system.

Up until the early 1980s, most publications on breastfeeding were descriptive. Studies such as those conducted by Lönnerdal, Forsum, Gebre-Medin, and Hambraeus (1976) investigated breast milk composition and contrasted the quality of breast milk from malnourished women in Africa to their better nourished counterparts in Europe, allaying fears that the quality and quantity of breast milk would be influenced by the mother's nutritional status. Some opinion editorials, such as a letter in the Lancet (1978) stimulated lively discussions (Baumslag 1978; Jelliffe & Jelliffe 1978) on the benefits of breastfeeding versus bottle-feeding and on the role of industry in providing artificial infant foods. There were increasing calls to regulate the infant formula industry to avoid marketing breast milk substitutes, particularly in health care settings.

10.2 Breastfeeding and HIV/AIDS in the 1980s

The United States Centers for Disease Control (CDC) used the term AIDS (Acquired Immune Deficiency Syndrome) in the early 1980s to describe a new disease that primarily affected young gay men (Centers for Disease Control 1982). The finding that AIDS could be transmitted from the mother to the child was surprising as AIDS had been considered a gay man's disease. It was not until the mid 1980s that it was confirmed that HIV, a retrovirus, could be transmitted through blood products or body fluids, including breast milk. By 1986, Luc Montagnier and Robert Gallo were credited with the discovery of the Human Immuno Deficiency Virus (HIV), proving it was the causative agent for AIDS.

In the United States, the CDC recommended that HIV-positive mothers should not breastfeed (Baumslag 1987) as did the Department of Health and Social Security (DHSS) in the United Kingdom (The Lancet 1988). There were controversial proposals to issue DHSS recommendations in the developing world (Munyakho 1988). However, formulating policy in the developing world posed a difficult dilemma. On one hand, breastfed infants risked illness and death if they acquired HIV. On the other hand, where access to clean water and hygienic conditions were problematic, the risk of illness and death when infants were not breastfed could outweigh the potential benefit of preventing HIV transmission (Logan, Newell, Ades, & Peckham 1988; see also Chapter 11 in this volume). There were, however, no studies providing hard data on the difference in morbidity and mortality for breastfed versus non-breastfed infants of HIV-infected mothers (Tedder 1988).

By the late 1980s, the World Health Organization (WHO) proposed the use of heat-treated donated breast milk, or the use of wetnurses where mothers chose not to breastfeed due to HIV infection (Global Program on AIDS 1992). Given the rising number of HIV-infected infants, who were estimated to constitute a quarter of the 2 million suspected cases of infection (World Health Organization 1992), fears about the risk of mother-to-child transmission of HIV (MTCT) through breast milk may have led to calls for HIV-positive women to abort their unborn infant, or to abstain from breastfeeding once the infant was born (The Times 1988). In countries such as Australia, pregnant women were now routinely offered HIV counselling and testing (Southward 1989). When a study conducted in eight centres in Europe (European Collaborative Study 1988), estimated that up to one quarter of infants of HIV-positive mothers acquired the virus, the controversial calls for HIV-positive women to abort and/or to abstain from breastfeeding intensified. The infant food company Nestle added to these controversies when a representative presumably claimed that 50 percent of African women were HIV-infected, and that they risked infecting their infants through breastfeeding (Erlichman 1989). This, coupled with continued aggressive marketing of infant formula in the developing world, contributed to the revival of the 1989 Nestle boycott (Erlichman 1989).

Despite the risk of breastfeeding HIV transmission, child survival advocates emphasised that, in resource-poor settings, breastfeeding was still preferable to infant formula, even when the mother was HIV infected (Bailey 1991). To avoid the growing calls for the promotion of infant formula in the developing world, the WHO and UNICEF issued a joint statement on 'protecting, promoting and supporting breastfeeding: the special role of maternity services' in 1989. The 'ten steps to successful breastfeeding', destined for facilities providing maternal and newborn health care services, were outlined in the joint statement (UNICEF 1989). These ten steps are described in the box 10.1 below.

Box 10.1 The ten steps to successful breastfeeding

(1) Have a written breastfeeding policy that is routinely communicated to all health care staff;
(2) Train all health care staff in skills necessary to implement this policy;
(3) Inform all pregnant women about the benefits and management of breastfeeding;
(4) Help mothers initiate breastfeeding within half an hour of birth;
(5) Show mothers how to breastfeed, and how to maintain lactation even if they should be separated from their infants;
(6) Give newborn infants no food or drink other than breast milk, unless medically indicated;
(7) Practise rooming-in – that is, allow mothers and infants to remain together – 24 hours a day;
(8) Encourage breastfeeding on demand;
(9) Give no artificial teats or pacifiers to breastfeeding infants;
(10) Foster the establishment of breastfeeding support groups and refer mothers to them on discharge from the hospital or clinic.

10.3 Breastfeeding and HIV/AIDS in the 1990s

The early 1990s was marked by additional policies enacted by UNICEF and the WHO. The first policy, enacted in 1990 was the Innocenti Declaration on the Protection, Promotion, and Support of Breast-feeding (UNICEF 1990). Prior to this declaration, breastfeeding policy had focused on 'any breastfeeding'. However, based on the results of several clinical trials, the Innocenti Declaration emphasised the importance of exclusive breastfeeding from 0 to 6 months, followed by complementary feeding well into the infant's second year. The second policy was the Baby Friendly Hospital Initiative (BFHI) of 1991–2 (UNICEF 1991). Through this initiative, health care facilities could become accredited as 'Baby Friendly' if they did not accept breast milk substitutes, feeding bottles or teats from commercial companies, whether free or at a subsidised price, and if they implemented the 'ten steps to successful breastfeeding'.

Despite these policy initiatives, throughout the 1990s, the scientific information regarding HIV and breastfeeding was increasingly uncertain and complex. According to the WHO, by 1996 there was a dearth of information regarding the timing of HIV transmission during the breastfeeding period, the exact risk of HIV infection that could be attributed to breastfeeding, risk factors for MTCT through breastfeeding, and the potential interventions that could be used to reduce the risk of MTCT (World Health Organization 1996). Given the difficulty of enacting blanket recommendations, the WHO proposed the provision of individualised information to HIV-positive mothers, which was based on a Human Rights approach. The WHO developed a statement outlining women's right to information and their rights to make informed decisions about the best way of feeding their infant, regardless of their HIV status (World Health Organization 1996). According to the statement: 'Counselling for women who are aware of their HIV status should include the best available information [...]. However, it is mothers who are in the best position to decide whether to breast-feed' (World Health Organization 1996, p. 291). Implicit in these recommendations was that HIV-infected mothers were expected to assume increasing responsibility for making their own infant feeding decisions in comparison to HIV-negative mothers for whom the decision to breastfeed was supported by international and national recommendations as well as long-standing cultural practices.

In the 1996 statement, the WHO emphasised the importance of empowering mothers to make informed decisions: 'It is therefore important that women be empowered to make fully informed decisions about infant feeding, and that they be suitably supported in carrying them out' (p. 291). In the statement, the WHO described the support as 'efforts to promote a hygienic environment, essentially clean water and sanitation, that will minimise health risks when a breast-milk substitute is used' (p. 291). By the end of the 1990s, it was clear that factors other than the presence of clean water and sanitation played an important role in empowering women to make informed infant feeding decisions. These included poorly organised health services, women's unwillingness to learn about their HIV status, health care providers' lack of knowledge about HIV and infant feeding and women's lack of authority in making decisions in environments which were often paternalistic.

10.4 Breastfeeding and HIV/AIDS in the New Millennium

While the 1980s and the 1990s were marked by a number of controversies as discussed previously, these were resolved by the early 2000s as the results of several clinical trials became available. Social and cultural studies on the topic also shed light on women's beliefs and practices. Together, these studies provided guidance for selecting the optimal mode of infant feeding for HIV-positive mothers in resource-poor settings. The epidemiological studies answered questions such as the risk of HIV infection when infants are breastfed (attributable risk), risk factors for MTCT through breastfeeding, the importance of the pattern of breastfeeding, the timing of HIV transmission during the breastfeeding period, which could be used to determine the optimal weaning period, and potential interventions that could be used to reduce the risk of MTCT. In contrast, the social and cultural studies shed light on issues such as the acceptability of various infant feeding options and mothers' infant feeding decision-making.

10.4.1 Breastfeeding Versus Replacement Feeding

The mechanisms through which HIV is transmitted through breast milk are not well understood (Kourtis, Butera, Ibegbu, Beled, & Duerr 2003). On one hand, some immune factors may protect infants who are exposed to breast milk from HIV infection. On the other hand, the infant is exposed to virus for as long as he breastfeeds and is, therefore, at risk of acquiring HIV.

In 2000, the results of a landmark study in a low-income Kenyan setting showed that 16 percent of infants become infected through breast milk HIV transmission before they are 24 months of age (Nduati et al. 2000). While there were no significant differences in infant mortality for replacement versus breastfed infants (Nduati et al. 2000), infants who were formula fed were more likely to have been hospitalised and to have suffered from sepsis (Mbori-Ngacha et al. 2001). By 2007, Becquet and colleagues (2007) had found similar results. The authors compared morbidity and mortality outcomes for infants who were breastfed and weaned at 4 months versus those who were replacement fed. Mothers of both groups of infants had received an intrapartum dose of Zidovudine. At 2 years, the rates of mortality were similar for both breastfed and replacement-fed infants. However, the rates of diarrhoea and acute respiratory infections were higher for formula-fed infants.

In 2000 and again in 2003, the WHO proposed exclusive breastfeeding, wet-nursing, the use of animal milk (such as cow and goat's milk), infant formula, heat-treating expressed breast milk and the use of banked milk as infant feeding options for HIV-positive mothers (UNICEF, UNAIDS, WHO & UNFPA 2003).

The results of a study conducted in Kenya by myself illustrate women's views about the infant feeding options recommended by the WHO (Thairu 2002). The study is described in the box 10.2 below.

Box 10.2 Study illustrating women's beliefs about various infant feeding options

About 70 women in the Kiambu district in 2000 were interviewed using a semi-structured questionnaire. The questionnaire was refined and translated in the field with the assistance of a research assistant. In the first part of the interview, women were asked to provide the following demographic information: date of birth, ethnic group, level of education, source of income, marital status, number of children and the last infant's demographic data. The next set of questions were related to the infant's dietary history (e.g., foods given to the infant and their preparation) followed by questions about breastfeeding and HIV/AIDS.

All women were presented with the following infant feeding options: cow's milk, goat's milk, infant formula, wetnursing, milk banks, heat-treating expressed breast milk, exclusive breastfeeding and breastfeeding 'as usual' (mixed feeding). For example, with regard to wetnursing, women were asked: 'let's assume your sister dies and leaves her 2 week old infant, you have a baby you are breastfeeding, would you also breastfeed your sister's infant?' Regarding heat-treating expressed breast milk, women were asked: 'if you had AIDS and your milk also had AIDS, would you express your milk and boil it to "kill" the disease?' A variety of questions were used to elicit information about exclusive breastfeeding. These included: 'if an infant is 2 weeks old, do you think he can survive on breastmilk alone-no water, no milk. . .only breastmilk?' and 'would you be willing to feed your infant in this way?' Interviews were conducted in Kikuyu (the local language) for the vast majority of respondents or in Kiswahili or English when respondents were not from the Kikuyu ethnic group. Demographic information and quantifiable responses were analysed using SPSS.

The women's mean age was 25 years, and the mean number of years of education was 12.4. 57 percent of the women were aware of the possibility of breast milk HIV transmission. Of the 25 women who were confronted for the first time with this knowledge (n=25), a minority (24 percent) chose not to breastfeed, possibly because this was new information. When women were asked what method they would select if they hypothetically tested positive for HIV/AIDS, 84 percent noted that they would select cow's milk as an infant feeding option, 50 percent selected infant formula, 57 percent would breastfeed if they were infected with HIV, 29 percent would use a wetnurse, 26 percent would consider goat's milk, 16 percent would use milk banks, and 13 percent would heat-treat expressed breast milk. Clearly, the majority of the women preferred not to breastfeed if they became infected with HIV/AIDS. However, since the study did not inquire about the women's HIV status, questions about HIV and infant feeding were hypothetical, and it was difficult to anticipate the choices women would have made if indeed they were HIV-positive.

Despite the risk of HIV transmission, various studies conducted over the past decade indicate that most HIV-positive mothers recognise the importance of breastfeeding and have difficulty changing their beliefs and practices. In the study by Nduati and colleagues (2000), even when women were provided with up-to-date information and with free or subsidised replacement foods, only 70 percent adhered to formula feeding in comparison with 96 percent in the breastfeeding arm. The results of a study conducted by myself in KwaZulu Natal, South Africa (Thairu et al. 2005), illustrate HIV-positive women's actual choices. Twenty-two HIV-positive women were interviewed. The study is described in the box 10.3 below.

Box 10.3 Infant feeding choices in a group of HIV-positive women participating in a PMTCT program in South Africa

The women were part of a larger cohort study investigating the impact of breastfeeding practices on mother-to-child transmission of HIV/AIDS. They had received counselling and information about HIV and infant feeding from nurses and counsellors in the cohort study. To be included in the qualitative study, they had to have an infant and to be HIV-positive. Interview schedules were developed and refined in the field. All interviews were conducted in Zulu, with the help of a Zulu research assistant. Interviews were tape-recorded, translated into English and transcribed. Some of the questions were open ended; key concepts were also written on index cards, and used to elicit supplementary information about HIV and breastfeeding.

All the women in the KwaZulu Natal study were of the Zulu ethnic group. They had received nevirapine as part of prophylaxis to prevent mother-to-child transmission of HIV/AIDS. However, none reported receiving anti-retroviral therapy to prevent their own disease from progressing to full-blown AIDS. Information about the women's level of education was not available. The mean age was 26. Despite the information they had received about the risk of breast milk HIV transmission, 77 percent of the women had selected breastfeeding while 23 percent had selected infant formula. Age, economic circumstances and other socio-economic variables influenced the women's infant feeding choices.

In epidemiological studies in low-income settings, there is a consistent finding that, breastfed infants of HIV-positive mothers are not significantly worse off with regard to health and survival outcomes compared to their replacement-fed peers (Nduati et al. 2000; Becquet et al. 2007). For this reason, it has been reasonable to consider alternative solutions to reduce the risk of breast milk transmission by making breastfeeding safer. The current consensus, based on a review of the available evidence, indicates that exclusive breastfeeding, coupled with antiretroviral therapy is the safest and most optimal mode of infant feeding (WHO 2006). The challenge for PMTCT programs will be to support mothers to exclusively breastfeed and to offer anti-retroviral therapy during lactation. See also Chapter 11 in this volume.

10.4.2 Pattern of Infant Feeding

By 2003, Rousseau and associates (2004) had observed changes in the quantity of virus, and provided convincing evidence that colostrum has the highest levels of virus in comparison to mature milk. The authors noted a dose-response relationship, such that the higher the viral load, the higher the infant's risk of transmission. They also noted that the rate of MTCT through breastfeeding decreased by about two times when maternal viral load decreased 10 times. Around the same time, various authors proposed immunological ways in which damage to infant mucosa may increase rates of HIV acquisition, such as increased mucosal permeability due to inflammation, thus explaining how HIV could be related to the pattern of infant feeding. By 2005, a study by Iliff and colleagues (2005) in Zimbabwe had indicated that, at 6 months postpartum, the rates of infant mortality were four times higher for mixed-fed infants compared to exclusively breastfed infants. The study did not find any significant differences in infant mortality when infants were predominantly versus exclusively breastfed. This indicates the importance of the pattern of infant feeding (mixed versus exclusive). A study conducted in Rwanda by myself (Thairu and Rwahungu 2005), described in the box 10.4 below, illustrates HIV-positive women's actual infant feeding patterns.

Box 10.4 Infant feeding choices in a nationally representative sample of HIV-positive women in Rwanda

Seven hundred and six HIV-positive mothers participating in PMTCT programs were surveyed. At the time of the study, there were 12 provinces in Rwanda, 3 PMTCT programs were randomly selected from each province, for a total sample of 36 clinics. Health workers were requested to invite HIV-positive women enrolled in the program prior to visiting each clinic. On the day the interviewers were at the clinic, all HIV-positive women enrolled in the program who had a child 18 months or younger and who were interviewed in Kinyarwanda, the local language. Most of the questions were closed-ended.

The mean age was 30, and 35 percent had never been to school. The majority of the women had chosen to breastfeed (84 percent). Because some of the infants whose mothers had chosen to replacement feed also received some breast milk, they were considered breastfed. 346 infants (51 percent) were still being breastfed. Of those breastfed infants who were <6 months of age, 72 percent were exclusively breastfed.

It is not surprising that the majority of HIV-positive Rwandan mothers described above had chosen to breastfeed. Mothers' difficulty in fully abstaining from breastfeeding or in significantly changing their infant feeding practices to avoid breast milk transmission has been noted in Kenya (Nduati et al. 2000) and in the Ivory Coast (Becquet et al. 2007). However, the finding that the majority of Rwandan mothers breastfed exclusively is unusual.

10.4.3 Weaning

Given the dangers of mixed feeding, by 2003, mothers were encouraged to rapidly transition from exclusive breastfeeding to replacement feeding (rapid weaning) (UNICEF, UNAIDS, WHO & UNFPA 2003). According to the 2003 WHO guidelines for health care managers and supervisors : '[. . .] ensure that mothers get support for exclusive breastfeeding and [. . .] early cessation of breastfeeding as soon as it is acceptable, feasible, affordable, sustainable and safe' (p. 18). These guidelines were revised in 2006 when various studies compared mortality outcomes for infants weaned early versus those breastfed for 6 months or more. Early breastfeeding cessation (before or at 6 months) was shown to lead to worse overall outcomes (increased mortality, decreased rates of HIV free survival) compared to longer periods of breastfeeding (WHO 2006). Gasteroenteritis was also more frequent (Onyango et al. 2007) even when infants were given ARV prophylaxis (Kafulafula et al. 2007; Kourtis et al. 2007). Controlling for HIV-status and when all mothers received HAART, early cessation led to higher mortality in infants and young children (Homsy, Moore, Barasa, & Mermin 2006). In a study in Zambia, there were no significant differences in HIV-free survival between a group of mothers who had been randomised to advice to stop breastfeeding at 4 months and a group that continued breastfeeding as long as they wanted to (Sinkala et al. 2006). Thirty five percent of the mothers assigned to stop breastfeeding at 4 months did not comply with the advice, and continued breastfeeding. An analysis based on actual practice (regardless of the group to which mothers had been randomised) also showed no significant difference in HIV-free survival for early versus late weaning.

While reports had indicated that early and rapid weaning was dangerous, it still remains unclear how to advise mothers to stop breastfeeding without endangering the infant. Currently, it is recommended that breast milk should be supplemented with other foods when infants are 4 months or older, and that infants should be weaned as soon as it is feasible to do so (see also Chapter 11). The World Health Organization has proposed the AFASS (Acceptability, Affordability, Safety and Sustainability) criteria for determining when it is feasible to introduce replacement foods.

In the Rwanda study previously described, the mean age for the 299 infants who had been weaned was 11.3 months. Of these, 73 infants (24 percent) were weaned before 6 months of age. A 12-h dietary recall for weaned infants indicated a monotonous diet of porridge (62 percent), milk (16 percent), biscuits and bread (6 percent) and other items such as fruit juices and teas. While the infants' health outcomes were not documented, it is likely that, in the long term, such a diet would not meet the infant's nutritional requirements.

10.5 Conclusion

Over the past two decades, information about breast milk HIV/AIDS transmission has evolved rapidly. The 1980s were marked with relatively limited information while the hallmark of the 1990s was uncertainty and fear. The results of epidemiological studies in the early part of the millennium have provided significant guidance on HIV and infant feeding. Now the challenge is to translate global recommendations into good practice in the field.

Currently, some HIV-positive women, such as those who participated in the studies in Rwanda and in South Africa conducted by myself, may have had access to this information through their participation in PMTCT programs. In contrast, women of unknown HIV status or those who were HIV-negative may have formed their opinions in the absence of specialised knowledge, such as in the study in Kenya. When Kenyan mothers were presented with hypothetical questions about HIV and infant feeding, the majority chose to support replacement feeding. In contrast, mothers who were HIV-positive (Rwanda and South Africa) and who had been provided with up-to-date information had chosen breastfeeding. Mothers in the South Africa study and in Rwanda had received nevirapine to prevent MTCT during delivery. However, to my knowledge, none of the HIV-positive mothers were receiving antiretroviral therapy to prevent progression to HIV/AIDS or to prevent MTCT through breast milk. With regard to weaning, about one quarter of the Rwandan women had done so before the infant was 6 months of age. The monotonous diets that their infants received were of concern.

Now that research has shown that exclusive breastfeeding is optimal for both HIV-positive and HIV-negative women, it is critical to provide this information to all women, regardless of their HIV status. Looking ahead, additional challenges for prevention of MTCT programs will include the provision of antiretroviral therapy to prevent transmission during delivery and treating mothers whose own disease has progressed to AIDS in order to prevent breast milk transmission. These interventions will have to be coupled with information for women to breastfeed exclusively, introduce appropriate complementary foods when the infant is 6 months or older and safe transition to non-breast milk foods (weaning). To be successful, PMTCT programs will also need to recruit women early, monitor response to treatment and promote drug adherence.

References

Bailey, M. (1991). Why breastfeeding is still best. *The Independent (London),* (September 2), p. 16.

Baumslag, N. (1978). The infant food industry. *The Lancet, 312*(8081), 166.

Baumslag, N. (1987). Breastfeeding and HIV infection. *The Lancet* (August 15), 400–401.

Becquet, R., Becquet, L., Ekouevi, D. K., Viho, I., Sarakovitch, C., Fassinou, P., et al. (2007). Two-year morbidity-mortality and alternatives to prolonged breast-feeding among children born to HIV-infected mothers in Cote d'Ivoire. *PLoS Medicine, 4*(1), e17, 139–151.

Brown, R. (1973). Breastfeeding in modern times. *The American Journal of Clinical Nutrition, 26,* 556–552.

Centers for Disease Control. (1982). Update on acquired immune deficiency syndrome (AIDS) – United States. *Morbidity and Mortality Weekly Report, 31*(34), 507–508.

Davis, W. (1912). Prevention of infant mortality by breastfeeding. *American Journal of Public Health, 2*(2), 67–71.

European Collaborative Study (1988). Mother to child transmission of HIV infection. *The Lancet* (Saturday November 5), 1039–1042.

Global Program on AIDS. (1992). Consensus statement from the WHO/UNICEF consultation on HIV transmission and breastfeeding. *Weekly Epidemiological Record, 67*(24), 177–178.

Homsy, J., Moore, D., Barasa, A., & Mermin, J. (2006). *Mother-to-child HIV transmission and infant mortality among women receiving highly active antiretroviral therapy (HAART) in rural Uganda.* Durban: The President's Emergency Plan for AIDS Relief Annual Meeting. The 2006 HIV/AIDS Implementers' Meeting. Building on Success: Ensuring Long-Term Solutions.

Iliff, P. J., Piwoz, E. G., Tavengwa, N. V., Zunguza, C. D., Marinda, E. T., Nathoo, K. J., et al. (2005). Early exclusive breastfeeding reduces the risk of postnatal HIV-1 transmission and increases HIV-free survival. *AIDS, 19*(7), 699–708.

James Erlichman, Consumer Affairs Correspondent (1989). Nestle accused of AIDS 'scare'. *The Guardian*, London, Nov 21, p. 6.

Jelliffe, D. B., & Jelliffe, E. F. P. (1978). The infant food industry. *The Lancet, 2*(8083), 263.

Kafulafula, G., Hoover, D., Li, Q., Kumwenda, N., Mipando, L., Taha, T., et al. (2007). *Post-weaning gastroenteritis and mortality in HIV-uninfected African infants receiving antiretroviral prophylaxis to prevent MTCT of HIV-1.* Los Angeles: Fourteenth Conference on Retroviruses and Opportunistic Infections.

Kourtis, A. P., Butera, S., Ibegbu, C., Beled, L., & Duerr, A. (2003). Breast milk and HIV-1: Vector of transmission or vehicle of protection? *Lancet Infectious Diseases, 12,* 786–793.

Kourtis, A. P., Fitzgerald, D., Hyde, L., Tien, H. C., Chavula, C. Mumba, N., et al. (2007). *Diarrhea in uninfected infants of HIV-infected mothers who stop breastfeeding at 6 Months: The BAN Study Experience.* Los Angeles: Fourteenth Conference on Retroviruses and Opportunistic Infections.

Lancet, T. (1978). The infant food industry. *The Lancet, 1*(8076), 1240–1241.

Logan, S., Newell, M. L., Ades, T., & Peckham, S. (1988). Breastfeeding and HIV infection. *The Lancet,* June 11, 1346.

Lönnerdal, B., Forsum, E., Gebre-Medin, M., & Hambraeus, L (1976). Breast milk composition in Ethiopian and Swedish mothers. II. Lactogen, nitrogen, and protein contents. *American Journal of Clinical Nutrition, 29,* 1134–1141.

Mbori-Ngacha, D., Nduati, R., John, G., Reilly, M., Richardson, B., Mwatha, A., et al. (2001). Morbidity and mortality in breastfed and formula-fed infants of HIV-1-infected women: A randomized clinical trial. *Journal of the American Medical Association, 286*(19), 2413–2420.

Munyakho, D. (1988). Breastfeeding and HIV. *The Lancet,* June 18, 1394–1395.
Nduati, R., John, G., Mbori-Ngacha, D., Richardson, B., Overbaugh, J., Mwatha, A., et al. (2000). Effect of breastfeeding and formula feeding on transmission of HIV-1: A randomized clinical trial. *Journal of the American Medical Association, 283*, 1167–1174.
Onyango, C., Bagenda, D., Mubiru, M., Musoke, P., Fowler, M., Jackson, J., et al. (2007). *Early breastfeeding cessation among HIV-exposed negative infants and risk of serious gastroenteritis: Findings from a perinatal prevention trial in Kampala, Uganda.* Los Angeles: Fourteenth Conference on Retroviruses and Opportunistic Infections (CROI).
Rousseau, C. M., Nduati, R. W., Richardson, B. A., John-Stewart, G. C., Mbori-Ngacha, D. A., Kreiss, J. K., et al. (2004). Association of levels of HIV-1–infected breast milk cells and risk of mother-to-child transmission. *Journal of Infectious Diseases, 10*(190), 1880–1888.
Sinkala, M., Kuhn, L., Kankasa, C., Kasonde, P., Vwalika, C., Mwiya, M., et al. (2006). *No benefit of early cessation of breastfeeding at 4 months on HIV-free survival of infants born to HIV-infected mothers in Zambia: The Zambia exclusive breastfeeding study*. Los Angeles: Fourteenth Conference on Retroviruses and Opportunistic Infections (CROI).
Southward, J. (1989). Breastmilk can spread AIDS. *The Sun Herald,* February 19, p. 27.
Tedder, R. S. (1988). Breastfeeding and HIV infection. *The Lancet,* August 20, 453.
Thairu, L. (2002). *Women's beliefs about infant feeding options for mothers with HIV: An ethnographic study in the Kiambu district of Kenya*. Ithaca: Division of Nutritional Sciences, Cornell University.
Thairu, L., & Rwahungu, J. (2005). *Evaluation des pratiques d'alimentation des nourrissons et des jeunes enfants dans le contexte du VIH/SIDA au Rwanda*. Kigali: UNICEF.
Thairu, L. N., Pelto, G. H., Rollins, N. C., Bland, R. M., & Ntshangase, N. (2005). Sociocultural influences on infant feeding decisions among HIV-infected women in rural Kwa-Zulu Natal, South Africa. *Maternal and Child Nutrition Journal, 1*, 2–10.
The Lancet. (1988). HIV infection, breastfeeding and human milk banking. *The Lancet,* July 16, 143–144.
The Times (Our Social Services Correspondent) (1988, May 20). AIDS test plan for pregnancy – Volunteer Aids tests for pregnant women. *The Times*, London. Retrieved January 4, 2010, from NewsBank on-line database (Access World News).
UNICEF. (1989). *Protecting, promoting and supporting Breastfeeding: The special role of maternity services. A joint WHO/UNICEF statement published by the World Health Organisation.* Geneva: UNICEF and WHO.
UNICEF. (1990). *Innocenti declaration on the protection, promotion and support of breastfeeding*. (UNICEF) Retrieved 20 July 2009, from http://www.unicef.org/programme/breastfeeding/innocenti.htm
UNICEF. (1991). The Baby Friendly Hospital initiative. Retrieved 20 July 2009, from http://www.unicef.org/programme/breastfeeding/baby.htm
UNICEF, UNAIDS, WHO and UNFPA. (2003). *HIV and infant feeding: A guide for health care managers and supervisors*, revised edition. Geneva: World Health Organization.
World Health Organization. (1981). *International code of marketing of breastmilk substitutes*. Retrieved 20 July 2009, from http://www.who.int/nutrition/publications/code_english.pdf
World Health Organization (1992). World AIDS cases: Update. *Weekly Epidemiological Record, 67*(26), 201–204.
World Health Organization (1996). HIV and infant feeding: An interim statement. *Weekly Epidemiological Record, 71*(39), 289–290.
World Health Organization (2006). *HIV and infant feeding technical consultation held on behalf of the Inter-agency Task Team (IATT) on prevention of HIV infections in pregnant women, mothers and their infants 2006*. Geneva: World Health Organization.

Chapter 11
Infant Feeding in the Era of HIV: Challenges and Opportunities

Tanya Doherty

Contents

11.1 Introduction

Transmission of HIV from mother-to-child after birth has become one of the greatest challenges in HIV prevention. The transmission of HIV through breast milk has created a dilemma; for each HIV-positive woman the benefits of breastfeeding, and the risks of not breastfeeding, have to be weighed against the risk of HIV transmission through breastfeeding. Whilst intrauterine and intrapartum transmission can be substantially reduced through improved drug regimens, modifying infant feeding practices in order to reduce postnatal transmission is complex and proving difficult to achieve. Mother-to-child transmission (MTCT) of HIV rates of less than

T. Doherty (✉)
Health Systems Research Unit, Medical Research Council, Francie van Zyl Drive, Parrow, Cape Town, South Africa
e-mail: tanya.doherty@mrc.ac.za

P. Liamputtong (ed.), *Infant Feeding Practices*, DOI 10.1007/978-1-4419-6873-9_11,
© Springer Science+Business Media, LLC 2011

2 percent are now reported from countries where antiretroviral prophylaxis, elective Caesarean section and refraining from breastfeeding can be applied (Newell 2006), whilst in settings where refraining from breastfeeding is not feasible or safe, programmes for prevention of MTCT need to focus not only on preventing HIV transmission but also on improving child survival.

The single most effective way of saving the lives of millions of young children in developing countries would be the promotion of exclusive breastfeeding (EBF). Over a period of 10 years, it could save the lives of an estimated 15 million children (Jones, Steketee, Black, Bhutta, & Morris 2003). Breastfeeding makes a major contribution to child health by protecting infants from morbidity and mortality associated with common infectious diseases. Breastfeeding is also said to provide a number of social, psychological, family spacing and economic benefits to both mother and baby (Victora et al. 1987; WHO Collaborative Study Team on the Role of Breastfeeding on the Prevention of Infant Mortality 2000). Black, Morris, and Bryce (2003, p. 2227) point out that: 'Infants aged 0–5 months who are not breastfed have seven-fold and five-fold increased risks of death from diarrhoea and pneumonia respectively, compared with infants who are exclusively breastfed. At the same age, non-exclusive rather than exclusive breastfeeding results in more than two-fold increased risks of dying from diarrhoea and pneumonia'.

This assertion and related comments and findings are set out by the Bellagio Child Survival Group in an article series in the *Lancet* (Black et al. 2003; Jones et al. 2003), summarising findings from international research of how best to reduce infant mortality in developing countries. The finding that HIV is present in breast milk has led to a re-assessment of the benefits of breastfeeding and a global decline in support for exclusive breastfeeding.

In order to guide health workers in assisting women to make appropriate infant feeding choices, WHO and United Nations Children's Fund (UNICEF) developed the Global Strategy for Infant and Young Child Feeding (WHO 2003). The recommendation for women known to be HIV-positive was avoidance of all breastfeeding if replacement feeding is acceptable, feasible, affordable, sustainable and safe (AFASS[1]). Otherwise, exclusive breastfeeding for the first months of life was recommended followed by early breastfeeding cessation as soon as feasible, when conditions for safe replacement feeding could be met. This guideline was revised in 2007, and now states that 'at six months, if replacement feeding is still not acceptable, feasible, affordable, sustainable and safe, continuation of breastfeeding with additional complementary foods is recommended' (WHO 2007, p. 7). Box 11.1 sets out the guidelines in great detail.

---

[1]The AFASS criteria are meant to guide health workers in assisting women to make infant feeding choices that are appropriate to their individual circumstances. The translation of this recommendation into operational settings is a challenge for health workers and counsellors as there is little guidance on what the terms 'acceptable', 'sustainable', 'safe' and 'feasible' mean in practice.

Box 11.1 WHO HIV and Infant Feeding Recommendations (WHO 2007)

- The most appropriate infant feeding option for an HIV-infected mother should continue to depend on her individual circumstances, including her health status and the local situation, but should take greater consideration of the health services available and the counselling and support she is likely to receive.
- Exclusive breastfeeding is recommended for HIV-infected women for the first 6 months of life, unless replacement feeding is acceptable, feasible, affordable, sustainable and safe for them and their infants before that time.
- When replacement feeding is acceptable, feasible, affordable, sustainable and safe, avoidance of all breastfeeding by HIV-infected women is recommended.
- At 6 months, if replacement feeding is still not acceptable, feasible, affordable, sustainable and safe, continuation of breastfeeding with additional complementary foods is recommended, while the mother and baby continue to be regularly assessed. All breastfeeding should stop once a nutritionally adequate and safe diet without breast milk can be provided.
- All HIV-infected mothers should receive counselling, which includes provision of general information about the risks and benefits of various infant feeding options and specific guidance in selecting the option most likely to be suitable for their situation. Whatever a mother decides, she should be supported in her choice.
- Adequate numbers of people who can counsel HIV-infected women on infant feeding should be trained, deployed, supervised and supported. Such support should include updated training as new information and recommendations emerge.
- When HIV-infected mothers choose not to breastfeed from birth or stop breastfeeding later, they should be provided with specific guidance and support for at least the first 2 years of the child's life to ensure adequate replacement feeding. Programmes should strive to improve conditions that will make replacement feeding safer for HIV-infected mothers and families.
- Information and education on mother-to-child transmission of HIV should be urgently directed to the general public, affected communities and families. HIV-infected mothers who breastfeed should be: (a) assisted to ensure that they use a good breastfeeding technique to prevent breast problems, which should be treated promptly if they occur; (b) provided with specific guidance and support when they cease breastfeeding to avoid harmful nutritional and psychological consequences and to maintain breast health.

- Whatever the mother's decision on infant feeding, health services should follow up all HIV-exposed infants, and continue to offer infant feeding counselling and support, particularly at key points when feeding decisions may be reconsidered, such as at the time of early infant HIV diagnosis and at 6 months of age.
- Breastfeeding mothers of infants and young children who are known to be HIV-infected should be strongly encouraged to continue breastfeeding as per the recommendations for the general population; that is up to 2 years or beyond.
- National programmes should provide all HIV-exposed infants and their mothers with a full package of child survival and reproductive health interventions with effective linkages to HIV prevention, treatment and care services. In addition, health services should make special efforts to support primary prevention for women who test negative in antenatal and delivery settings, with particular attention to the breastfeeding period.
- Governments should ensure that the package of interventions referenced above, as well as the conditions described in current guidance, are available before any distribution of free commercial infant formula is considered.
- Governments, other stakeholders and donors should greatly increase their commitment and resources for implementation of the Global Strategy for Infant and Young Child Feeding and the United Nations HIV and Infant Feeding Framework for Priority Action in order to effectively prevent postnatal HIV infections, improve HIV-free survival and achieve relevant United Nations. General Assembly Special Session goals.

This chapter will summarise the scientific literature on infant feeding and HIV and present some of the challenges to implementation of infant feeding recommendations in programmatic settings. It will also present interventions and strategies for supporting women in their feeding choices and opportunities to strengthen infant nutrition in the general population.

11.2 Overview of the Scientific Evidence

HIV infection can be transmitted from a mother to her child during pregnancy, peripartum or during the postnatal period via breastfeeding (MTCT). In the absence of antiretroviral therapy or prophylaxis for the mother or baby, rates of MTCT range from 15 to 25 percent amongst mothers are not breastfeeding to 30 to

45 percent in children who are subsequently breastfed up to 24 months of age (WHO/UNAIDS/UNICEF/UNFPA 2008).

Breastfeeding has been described as a route for transmission of the HIV virus from the mother to her infant since 1985 (Dunn, Newell, Ades, & Peckham 1992; see also Chapter 10 in this volume). Breastfeeding transmission is estimated to represent approximately one third to one half of vertical (mother-to-child) transmission in breastfeeding populations who are not treated with antiretroviral treatment or prophylaxis (De Cock et al. 2000). However, recent advances and policy changes globally have seen an increasing number of HIV-positive women gaining access to antiretroviral drug regimens, shown to be effective in reducing mother-to-child-transmission of HIV during pregnancy and delivery (WHO/UNAIDS/UNICEF/UNFPA 2008). These options range from single-dose nevirapine prophylaxis to the mother in labour and child after birth to full highly active antiretroviral therapy (HAART) to the mother for her own health and also to reduce HIV transmission. These regimens range in efficacy. Single-dose nevirapine reduces MTCT to 13 percent in breastfeeding populations (Guay et al. 1999) even in very poor developing countries, while HAART and infant feeding with breast milk substitutes has now reduced MTCT in developed countries to less than 1–2 percent (Dorenbaum et al. 2002). WHO (2008) notes that MTCT can be reduced to below 5 percent, even with continued breastfeeding, with effective perinatal antiretroviral prophylaxis programs.

While operational challenges continue to exist in the implementation of prevention of mother-to-child-transmission (PMTCT) programs (Jackson et al. 2007), the gains in the reduction of MTCT during pregnancy and peripartum have been significant in both developed and developing countries. However, substantial disparities currently exist between developed and developing countries for evidenced-based safe options for prevention of breastfeeding transmission of HIV. As a result, breastfeeding transmission is becoming an increasing percentage of MTCT in developing countries as antenatal and perinatal transmission are reduced, making this issue the major challenge in reducing paediatric HIV infections.

It is important to point out several factors which have been known to increase the risk of HIV transmission through breast milk (John-Stewart et al. 2004). The maternal factors include high plasma viral load, low CD4 count, breast pathology (including mastitis and abscesses), mode of infant feeding and prolonged duration of breastfeeding (more than 6 months). In particular, recent HIV infection is an important risk factor for HIV transmission through breast milk as it doubles the risk compared to a woman with earlier established infection due to the high viral load associated with recent infection (Dunn et al. 1992). Infant factors known to increase the risk of transmission through breastfeeding include damage to the mucous membranes (e.g. by oral thrush), damage to the intestinal mucosa by cow's milk or allergic reactions to complementary foods, and mixed feeding which may affect intestinal permeability (Rollins, Filteau, Coutsoudis, & Tomkins 2001). A summary of the key scientific knowledge on HIV and infant feeding is given in Box 11.2.

Box 11.2 Summary of Key Scientific Evidence on HIV and infant feeding

- Exclusive breastfeeding for up to 6 months was associated with a three- to fourfold decreased risk of transmission of HIV compared to non-exclusive breastfeeding in three large cohort studies conducted in Côte d'Ivoire, South Africa and Zimbabwe.
- Low maternal CD4+ count, high viral load in breast milk and plasma, maternal seroconversion during breastfeeding and breastfeeding duration are confirmed as important risk factors for postnatal HIV transmission and child mortality.
- In settings where antiretroviral prophylaxis and free infant formula were provided, the combined risk of HIV infection and death by 18 months of age was similar in infants who were replacement fed from birth and infants breastfed for 3–6 months (Botswana and Côte d'Ivoire).
- The sharp increase in deaths from diarrhoea and malnutrition in non-breastfed infants and young children during a diarrhoeal disease outbreak in one country emphasizes the vulnerability of replacement-fed infants and young children, and the need for adequate follow-up for all infants.
- Early cessation of breastfeeding (before 6 months) was associated with an increased risk of infant morbidity (especially diarrhoea) and mortality in HIV-exposed children in studies in Malawi, Kenya, Uganda and Zambia.
- Early breastfeeding cessation at 4 months was associated not only with reduced HIV transmission but also with increased child mortality from 4 to 24 months in a randomised trial in Zambia. Mortality was highest amongst those infants already infected with HIV at the time of weaning.
- Breastfeeding of HIV-infected infants beyond 6 months was associated with improved survival compared to stopping breastfeeding in Botswana and Zambia.
- Weak and poorly organised health services affect the quality of infant feeding counselling and support. Inaccurate, insufficient or non-existent infant feeding counselling has led to inappropriate feeding choices by both HIV-infected and HIV-uninfected women.
- Improved adherence and longer duration of exclusive breastfeeding up to 6 months were achieved in HIV-infected and HIV-uninfected mothers when they were provided with consistent messages and frequent, high-quality counselling in South Africa, Zambia and Zimbabwe.

11.3 Mode of Feeding and HIV Transmission

Current approaches to reducing or preventing postnatal transmission through breastfeeding in resource-poor settings include the avoidance of all breastfeeding (exclusive replacement feeding) or exclusive breastfeeding (breast milk feeding and medications only) (see Box 11.1).

11.3.1 Exclusive Replacement Feeding

While exclusive replacement feeding eliminates the risk of postnatal HIV transmission, in low- and middle-income countries replacement feeding is not considered to be the automatic choice for HIV-positive women as poor socio-economic environments threaten the safety of replacement feeding.

In developing countries, the risks of formula feeding in the general population are well described. A pooled-meta analysis (WHO Collaborative Study Team on the Role of Breastfeeding on the Prevention of Infant Mortality 2000) of studies in developing countries in populations with a low HIV prevalence found that infants who are not breastfed and receive formula milk or other replacement feeding have a 6-fold increased risk of dying in the first 2 months of life, a 4-fold increase between 2 and 3 months, and a 2.5 fold increase between 4 and 5 months compared with those who are breastfed. There is increasing data on the risks of replacement feeding in the context of PMTCT, and this data suggest that replacement feeding is not giving the results that were expected even in fairly resource-intensive settings.

One randomised controlled trial conducted in urban Kenya found that infants in the formula feeding group, whose mothers had access to clean water, free formula and frequent support by health workers, had a 40 percent lower risk of HIV transmission, but their 24 month mortality was similar to that in the breastfed group (Mbori-Ngacha et al. 2001). A more recent study from Kenya (Obimbo et al. 2004) followed HIV-infected infants in order to determine predictors of mortality during the first 2 years of life. One of the predictors of infant mortality in addition to biological factors, such as low birth weight, was formula feeding (HR 4.0, $p = 0.01$). All deaths amongst the non-breastfed infants occurred during the first 6 months of life and these infants were more likely to be of low weight for age at age 1 month compared to breastfed infants.

The MASHI (meaning milk in Setswana) study in Botswana (Thior et al. 2006) was a randomised controlled trial that compared the efficacy of exclusive breastfeeding plus 6 months of infant zidovudine (ZDV) prophylaxis versus formula feeding plus 1 month of infant ZDV. Cumulative HIV transmission rates at 7 months were 5.6 percent in the formula group and 9.0 percent in the breastfed plus ZDV group. The cumulative incidence of infant death by month 7 was significantly higher in the formula fed group than in the breastfed plus ZDV group (9.3 percent vs.

4.9 percent; $p = 0.003$). However, by 18 months there were no significant differences between the formula fed and breastfed plus ZDV group in the combined outcome HIV infection or mortality (13.9 percent vs. 15.1 percent; $p = 0.60$).

A recent study that followed formula feeding and breastfeeding HIV-positive mother infant pairs in a programmatic setting in Uganda (Kagaayi et al. 2008) found considerably higher mortality at 12 months amongst the formula fed infants (18 percent) compared to the breastfed infants (3 percent) (unadjusted hazard ratio (HR) = 6.1(95 percent CI = 1.7–21.4, P-value, 0.01). The results of this study led to a change in the policy of this district of providing formula milk as part of the PMTCT programme.

The Diminution De La Transmission Mere-Enfant (DITRAME) PLUS study (Bequet et al. 2007) conducted in Ivory Coast found a more positive outcome with formula feeding in an urban setting with high levels of support. This study found no significant difference in rates of infant illness and death at 24 months between breastfed and formula fed infants, and suggests that safe formula feeding can be achieved in settings where women have regular access to electricity, clean water, free health care, free transport to health facilities, free formula milk and formula feeding supplies.

Current data on the risks of formula feeding reinforce the importance of individual assessments of home circumstances in the process of decision-making. Based on available evidence, formula feeding may be an appropriate feeding choice for women who have uninterrupted access to safe water, electricity and adequate quantities of formula milk supplies, and who receive intensive counselling and follow-up support. However, in rural or urban settings with a poor infrastructure, limited counselling and support from the health system and those without access to safe water supplies and regular fuel, exclusive breastfeeding is the preferred option.

11.3.2 Exclusive Breastfeeding

There is now substantial evidence that exclusive breastfeeding (feeding an infant on breast milk alone with no other liquids or solid foods except for medicines and vitamin-mineral supplements) has substantial child survival benefits – even in the context of HIV. The Lancet Child Survival series (Jones et al. 2003) showed that, notwithstanding HIV, universal coverage with exclusive breastfeeding (EBF) for the first 6 months and continued breastfeeding (BF) until at least 11 months may prevent 13 percent of under-five deaths globally.

More recently, exclusive breastfeeding has been found to result in a three- to fourfold decrease in HIV transmission compared to non-exclusive breastfeeding in several large prospective studies in South Africa (Coovadia et al. 2007; Coutsoudis, Pillay, Spooner, Kuhn, & Coovadia 1999), Zimbabwe (Iliff et al. 2005), Zambia (Kuhn et al. 2007), and Ivory Coast (Becquet et al. 2008).

Early cessation of breastfeeding, at around 6 months of age, whereas previously recommended by the World Health Organisation (WHO 2003) as a strategy to limit the exposure to HIV through breast milk, is now only recommended if avoiding all breastfeeding is acceptable, feasible, affordable, sustainable and safe (AFASS) and if the benefits of stopping breastfeeding as a strategy to reduce HIV transmission far outweighs its child survival risk. Recent data have highlighted the dangers of early cessation of breastfeeding under conditions of underlying poor socio-economic status and food insecurity. A cross-sectional study in Mozambique (Johnson et al. 2006) found that most (78 percent) HIV-positive women had stopped breastfeeding their infants by 6 months of age and that commonly consumed, locally available foods would not meet the nutritional needs of non-breastfed infants between 6 and 12 months of age. Furthermore, replacing breast milk with local foods would double the estimated daily cost of feeding a 6–12 month old infant.

The Zimbabwe Vitamin A for Mothers and Babies (ZVITAMBO) study, a randomised trial to assess the impact of Vitamin A supplementation on MTCT, also found inadequate feeding of infants weaned early from breastfeeding (Lunney et al. 2008). During in-depth interviews with a sub-sample of HIV-positive mothers who had weaned their infants at around 6 months of age, women were asked about their infants' diet using food frequency assessments. The same assessment was undertaken with a group of HIV-negative women who were still breastfeeding their 6–9 month old infants. Median energy intake (percent requirement) was 1382 kJ (54 percent) among weaned infants compared with 2234 kJ (87 percent) among breastfeeding infants. Food unavailability was the primary barrier to early weaning suggesting that it is difficult for HIV-positive women in Zimbabwe to safely wean their infants from breast milk.

A cohort study of HIV-positive mother infant pairs in South Africa (Goga et al. 2009) found that, despite a national recommendation of early weaning at 6 months, only 39 percent of women had ceased breastfeeding at 6 months. Amongst women who were able to stop breastfeeding, 39 percent reported being criticized for not breastfeeding, mainly by their mother, mother-in-law, and the father of the child, and 61 percent experienced self-reported breast health problems (engorged and inflamed breasts).

The Zambian Exclusive Breastfeeding Study (ZEBS) sought to answer the question of whether early weaning is safe in an African setting with a high background infant mortality rate. The study randomised HIV-positive women to early abrupt weaning at 4 months or continued breastfeeding for as long as the women chose. In the overall cohort, there was no significant difference between the groups in the rate of HIV-free survival among the children; 68.4 percent and 64.0 percent survived to 24 months without HIV infection in the intervention and control groups, respectively ($p = 0.13$).

Children who were infected with HIV by 4 months had a higher mortality by 24 months if they had been assigned to the intervention group than if they had been assigned to the control group (73.6 percent vs. 54.8 percent, $p = 0.007$) (Kuhn et al. 2008). This study has shown that there is no child survival benefit to early weaning and that it can be extremely harmful for infants already infected with HIV. These results led WHO to change their recommendations (see Box 11.1) from supporting early weaning at 6 months to continued breastfeeding if the mother does not meet the AFASS criteria (WHO 2007).

11.4 Implementing Infant Feeding Choices: Experiences of HIV-Positive Mothers

Most women in sub-Saharan Africa have their HIV status diagnosed during pregnancy because of testing available through programmes for the prevention of mother-to-child transmission (PMTCT) of HIV. A diagnosis of HIV during pregnancy necessitates complex decision-making about participation in PMTCT programmes and infant feeding methods. Women usually make these decisions alone, as disclosure rates remain very low in sub-Saharan Africa (Medley, Garcia-Moreno, McGill, & Maman 2004). The purpose of infant feeding counselling is to prepare a mother to make an informed choice of a feeding method that is appropriate to her particular situation. The concept of choice is new in the infant feeding discourse in resource-poor settings where how to feed a baby has not previously been a subject of choice (Seidel, Sewpaul, & Dano 2000). Breastfeeding has, by and large, been considered the 'only way to feed an infant' with alternative methods only being used under specific situations such as the death of a mother. However, the PMTCT programme promotes alternative infant feeding methods as safe or safer in an HIV context and presents HIV-positive women with a choice. In sub-Saharan Africa, breastfeeding is normative and prolonged breastfeeding and early supplementation are also normative; any alteration in infant feeding practice poses significant challenges for women. Thus, adherence to a chosen infant feeding method is especially challenging for women with HIV. Breastfeeding involves more than infant nutrition and attempts to deviate from established infant feeding practices will engage power relations, social obligations and customary ideas and values surrounding motherhood.

A qualitative study undertaken in South Africa (Doherty, Chopra, Nkonki, Jackson, & Greiner 2006a) to explore the experiences of HIV-positive mothers in relation to infant feeding found that these HIV-positive mothers were struggling to protect their decision-making autonomy. Uncertainty about the safety of breastfeeding appeared to have increased the power and influence of health workers, who now acted as gatekeepers to not only this new knowledge but also to essential resources such as formula milk. Fear of disclosure of HIV status and stigma had also weakened the ability of mothers to resist entrenched family and community norms that encourage early introduction of fluids and foods and that question non-breastfeeding. Women who chose to exclusively formula feed had difficulties accessing formula milk because of inflexible clinic policies and a lack of supplies at clinics. Limited postpartum support led to social isolation and mothers doubting their ability to care for their children.

The HIV epidemic appears to have changed the interactions between women and health workers in the context of infant feeding. There is already a very hierarchical relationship between health workers and women, which has been described in the literature in different settings (Jewkes, Abrahams, & Mvo 1998; Seidel et al. 2000;

Manuela de Paoli, Manongi, & Klepp 2004). Uncertainties about the risk of HIV transmission through breastfeeding and control of the provision of formula feeds in certain settings further accentuate this power divide. Thus, it is not surprising that HIV-positive women may feel confused and unsure about the best infant feeding choice and, therefore, choose whatever they are told will provide the best protection for their child.

A longitudinal qualitative study undertaken in South Africa to explore characteristics of HIV-positive women who were able to sustain exclusive infant feeding (Doherty, Chopra, Nkonki, Jackson, & Persson 2006b) found that women who achieved success in exclusivity were able to resist pressure from family to introduce other fluids and to recall key messages on mother-to-child transmission risks and mixed feeding. Among women who maintained exclusive breastfeeding, a strong belief in the benefits of breastfeeding and a supportive home environment was important. For women using formula milk, having resources such as electricity, a kettle and flask made feeding at night easier. This study has highlighted the importance of support for infant feeding that extends beyond the antenatal period to enable mothers to cope with new challenges and pressures at critical times during the early postpartum period

A qualitative study undertaken in Tanzania, which used case studies to explore infant feeding experiences of 20 HIV-positive women (Leshabari, Blystad, & Moland 2007), described the gap between intentions and infant feeding practice in a context where the social expectations to breastfeed are high and where family and neighbours are part of the decision-making team surrounding infant feeding.

The international guidelines on HIV and infant feeding, which require that an HIV-positive woman be provided with adequate information about the recommended feeding options, are based on the principle of 'informed choice' (see also Chapter 4 in this volume). Decision-making on infant feeding is not only based on knowledge about medical risks but also on the social risks regarding disclosure, rejection and stigma. In the context in which most HIV-positive women in Africa find themselves truly informed, choice is seldom a reality either due to social or economic constraints. As a result, translating international guidelines into operational settings remains a challenge, and the gap between intentions and actual practices is proving difficult to bridge. For the HIV-positive mother, infant feeding choices carry a burden of responsibility, which is mostly carried alone. Furthermore, the practice of infant feeding takes place largely at home out of reach of continuous health care surveillance. International guidelines need to take this into account with practical recommendations that incorporate the social reality for largely isolated and vulnerable HIV-positive women. For an individual mother, to modify deeply meaningful nurturing practices without being the victim of close unwanted scrutiny will require programmes that include community involvement and mobilisation for exclusive breastfeeding so that this becomes a normative practice for all mothers.

11.5 What Is Required to Increase Optimal Infant Feeding Practices in the Context of HIV?

11.5.1 Improving Infant Feeding Practices in the General Population

The challenge of improving infant feeding practices for HIV-positive women needs to be understood within a context of poor infant feeding in the general population. In most parts of the world, and especially in Sub-Saharan Africa settings, more than 95 percent of mothers initiate breastfeeding after birth, and most of them continue to breastfeed for more than a year (UNICEF 2005). However, exclusive breastfeeding is rare and has even been noted to be an alien concept in most African cultures (Magoni et al. 2005), the prevailing form of breastfeeding worldwide being mixed breastfeeding (WHO 2001).

It is against this background that infant feeding recommendations for women with HIV are being implemented. If women with HIV are to succeed in practicing exclusive infant feeding, then improvements in infant feeding practices in the general population are necessary to ensure that exclusive breastfeeding is a norm rather than an exception and that women opting for formula feeding are not stigmatised.

Research conducted in study (rather than operational) sites have shown that in the presence of intensive support and home visits exclusive breastfeeding rates can be increased in the general population and in the context of HIV.

Coovadia and colleagues (2007), in an infant feeding intervention in South Africa, reported exclusive breastfeeding rates of 82 percent, 67 percent and 40 percent in HIV-positive women at 6 weeks, 3 months and 6 months, respectively, amongst their study population. The intervention was intense and included improved counselling at health facilities and home visits by infant feeding counsellors three or four times in the first 2 weeks of life and every 2 weeks thereafter until the infant was 6 months old (Coovadia et al. 2007). Counselling visits were strongly associated with adherence to cumulative exclusive breastfeeding at 4 months; those who had received the scheduled number of visits were more than twice as likely to still be exclusively breastfeeding than those who had not (HIV-negative women: adjusted odds ratio: 2.07, 95 percent CI: 1.56–2.74, $p<0.0001$; HIV-positive women: adjusted odds ratio: 2.86, 95 percent CI 2.13– 3.83, $p<0.0001$) (Bland et al. 2008).

Quinn and colleagues (2005) demonstrated improved feeding practices on a programmatic level when a multi-pronged intervention was implemented in Africa and Latin America. This intervention included the appointment of focal infant feeding persons, the strengthening of partnerships, the integration of appropriate feeding messages into routine child health care services, capacity building through training, formative research leading to the development of behaviour-change communication materials and community activities such as breastfeeding-promotion songs.

One intervention that has been shown in a variety of settings to increase exclusive breastfeeding is peer counselling. Peer counselling is a proven cost-effective approach for changing behaviour, and several studies have examined its impact on breastfeeding behaviour. Studies in developing country settings have shown that intensive counselling and support can increase the proportion of women who breastfeed exclusively. However, there are considerable variations on the type of counselling support provided. Haider and colleagues in Bangladesh, in a trial randomised by community (Haider, Ashworth, Kabir, & Huttly 2000), and Morrow and colleagues in a trial randomised at individual level in Mexico (Morrow et al. 1999) obtained substantial increases in exclusive breastfeeding. A study in Ghana (Aidam, Perez-Escamilla. & Lartey 2005) randomised women to one of two intervention groups or a control group. The intervention groups were exclusive breastfeeding support pre-, peri- and postnatally, or only peri- and postnatally, and the control group received non-breastfeeding-related health education with an equal amount of contact from counsellors as the intervention groups. Mothers received nine postnatal home visits in the first 6 months postpartum and infant feeding data were collected monthly. By 6 months postpartum, 90 percent of women in the intervention group 1 and 74 percent of women in the intervention group 2 had exclusively breastfed in the previous month; only 48 percent of women in the control group were doing so.

The challenge is to take the lessons learnt from these projects and implement them on a large scale within the context of investments in PMTCT programs in Africa and other developing regions. Revitalisation is also needed of the Baby Friendly Hospital Initiative of WHO (WHO 1998) so that mothers start out with good quality support for exclusive breastfeeding in hospital. Furthermore, governments need to ensure up-to-date policies on Infant and Young Child Feeding, which can be implemented by health workers in operational settings.

11.5.2 Good Quality Infant Feeding Counselling and Support

Reducing MTCT through improved infant feeding requires greater attention to the quality of counselling and support provided to mothers. International guidelines (WHO 2007) recommend that all HIV-positive women should receive counselling, which includes general information about the risks and benefits of various infant feeding options and specific guidance in selecting the option most likely to be suitable for their situation. In developing countries, this counselling role is mainly the responsibility of maternity and paediatric nurses and midwives as well as lay counsellors.

In many countries, shortcomings in the implementation of these guidelines have been found. Inadequate training of health workers, particularly infant feeding counsellors, about the relative risks associated with infant feeding in the context of HIV, lack of culturally sensitive counselling tools and the stigma associated with replacement feeding, all make appropriate and effective infant feeding counselling difficult. Even after training, health workers are often unsure of the risks of different feeding options. For example, an evaluation of the WHO/UNICEF infant feeding training in South Africa (Tint, Doherty, Nkonki, Witten, & Chopra 2003) found low levels of knowledge amongst both participants and trainers. Most participants (88 percent) over-estimated the risks of breastfeeding for HIV-positive women and very few (10 percent) knew of the health risks of formula feeding. Participants' confidence in counselling following training was also disappointing with 44 percent being uncomfortable counselling women experiencing breastfeeding difficulties.

A similar cross-sectional assessment of health worker knowledge was undertaken in a rural area of KwaZulu Natal, South Africa (Shah, Rollins, & Bland 2005). This study found that 71 percent of doctors would recommend water and 50 percent solids to breastfed infants under 6 months of age. The most common response by all health workers to problems of infants being thirsty or unsatisfied was to supplement with other fluids or feeds.

It is not surprising that health workers are generally unsure of how to guide the mother in making her feeding choice (Chopra et al. 2002). Providing full information to achieve empowered decision-making in this context requires skilled counselling and additional time, which is often not available in busy health facilities. As a result, the quality of infant feeding counselling is poor. For example, one observational study (Chopra, Doherty, Jackson, & Ashworth 2005) across three facilities in South Africa found that only 9 percent of HIV-positive women were asked about access to clean water, fuel and a fridge before deciding upon an feeding option. For women who opted to formula feed, there was no discussion about how the mother would explain the lack of breastfeeding to others. For women who chose to breastfeed, only 17 percent were asked if they understood the practice of exclusive breastfeeding and no one was asked if they thought it was feasible.

In the context of poor counselling, many HIV-positive mothers are making inappropriate choices, such as choosing to avoid breastfeeding when the safety of replacement feeding cannot be assured and choosing to breastfeed when conditions for safe formula feeding are present. Recent work in South Africa has described inappropriate choices of intended infant feeding in a cohort of HIV-positive mothers (Doherty et al. 2007). The research noted that when a choice to formula feed was made in the absence of piped water, sustainable cooking fuel or disclosure of HIV status, infants were 3.45 times more likely to die or become HIV-positive by 9 months of age when compared to formula feeding in women who met all three criteria. This suggests that inappropriate choice of infant feeding method places the child at risk.

It is also clear that health workers are having a significant influence on mothers' feeding decisions and that individual circumstances are not being taken into account during counselling. For example, despite cultural and socio-economic similarities, the uptake of formula feeding was 65 percent in a relatively rural site in South Africa compared with 40 percent a hundred kilometres away in an urban Durban site (Doherty, McCoy, & Donohue 2005).

In contrast, an intervention study in a rural area in KwaZulu-Natal, South Africa (Bland, Rollins, Coovadia, Coutsoudis, & Newell 2007), which provided intensive training and support to counsellors, found that the HIV-positive women who did not have the resources to safely formula feed appropriately chose to exclusively breastfeed. This study suggested that well-trained and supported counsellors are able to provide high-quality infant feeding counselling according to international guidelines.

Infant feeding counselling is one of the most important components of PMTCT programs. If it is done well, it could result in significant reductions in child mortality through decreased postnatal HIV transmission and improved infant feeding practices. But if it is done badly, it could lead to deaths from diarrhoea and other infections, and the spread of poor infant feeding practices into the general population. High-quality training for counsellors that addresses attitudes and interpersonal relations can lead to greater support for women, increased disclosure rates and greater confidence for mothers in their ability to carry out infant feeding decisions. See also Chapter 12 in this volume.

11.6 Conclusion

International approaches for preventing mother-to-child transmission of HIV are now focusing on child survival, not just HIV transmission, as the appropriate health outcome to measure success of PMTCT programs (Rollins & Mphatswe 2008). Ultimately, the goal is a live and healthy, HIV-negative child, and an alive and healthy mother to care for that child. This goal is universal whether in a developed or developing country. While the goal is universal, policies and recommendations to promote this goal vary across settings.

In developed countries, treatment and prevention guidelines and choices regarding infant feeding in the context of maternal HIV infection are fairly straightforward and avoidance of breastfeeding by HIV-positive women is universal in these settings. In developing countries, infant feeding policies are guided by the local context. In most contexts in sub-Saharan Africa, it is clear that even for HIV-positive women avoidance of breastfeeding causes more harm for infants. In some settings such as South Africa and Botswana, the governments have chosen to provide HIV-positive women with an alternative to breastfeeding by providing free formula milk. However, research has found that even with the provision of free milk, the risks of replacement feeding can outweigh the risks of breastfeeding in terms of child survival (Creek, Luo, & Quick 2006; Thior et al. 2006; Doherty et al. 2007). Increased access to antiretroviral drugs for mothers has been shown to markedly decrease breastfeeding HIV transmission, shifting the balance to make replacement feeding less beneficial. A way forward for PMTCT, which would optimise child survival in developing country contexts, would be to remove the illusionary choices of infant feeding method and to reintroduce exclusive breastfeeding as the optimal approach for all women. This approach is now recommended in the latest WHO Guidelines on HIV and Infant Feeding, as it has the benefit of reducing the risk of HIV transmission while maintaining support for breastfeeding as the single most effective child survival strategy. This approach would also move the attention and responsibility away from the HIV-positive woman and shift the focus onto developing ways to promote exclusive breastfeeding on a large scale. The challenge of HIV and breastfeeding and the research conducted over the past decade now open up an opportunity to use this knowledge to revitalise support for exclusive breastfeeding. We need to seize this opportunity and use it to turn the tide of child mortality in Africa.

References

Aidam, B. A., Perez-Escamilla. R., & Lartey, A. (2005). Lactation counseling increases exclusive breast-feeding rates in Ghana. *Journal of Nutrition, 135*, 1691–1695.

Becquet, R., Bequet, L., Ekouevi, D. K., Viho, I., Sakarovitch, C., Fassinou, P., et al. (2007). Two-year morbidity-mortality and alternatives to prolonged breast-feeding among children born to HIV-infected mothers in Cote d'Ivoire. *PLoS Medicine, 4*, e17.

Becquet, R., Ekouevi, D. K., Menan, H., Amani-Bosse, C., Bequet, L., Viho, I., et al. (2008). Early mixed feeding and breastfeeding beyond 6 months increase the risk of postnatal HIV transmission: ANRS 1201/1202 Ditrame Plus, Abidjan, Cote d'Ivoire. *Preventive Medicine, 47*, 27–33.

Black, R. E., Morris, S. S., & Bryce, J. (2003). Where and why are 10 million children dying every year? *Lancet, 361*, 2226–2234.

Bland, R. M., Rollins, N. C., Coovadia, H. M., Coutsoudis, A., & Newell, M. L. (2007). Infant feeding counselling for HIV-infected and uninfected women: Appropriateness of choice and practice. *Bulletin of the World Health Organisation, 85*, 289–296.

Bland, R. M., Little, K. E., Coovadia, H. M., Coutsoudis, A., Rollins, N. C., & Newell, M. L. (2008). Intervention to promote exclusive breast-feeding for the first 6 months of life in a high HIV prevalence area. *AIDS, 22*, 883–891.

Chopra, M., Piwoz, E., Sengwana, J., Schaay, N., Dunnett, L., & Saders, D. (2002). Effect of a mother-to-child HIV prevention programme on infant feeding and caring practices in South Africa. *South African Medical Journal, 92*, 298–302.

Chopra, M., Doherty, T., Jackson, D., & Ashworth, A. (2005). Preventing HIV transmission to children: Quality of counselling of mothers in South Africa. *Acta Paediatrica, 94*, 357–363.

Coovadia, H. M., Rollins, N. C., Bland, R. M., Little, K., Coutsoudis, A., Bennish, M. L., et al. (2007). Mother-to-child transmission of HIV-1 infection during exclusive breastfeeding in the first 6 months of life: An intervention cohort study. *Lancet, 369*, 1107–1116.

Coutsoudis, A., Pillay, K., Spooner, E., Kuhn, L., & Coovadia, H. M. (1999). Influence of infant-feeding patterns on early mother-to-child transmission of HIV-1 in Durban, South Africa: A prospective cohort study. South African Vitamin A Study Group. *Lancet, 354*, 471–476.

Creek, T., Luo, C., & Quick, T. (2006). *HIV-exposed children highly affected by deadly outbreak of diarrhea and severe acute malnutrition – Botswana, 2006*. Durban: 2006 HIV/AIDS Implementers Meeting of the President's Emergency Plan for AIDS Relief.

De Cock, K. M., Fowler, M. G., Mercier, E., de Vincenzi, I., Saba, J., Hoff, E., et al. (2000). Prevention of mother-to-child HIV transmission in resource-poor countries: Translating research into policy and practice. *Journal of the American Medical Association, 283*, 1175–1182.

Doherty, T. M., McCoy, D., & Donohue, S. (2005). Health system constraints to optimal coverage of the prevention of mother-to-child HIV transmission programme in South Africa: Lessons from the implementation of the national pilot programme. *African Health Sciences, 5*, 213–218.

Doherty, T., Chopra, M., Nkonki, L., Jackson, D., & Greiner, T. (2006a). Effect of the HIV epidemic on infant feeding in South Africa: "When they see me coming with the tins they laugh at me". *Bulletin of the World Health Organisation, 84*, 90–96.

Doherty, T., Chopra, M., Nkonki, L., Jackson, D., & Persson, L. A. (2006b). A longitudinal qualitative study of infant-feeding decision making and practices among HIV-positive women in South Africa. *Journal of Nutrition, 136*, 2421–2426.

Doherty, T., Chopra, M., Jackson, D., Goga, A., Colvin, M., & Persson, L. A. (2007). Effectiveness of the WHO/UNICEF guidelines on infant feeding for HIV-positive women: Results from a prospective cohort study in South Africa. *AIDS, 21*, 1791–1797.

Dorenbaum, A., Cunningham, C. K., Gelber, R. D., Culnane, M., Mofenson, L., Britto, P., et al. (2002). Two-dose intrapartum/newborn nevirapine and standard antiretroviral therapy to reduce perinatal HIV transmission: A randomized trial. *Journal of the American Medical Association, 288*, 189–198.

Dunn, D. T., Newell, M. L., Ades, A. E., & Peckham, C. S. (1992). Risk of human immunodeficiency virus type 1 transmission through breastfeeding. *Lancet, 340*, 585–588.

Goga, A. E., Van Wyk, B., Doherty, T., Colvin, M., Jackson, D. J., & Chopra, M. (2009). Operational effectiveness of guidelines on complete breast-feeding cessation to reduce mother-to-child transmission of HIV: Results from a prospective observational cohort study at routine prevention of mother-to-child transmission sites, South Africa. *Journal of Acquired Immune Deficiency Syndromes, 50*, 521–528.

Guay, L. A., Musoke, P., Fleming, T., Bagenda, D., Allen, M., Nakabiito, C., et al. (1999). Intrapartum and neonatal single-dose nevirapine compared with zidovudine for prevention of mother-to-child transmission of HIV-1 in Kampala, Uganda: HIVNET 012 randomised trial. *Lancet, 354*, 795–802.

Haider, R., Ashworth, A., Kabir, I., & Huttly, S. R. (2000). Effect of community-based peer counsellors on exclusive breastfeeding practices in Dhaka, Bangladesh: A randomised controlled trial. *Lancet, 356*, 1643–1647.

Iliff, P. J., Piwoz, E. G., Tavengwa, N. V., Zunguza, C. D., Marinda, E. T., Nathoo, K. J., et al. (2005). Early exclusive breastfeeding reduces the risk of postnatal HIV-1 transmission and increases HIV-free survival. *AIDS, 19*, 699–708.

Jackson, D. J., Chopra, M., Doherty, T. M., Colvin, M. S., Levin, J. B., Willumsen, J. F., et al. (2007). Operational effectiveness and 36 week HIV-free survival in the South African programme to prevent mother-to-child transmission of HIV-1. *AIDS, 21*, 509–516.

Jewkes, R., Abrahams, N., & Mvo, Z. (1998). Why do nurses abuse patients? Reflections from South African obstetric services. *Social Science and Medicine, 47*, 1781–1795.

John-Stewart, G., Mbori-Ngacha, D., Ekpini, R., Janoff, E. N., Nkengasong, J., Read, J. S., et al. (2004). Breast-feeding and transmission of HIV-1. *Journal of Acquired Immune Deficiency Syndromes, 35*, 196–202.

Johnson, W., Alons, C., Fidalgo, L., Piwoz, E., Kahn, S., Macombe, A., et al. (2006). The challenge of providing adequate infant nutrition following early breastfeeding cessation by HIV-positive, food insecure Mozambican mothers. *International AIDS Conference,* 13–18 August, Toronto.

Jones, G., Steketee, R. W., Black, R. E., Bhutta, Z. A., & Morris, S. S. (2003). How many child deaths can we prevent this year? *Lancet, 362*, 65–71.

Kagaayi, J., Gray, R. H., Brahmbhatt, H., Kigozi, G., Nalugoda, F., Wabwire-Mangen, .F, et al. (2008). Survival of infants born to HIV-positive mothers, by feeding modality, in Rakai, Uganda. *PLoS One, 3*, e3877.

Kuhn, L., Sinkala, M., Kankasa, C., Semrau, K., Kasonde, P., Scott, N., et al. (2007). High uptake of exclusive breastfeeding and reduced early post-natal HIV transmission. *PLoS One, 2*, e1363.

Kuhn, L., Aldrovandi, G. M., Sinkala, M., Kankasa, C., Semrau, K., Mwiya, M., et al. (2008). Effects of early, abrupt weaning on HIV-free survival of children in Zambia. *New England Journal of Medicine, 359*, 130–141.

Kuhn, L., Reitz, C., & Abrams, E. J. (2009). Breastfeeding and AIDS in the developing world. *Current Opinion in Pediatrics, 21*, 83–93.

Leshabari, S. C., Blystad, A., & Moland, K. M. (2007). Difficult choices: Infant feeding experiences of HIV-positive mothers in northern Tanzania. *Journal of Social Aspects of HIV/AIDS Research Alliance, 4*, 544–555.

Lunney, K. M., Jenkins, A. L., Tavengwa, N. V., Majo, F., Chidhanguro, D., Iliff, P., et al. (2008). HIV-positive poor women may stop breast-feeding early to protect their infants from HIV infection although available replacement diets are grossly inadequate. *Journal of Nutrition, 138*, 351–357.

Magoni, M., Bassani, L., Okong, P., Kituuka, P., Germinario, E. P., Giuliano, M., et al. (2005). Mode of infant feeding and HIV infection in children in a program for prevention of mother-to-child transmission in Uganda. *AIDS, 19*, 433–437.

Manuela de Paoli, M., Manongi, R., & Klepp, K. I. (2004). Are infant feeding options that are recommended for mothers with HIV acceptable, feasible, affordable, sustainable and safe? Pregnant women's perspectives. *Public Health Nutrition, 7*, 611–619.

Mbori-Ngacha, D., Nduati, R., John, G., Reilly, M., Richardson, B., Mwatha, A., et al. (2001). Morbidity and mortality in breastfed and formula-fed infants of HIV-1-infected women: A randomized clinical trial. *Journal of the American Medical Association, 286*, 2413–2420.

Medley, A., Garcia-Moreno, C., McGill, S., & Maman, S. (2004). Rates, barriers and outcomes of HIV serostatus disclosure among women in developing countries: Implications for prevention of mother-to-child transmission programmes. *Bulletin of the World Health Organisation,* April, 299–307.

Morrow, A. L., Guerrero, M. L., Shults, J., Calva, J. J., Lutter, C., Bravo, J., et al. (1999). Efficacy of home-based peer counselling to promote exclusive breastfeeding: A randomised controlled trial. *Lancet, 353*, 1226–1231.

Newell, M. L. (2006). Current issues in the prevention of mother-to-child transmission of HIV-1 infection. *Transactions of the Royal Society of Tropical Medicine and Hygiene, 100*, 1–5.

Obimbo, E. M., Mbori-Ngacha, D. A., Ochieng, J. O., Richardson, B. A., Otieno, P. A., Bosire, R., et al. (2004). Predictors of early mortality in a cohort of human immunodeficiency virus type 1-infected African children. *Pediatric Infectious Diseases Journal, 23*, 536–543.

Quinn, V. J., Guyon, A. B., Schubert, J. W., Stone-Jimenez, M., Hainsworth, M. D., & Martin, L. H. (2005). Improving breastfeeding practices on a broad scale at the community level: success stories from Africa and Latin America. *J Hum Lact, 21*, 345–354.

Rollins, N., & Mphatswe, W. (2008). From prevention of mother-to-child transmission to child survival and back. *Current Opinion in HIV and AIDS, 3*, 180–185.

Rollins, N. C., Filteau, S. M., Coutsoudis, A., & Tomkins, A. M. (2001). Feeding mode, intestinal permeability, and neopterin excretion: A longitudinal study in infants of HIV-infected South African women. *Journal of Acquired Immune Deficiency Syndromes, 28*, 132–139.

Seidel, G., Sewpaul, V., & Dano, B. (2000). Experiences of breastfeeding and vulnerability among a group of HIV-positive women in Durban, South Africa. *Health Policy & Planning, 15*, 24–33.

Shah, S., Rollins, N. C., & Bland, R. (2005). Breastfeeding knowledge among health workers in rural South Africa. *Journal of Tropical Pediatrics, 51*, 33–38.

Thior, I., Lockman, S., Smeaton, L. M., Shapiro, R. L., Wester, C., Heymann, S. J., et al. (2006). Breastfeeding plus infant zidovudine prophylaxis for 6 months vs formula feeding plus infant zidovudine for 1 month to reduce mother-to-child HIV transmission in Botswana: a randomized trial: The Mashi Study. *Journal of the American Medical Association, 296*, 794–805.

Tint, K., Doherty, T., Nkonki, L., Witten, C., & Chopra, M. (2003). *An evaluation of PMTCT and infant feeding training in seven provinces of South Africa*. Durban: Health Systems Trust.

UNICEF (2005). *The state of the world's children 2005*. New York: UNICEF.

Victora, C. G., Smith, P. G., Vaughan, J. P., Nobre, L. C., Lombardi, C., Teixeira, A. M., et al. (1987). Evidence for protection by breast-feeding against infant deaths from infectious diseases in Brazil. *Lancet, 2*, 319–322.

World Health Organization. (1998). *Ten steps to successful breastfeeding*. Geneva: World Health Organization.

World Health Organization. (2001). *The optimal duration of exclusive breastfeeding: Report of an expert consultation*. Geneva: World Health Organization.

World Health Organization. (2003). *Global strategy for infant and young child feeding*. Geneva: World Health Organization.

World Health Organization. (2007). *HIV and infant feeding: New evidence and programmatic experience*. Geneva: World Health Organization.

World Health Organization. (2010). *Guidelines on HIV and infant feeding 2010: Principles and recommendations for infant feeding in the context of HIV and a summary of evidence.* Geneva, World Health Organization.

World Health Organization Collaborative Study Team on the Role of Breastfeeding on the Prevention of Infant Mortality. (2000). Effect of breastfeeding on infant and child mortality due to infectious diseases in less developed countries: A pooled analysis. *Lancet, 355*, 451–455.

WHO/UNAIDS/UNICEF/UNFPA. (2008). *HIV transmission through breastfeeding: A review of available evidence 2007 update*. Geneva: World Health Organization.

Chapter 12
Facing Competing Cultures of Breastfeeding: The Experience of HIV-Positive Women in Burkina Faso

Alice Desclaux and Chiara Alfieri

Contents

12.1 Introduction

It is commonly assumed that in all societies the HIV pandemic has revealed and transformed social practices and their symbolic underlying logics. Its dimension of revelation is related to the link between HIV modes of transmission and the circulation of biological fluids among individuals: HIV management gives public exposure to practices that are usually intimate or hidden. It also appears when epidemiological discrepancies in HIV prevalence rates among populations reveal underlying structural inequities. Its dimension of transformation is related, among other aspects, to the extent of the epidemic's social and cultural impact and the public health measures to fight it, with consequences at micro- and macro-social levels. Which significations might these notions hold regarding infant feeding practices in West Africa: were these practices or related norms, perceptions, social roles and relationships revealed or transformed by HIV?

A. Desclaux (✉)
Hôpital de Fann, Institut de Recherche pour le Développement (UMR 145), Université Paul Cézanne d'Aix-Marseille, BP 1386, 18524 Dakar, Sénégal
e-mail: alice.desclaux@ird.fr

P. Liamputtong (ed.), *Infant Feeding Practices*, DOI 10.1007/978-1-4419-6873-9_12,
© Springer Science+Business Media, LLC 2011

Despite high numbers (several hundred thousand infants becoming HIV-positive every year in Africa due to transmission through breastfeeding),[1] it was only at the end of the 1990s[2] that this issue became a worldwide public concern beyond specialists' circles, when UN agencies published a policy (WHO/UNAIDS/UNICEF 1998). Until then, several factors had hindered the definition of preventive strategies, including the lack of easily available and low-cost technical measures and the difficulty in implementing measures that could fit in with varied social, economic, educational and material environments, when all HIV-positive women had turned to replacement feeding in developed countries. Other factors included concerns about the spread of formula feeding in resource-poor settings (see Chapters 10 and 11 in this volume) and the conceptual and organisational difficulty for health agencies that promoted breastfeeding as a healthy behaviour when considering HIV transmission (Desclaux 2000). This situation of 'secrecy and ignorance' about HIV transmission through breastfeeding and consequences regarding paediatric AIDS, while other aspects of the pandemic such as HIV sexual transmission and clinical aspects of AIDS in adults were fully acknowledged at the public level, had a particular effect on the course of HIV/AIDS public policies regarding this mode of transmission, which first prevented any 'revelation' or 'transformation'.

Over the next 11 years,[3] strategies proposed in 1998 were implemented, promoting particular infant feeding practices among HIV-positive women – exclusive breastfeeding with early weaning[4] or replacement feeding – that fit in with local norms and habits among general populations. The decision to implement one of these two feeding patterns was 'left' to women, and should have resulted from an interaction with health workers during counselling sessions before the infant's birth. In this era of 'HIV particularism', health administrations were requested to set vertical programs for Prevention of Mother-to-Child Transmission of HIV (PMTCT), responsible for making prevention available and sustainable for all women at an individual level. In countries where preventive infant feeding options did not fit in with local habits, HIV-positive women were supposed to adopt 'new' patterns recommended by the health system. Their experiences at this intersection between two sets of norms would depend on the nature and extent of divergences between locally and medically defined feeding patterns, the adaptability of each

[1]The first estimates of global figures for Africa by UN agencies remained unpublished until the 2000s.

[2]This was 17 years after the identification of HIV and 8 years after the quantification of HIV transmission through breastfeeding in Africa.

[3]New recommendations have been published in November 2009 that, using antiretroviral treatments, propose that norms regarding infant feeding pattern for all HIV-positive mothers be defined at the national level, choosing between exclusive prolonged breastfeeding or replacement feeding (WHO 2009).

[4]Categories for breastfeeding practices, which have different rates for HIV transmission, include: exclusive breastfeeding, predominant breastfeeding, complementary feeding, breastfeeding, and (WHO 2008: 4).

pattern to the local environment, the meanings conveyed by 'new' feeding patterns at the local level and the social consequences of adopting particular feeding patterns.

This era of 'HIV particularism' may end, replaced by an era of 'normalisation' when recent WHO recommendations will be implemented, since they request HIV-positive mothers to use preventive antiretroviral treatment and apply an infant feeding pattern defined at the national level. HIV-positive women's experience regarding infant feeding choice and implementation in the 2000s may remain unique. Although public health studies mostly assessed them through successes or failures in achieving safe practices, these experiences may be considered as experiments of a social innovation, revealing the capacity for change and underlying deep cultural trends in social contexts. Was this innovation endorsed in West Africa? What do HIV-positive women's experiences reveal about the local and medical cultures of infant feeding? Has the HIV epidemic jeopardised local cultures of infant feeding and brought about changes, opposition or resistance in practices, meanings or discourses?

Burkina Faso is a particularly relevant site to study these issues. The prolonged breastfeeding is applied by most women and is hardly ever 'exclusive'.[5] The HIV prevalence rate was 8.5 percent among adults at the beginning of the 2000s, which meant that the epidemic was 'generalised' beyond vulnerable groups and every family had or was related to a person living with HIV or an 'AIDS case'.[6] In Burkina Faso, WHO recommendations proposed that a very high percentage of women known to be HIV-positive adopt infant feeding practices that differed from local habits; the recommendations also outlined that feeding patterns should be defined based on each individual woman's decision.

Transformations in infant feeding were experienced by HIV-positive women at the intersection of two 'sub-cultures' – defined as systems of values, beliefs and behaviours associated with a social group: (1) the local culture of infant feeding related to infant care provision and perceptions of motherhood in a multiethnic, mostly patrilinear society with polygamous households[7]; and (2) the medical culture of health services that implement PMTCT programs based on global biomedical norms, techniques and knowledge. This 'entrance' through culture does not mean that we assume that culture explains the behaviour of all women and health workers. On the contrary, we will show in the following pages that feeding practices are greatly determined by material and economic constraints. However, shifts and

[5]Some 85 percent of children are still breastfed at the age of 20–23 months; 7 percent are exclusively breastfed at 0–7 months; 50 percent get complementary food at 6–9 months (DHS 2003).

[6]The prevalence rate among adults at the national level decreased to 2.0 percent in 2005, mainly because of the deaths of people living with HIV before antiretroviral treatments were accessible and available on a national level.

[7]Burkinabe population is multiethnic (64 ethnic groups have been identified by national institutions) with a predominance of Mossi, Bobo, Dioula and Peulh categories. The main religion is Islam, followed by Christianity and African cults.

resistances experienced by women reveal underlying patterns of roles and relationships, as well as strong beliefs and values regarding infant care, which this chapter analyses.

This analysis is based on a rich amount of empirical data. Between 2003 and 2007, we conducted a research program on social and cultural aspects of prevention of HIV transmission in Burkina Faso, using a comparative approach with four other resource-poor countries (Cameroon, Cambodia, Kenya and Cote d'Ivoire).[8] Ethnographic method was adopted combining non-structured data collection by immersion in health services and associations supporting people living with HIV, 84 structured interviews with 45 HIV-positive mothers (with infants aged between 1 and 3 months, then again between 6 and 9 months), interviews with 7 health and social workers or NGO members, focus group discussions with the same populations and a 1-month observation and recording of individual and collective counselling sessions. Data collection was implemented in Ouagadougou and Bobo-Dioulasso in public health services applying the national program and in services where a PMTCT program was supported by an NGO, an association or a clinical trial. The results were compared to previous results from a study on infant feeding perceptions, stakeholders and practices in Burkina Faso and Côte d'Ivoire before the AIDS epidemic, in 1998–1999 (Desclaux & Taverne 2000). This enabled us to identify the main trends in perceptions and practices, changes over a 5–8 year time span and variations between pilot sites hosting PMTCT programs receiving external support and 'ordinary' sites from the national program. It also enabled us to identify common situations across countries and local cultural particularities regarding counselling (Desclaux & Alfieri 2009), interactions between mothers and health workers (Desclaux, Crochet, Querre, & Alfieri 2006), roles of fathers and feasibility and acceptability of preventive strategies (Desclaux & Alfieri 2008).

12.2 The Cultural Landscape of Infant Feeding in Burkina Faso in the Early 2000s

In the early 2000s, feeding patterns most resembled those described in the 1980s in neighbouring Mali (Dettwyller 1987). The population considers prolonged breastfeeding as the best infant feeding pattern for material reasons – to feed infants based on their needs and free of cost – and for social and symbolic reasons – to integrate infants into the kinship and finish forming the persona (Dieterlein 1993). The perpetuation of breastfeeding also results from women's living conditions. With very limited industrialisation in Burkina Faso, a 'Least Developed Country',[9] most

[8]ANRS 1271 (Social Science) Research Program, conducted by CReCSS (Centre de Recherche Cultures, Santé, Sociétés, JE 2424) Université Paul Cézanne d'Aix-Marseille and funded by Agence Nationale (française) de Recherches sur le Sida et les hépatites virales. For details about ethical approval by the National Ethics Committee, see Desclaux and Alfieri 2009.

[9]According to this United Nations categorization, these countries (49 in 2009) meet the following criteria: low income, human resources weakness and economic vulnerability. According to the

women do agricultural work and handicrafts or have small businesses in the informal sector, often as individual entrepreneurs. This situation allows them to keep infants '*au dos*' (keeping them on their backs), while doing their work and breastfeeding at any time; situations of incapacity to breastfeed in the workplace are infrequent.

Infants are breastfed about 2 years: it may be much later, sometimes up to 5 years, or less if the mother becomes pregnant again. Water and herbal teas are given as early as the first days of life, considered as cleansing or preventive liquids rather than as nutritive (cf Chapter 8, 9, 12, 14 and 18 in this volume). This includes lustral water produced by using water to rinse Koranic verses written on a slate and retaining the water as an 'indigenous vaccine'. Mothers start giving small pieces of various foods and millet gruel when the infant is 3–4 months or when teeth appear. This gruel may be enriched with sugar and salt, a piece of smoked fish or an egg, as advised by Mother-and-Child Health Services or elder women. Concentrated or powdered milk is also often added, and this gruel is used until the infant is 6 or 7 months old, progressively becoming the predominant food. Fruits such as bananas or oranges are also given squashed. Infants are weaned rather rapidly when they gain a certain level of autonomy and may receive food from the family dish. However, weaning remains an important stage in local perceptions of infant development and is not considered before the child looks healthy and strong enough.

Infant feeding practices are firstly a matter of inter-generational transmission between women at the household level. The influence of 'health education' in Mother-and-Child Health Services is also perceptible in women's words when they explain the advantages of breastfeeding in nutritional terms and when they state that breastfeeding is 'the best way to care for one's baby', shifting to normative statements. These perceptions are shaped by the discourses of breastfeeding promotion, which developed in West Africa during the 1990s (Desclaux 2000). Though Burkina Faso was never affected by the extension of formula feeding, programs were developed by UNICEF and the Ministry of Health to promote breastfeeding (Programme Hôpitaux Amis des Bébés, Programme national de promotion de l'allaitement maternel) with the help of a national association (APAIB: Association pour la promotion de l'Alimentation Infantile au Burkina Faso) and an international non-governmental organisation based in Ouagadougou (IBFAN-FAN: International Baby Food Action Network-French speaking African Network). APAIB brought together mostly health workers who were also experienced mothers and worked to set up a technical discourse and 'best practices' regarding breastfeeding, focusing on feeding positions, duration, mastitis prevention and treatment and exclusive breastfeeding, among other topics. However, besides this attempt to 'professionalise' infant feeding care, breastfeeding remains mostly a matter of folk healing and household care. Exclusive breastfeeding was mainly adopted by women who were influenced by health workers – often as friends or relatives – or NGO members.

GPI, Burkina Faso ranked 164 for Gross National Income per capita with 480 USD and ranked 177 for the Human Development Index in 2008 (World Bank, see UNICEF 2007).

Moreover, the social uses of breastfeeding promotion went beyond the limitations of the health system: a growing number of stakeholders felt they had something to say regarding breastfeeding, whenever their discourse was limited to a normative assertion when directing mothers to breastfeed. This was the case for political and religious authorities locally involved in pro-breastfeeding activities, particularly during Breastfeeding World Week (Desclaux 2000). Overall, the promotion of breastfeeding has seldom introduced new concepts,[10] techniques or practices at the community level, but it has introduced notions that converge with local perceptions in favour of breastfeeding and has given breastfeeding a moral content and a strong normative value. These notions put forward biological (nutritional) and social (pro 'interaction between mother and infant') advantages and turned breastfeeding into a symbol of 'a mother's love' – a notion rooted in a Western cultural understanding of individual relationships in nuclear families. Women combine these notions with body perceptions that are based on local ethnophysiology and the actual inscribing of mother–child relationship into the family, as defined by kinship structures.[11]

Infant feeding practices have undergone recent changes in other aspects. For instance, two decades ago, it was still common to encounter an infant breastfed by a woman who was not his/her biological mother. A classificatory mother in the local kinship system, whether it be a biological grand-mother or a mother's sister, or any woman, might replace the mother by chance if the infant was found crying from hunger or fatigue, or in case of the mother's unavailability for either short or prolonged periods due to illness, absence or disqualification by an ethnomedical diagnosis of insanity. These practices seem to have disappeared in urban settings, except for a few hours after birth when a mother's sister may feed the infant until the mother gets enough milk to do it herself; replacement breastfeeding is now limited to situations of replacement mothering – such as fostering. This evolution seems to result from the influence of health workers that discouraged breastfeeding by women who were not the biological mother, even before the HIV pandemic outbreak – which reinforced this trend.

12.3 The HIV Outbreak: Introducing 'Choice' in Infant Feeding

The UN agencies' recommendations regarding prevention of HIV transmission through breastfeeding were first applied in Burkina Faso within pilot projects either supported by NGOs or implemented in conjunction with clinical trials. It took a few years to adapt a strategy beyond these sites in an environment that lacked nutritional security and adequate sanitation. In 2000, the National PMTCT program adopted the international recommendations that promoted 'informed choice' by women. After undergoing a collective and (at least one) individual counselling session during antenatal visits after her HIV status was disclosed, a woman should opt either

[10] For instance those mentioned in footnote 4.

[11] For more information on these aspects see Desclaux and Taverne (2000).

for exclusive breastfeeding with early and rapid weaning between 4 and 6 months, or for replacement feeding if feasible, accessible, acceptable, sustainable and secure.[12]

In practice, many women had the feeling that what was labelled as 'choice' by health workers was instead a decision made under constraints, since the cost of formula and its preparation prevented many of them from considering this option. The second main constraint was the social risk due to HIV stigma related to formula feeding, since, as one mother said about people in Bobo-Dioulasso: 'They say that all mothers who do not breastfeed are HIV-positive'. The ability to 'have a choice' depended essentially on the context: an actual 'choice' occurred in services supported by an NGO or a research project that could provide long-term material and psychological support to women. In other facilities, women were compelled to turn to exclusive breastfeeding, except those who could get economic support from the child's father. Besides these structural – economic and social – factors, women's changes in infant feeding patterns were also influenced by the way 'counselling for infant feeding' was interpreted by health workers. Some of them decided which option would be the best for women, based on their social and economic status. In other health services, however, where formula and equipment were provided, women reported discussions with counsellors on the advantages and inconveniences of each feeding option. Interviews show that in most cases, women would prefer replacement feeding, since any risk of HIV transmission seems unbearable for a mother to consciously take for her infant. In the 'balance of risks', compared to HIV infection, the seriousness of diarrhoea or malnutrition related to formula feeding was considered insignificant, since these diseases are common in Burkina Faso and curable.[13]

Observations of counselling sessions and narratives of infant feeding decisions by women showed that fathers were often consulted before the decision, which might involve women's HIV status disclosure. Health workers encouraged this disclosure, but it was not always planned and might be unavoidable when a father's suspicion was aroused by unusual discussion about infant feeding, normally a banal infant care practice, or when the father had some knowledge about HIV transmission through breastfeeding and personal reasons to suspect the woman's HIV-positive status. In any case, despite the efforts of the health system to support a rational decision based on the respective advantages and risks of every feeding option, this 'choice under constraints' of an infant feeding option involved relational aspects with a strong emotional content for women who frequently had limited time to

[12]In both cases, psychosocial and nutritional counselling should be provided regularly in post-natal clinics and the woman should get help in non-governmental organisations and associations supporting people living with HIV. In addition, other measures were progressively set up to consider mothers' care for HIV, based on the scaling-up of HIV care and antiretroviral treatment availability.

[13]However, breastfeeding was sometimes chosen for its contraceptive effects by women who could not access other contraceptive means. The rate of contraceptive coverage in Burkina Faso is low. Moreover, access and information about contraception among persons living with HIV, as a component of HIV care, are poorly managed in many countries. It is a concern of UN agencies.

plan for their infant feeding decision after they were informed about their own HIV status.

Regarding practices, some women managed to implement formula feeding, mostly in pilot sites and when living with a certain level of social and economic autonomy or education. Many mothers faced difficulties for implementation in their household due to the economic and social constraints mentioned above, particularly in cases of shortages of formula provided by the national program. Contrary to what some health workers had anticipated, exclusive breastfeeding was not easy, due to the discrepancies between this feeding pattern and usual ones, for instance, a mother applying a different one from the one used with a previous child. Among the women we met, many made a 'default choice' to breastfeed exclusively, then practised mixed feeding (giving liquids in addition to breastfeeding). This situation[14] resulted from their inability to constantly avoid the introduction of liquids or food other than breast milk for 6 months. However, women set up various strategies to comply with recommendations and to hide their unusual 'choice' on matters previously managed by family and community 'know-how'.

12.4 HIV-Positive Mothers' Strategies in the Community

The strategies set up by women to avoid the social consequences of discrepancies between preventive patterns and the local sub-culture of infant feeding are particularly noticeable for three aspects: avoidance of HIV stigma, implementation of 'proper' breastfeeding and the relationship with the father. Some mothers invented infant feeding patterns that had not been proposed during counselling but that allowed them to minimise the social risks, the economic cost and the biological risks of HIV transmission while preserving infant health.

Since infant breastfeeding is a common public practice when infants are carried on their mothers' backs until the children can walk alone, or even later when they are tired, comments on avoidance of breastfeeding practice may come from the family and kinship, neighbourhood, mothers' friends or women encountered in public places like the market, the field or other work places. The use of formula or early weaning may be equivalent to public disclosure about a mother's HIV-infection and arouse interpretations about the woman's ability to be a 'good mother' (cf Chapters 7 and 9 in this volume). Some mothers would combine options on a sequential mode, applying breastfeeding for a few days or weeks after birth to be acknowledged as a 'good mother' and to avoid being labelled as HIV-positive then turning to formula feeding to prevent transmission. This use of breastfeeding as 'complementary feeding' was also adopted by mothers who maintained or re-started breastfeeding instead of replacement feeding if formula became unavailable or was provided in quantities perceived as insufficient; it also allowed women to avoid suspicion of being HIV-positive. In both cases, the use of breastfeeding for social reasons was not an easy experience for women who feared HIV transmission, since they felt, as

[14]Mixed feeding carries the highest level of risk for HIV transmission.

one mother stated: 'Every time I feed my baby I tell myself I may be transmitting the virus'. Their strategy to reduce the overall proportion of breastfeeding in infant feeding was their interpretation, which was not considered by the PMTCT program.

HIV stigma was especially difficult to avoid for poorer women whose formula was provided by the national program or in pilot sites. In their cases, their supposed ability to meet this cost was questioned by the household or neighbors; women had to provide believable reasons for using expensive food instead of free mother's milk. Some of them evoked medical reasons that protected them from being considered HIV-positive: inadequate lactation, a breast pathology such as mastitis, breast cancer, and so on, which some health workers helped to put into convincing words.

For many mothers the greatest difficulty was avoiding 'herbal teas', which is considered essential by elder women who have authority on infant care in the household. On this matter as on others, the mother's ability to ignore or contradict elder women, whose expertise should be acknowledged by all young women, depends on her relative status in the household and relationship with the infant's father, since an elder woman could easily get a young mother rejected. In this case too, some women managed social and biological risks in a diachronic way: they would start with non-exclusive breastfeeding by letting their mothers-in-law perform ritual bathing on the infant despite the possibility that this includes feeding liquids, then turn to exclusive breastfeeding for the remaining months.

Water is also often given to infants by female relatives or neighbours, for instance, as a 'greeting present' for a mother and her infant when they visit a household. One way to comply with preventive recommendations according to mothers' emic perceptions is to request that only bottled water be given to their infants, since they consider it purer than other kinds of water.[15] Lastly, the ultimate strategy to avoid confrontation, which was adopted by many women to varying degrees, was to remain secluded with their infants, protecting them from any social contact that could jeopardise the exclusiveness of breastfeeding or lead to criticism and questioning. For this reason, some women avoided being helped by young family housekeeping assistants who usually take care of infants. Others would adopt a less extreme strategy, for instance, by returning for a few months to their parents' household where they could more easily limit social contact for their infants.

Regarding fathers' attitudes towards mothers, our study shows a slight change between 1999 and 2007. In initial investigations, mothers generally considered fathers as obstacles to changes in infant feeding practices, since they were reluctant about women's unusual feeding practices except in cases of a medically defined reason. They played an active role in feeding choices for their infants only when mothers were too ill to do so (or were dead) and when family support from women was lacking. At that time, few women disclosed their HIV status to their partners: in our first study only one-third had told them 6 months after the infant's birth. Most

[15]There is no epidemiological evidence for the relative safety of bottled water compared to water from other sources regarding the risk of HIV transmission when breastfeeding is no longer exclusive.

women feared rejection, when being the first one in the couple to be diagnosed with HIV often meant her being considered as the one who had brought HIV to the couple. In recent interviews, women describe most fathers as supportive or indifferent, which is often interpreted by mothers as tolerance about their HIV status and perpetuation of ascribed social roles that give mothers full responsibility for infant care. Fewer women than in our previous study (about one-third) maintained secrecy about their HIV status as a strategy to avoid fathers' adverse reactions. In most cases, they used many precautions when communicating with them: carefully choosing the time to discuss this matter; relying on significant others such as a father's relative to show support or to act as an intermediary; requesting health workers to disclose their HIV status for them; or using means in the interaction that allowed denial in case of violent reaction – such as using 'half words', speaking of HIV-positive persons in general before coming to their own case or using euphemistic words. These aspects are not secondary matters regarding infant feeding, since rejection of a mother by her husband may completely disable her from providing proper and safe care to her infant.

Fathers' attitudes about infant feeding varied, depending on their perceptions of feeding options and their trust in preventive strategies when considering the cost for the household (cf Chapter 3 in this volume). The father's own experience with his HIV status, whether denial, ignorance or awareness, and his relationship to the mother will determine whether she must handle things alone or whether he will help her with child care after the disclosure. In some cases she will implement a strategy that also meets the needs of her other children. Recent investigations showed that more fathers supported women in their preventive decisions, which made it easier for mothers to handle questions from their families. This was especially the case when fathers knew that they were HIV-positive themselves. In some cases, fathers shared the decision about infant feeding; they would often be more cautious than women in avoiding any exposure to HIV whatever the benefits of breastfeeding and advice from health workers on that topic may be.

12.5 HIV-Positive Mothers' Strategies in Health Services

Contrary to what might be expected, women's interviews showed that their situations were not totally secure to implement preventive infant feeding options in health services settings.

The first reason is related to the institutional organisation of the management of infant feeding and HIV issues. Since relevant programs – the program for the promotion of breastfeeding and the AIDS program – are both vertically designed; and despite the political will to 'integrate' them at the local level during the 2000s, their implementation in health services never underwent consistent integration. As a result, the particular needs of HIV-positive women, for instance, regarding preventive feeding patterns, were still treated as contradicting and endangering the promotion of breastfeeding. HIV-positive mothers found this to be especially true when they were in Mother-and Child-Health services and confronted by posters claiming that 'Breast is Best', even though PMTCT programs were housed in the same services. Women would also receive contradictory messages, for instance, between Mother-and-Child Health workers unaware of a mother's HIV-positive status encouraging her to breastfeed as soon and as long as possible, when other health workers assigned to the PMTCT program advised her to do early weaning or replacement feeding. In this case, silence was the most frequently used strategy, whatever the uneasiness generated by the contradictions between health workers' messages.

Women experienced the risk of being labelled as HIV-positive, which has not totally disappeared in health services. Although stigma and rejection are now less common, some health workers still avoid relationships with HIV-positive persons, fearing they would not act properly or may breach confidentiality about their HIV status. In maternity wards where health workers considered promotion of breastfeeding as their priority, some women were compelled to reveal their HIV status to defend their withdrawal of colostrum or their refusal to place the infant on the breast immediately after birth. Women sometimes used strategies that could be dangerous for themselves or their babies, as in the case of one woman who only gave water to her baby for three days pretending that she was breastfeeding him, fearing both HIV transmission if she breastfed and being labelled as HIV-positive if she needed formula.

HIV-positive women also create strategies to work around follow-up by health workers. In terms of counselling, follow-up for nutritional purposes might be fairly prescriptive or comprehensive, depending on the health workers' knowledge and experience regarding HIV and counseling (see also Chapter 11 in this volume). Health workers' attitudes were also different among those who had strong opinions in favour of breastfeeding and advised it in any situation and others who considered respective HIV levels of risk and thought that formula was feasible in the local context. There were also differences in discourses between health workers who were 'optimistic' about women's ability to stick to the option she had chosen and those who were 'realistic' and considered that each choice might entail challenges in an evolving context. In many cases, women were criticised for being unable to apply preventive patterns that were beyond their scope, since this depended on the unpredictable attitudes of persons such as husbands or elder women who had authority in the household. Thus, the easiest strategy to avoid this undeserved treatment was lying to health workers about the feeding pattern used or how it was implemented. Some health workers would respond by using their own strategies to verify the mothers' statements, observing the infant's body language in proximity of the breast of a mother who pretended not to breastfeed or by pinching the mother's nipple to see if she was still breastfeeding after the prescribed weaning date.

As a result of HIV stigmatisation, women who feared being identified as HIV-positive also had to set strategies to avoid being seen in HIV-related places such as associations for people living with AIDS, pretending to go to Mother-and-Child Health Services or elsewhere. Yet, women who were supported by an NGO or PLHIV group or by counsellors from a research team managed to comply more easily with their chosen feeding option. Material means, free provision of substitutes and equipment and the delivery of more individualised information are not the only factors involved. In the 'space of confidentiality' of a support group, they are not compelled, as in health services and at home, to avoid certain subjects or justify their actions. They appreciate the opportunity to talk freely about various psychological and social aspects of HIV infection related to managing relationships with significant others, since these aspects are important for the feasibility of preventive options. They also find more coherent and contextualised discourses regarding infant feeding and HIV than in some health services, where partially different and non-articulated discourses for HIV-positive and HIV-negative mothers are confusing. Yet, many women did not take full advantage of these possibilities when they were unable to justify to their husbands why they were leaving the household for an indisputable medical reason, as is the case for going to health services.

12.6 Conclusion: The Evolving Culture of Infant Feeding in the Age of HIV

Women's experiences and the strategies they must set up to apply preventive feeding patterns reveal several aspects of local cultures that are not exclusively related to either health services or the community.

HIV-positive women who are literate and have a certain level of social and economic autonomy may assert their decision and manage implementing any infant feeding option, including formula feeding, whatever criticisms may arise in either health services or households. This is also the case for women who share the management of HIV with their husbands. This observation, which stresses the importance of personal autonomy or support in the couple, is consistent with observations made about HIV prevention in other settings (Buskens, Jaffe, & Mkhatshwa 2007; Leshabari, Blystad, & Moland 2007; Hofmann, de Allegria, Sarker, Sanon, & Böhler 2009) or for other kinds of challenges in women's lives, whatever the cultural setting.

Their experiences also show that most women may apply preventive recommendations fully and with ease only when they are alone with their infants. They often are compelled to 'maintain distance' from the actors of infant feeding in order to avoid the risk of being labelled as HIV-positive or as a 'bad mother'. This explains situations of psychological distress among some women who bear these constraints alone in addition to planned isolation. It also reveals to what extent infant feeding is a social behaviour, involving several protagonists, many of whom feel they have the legitimacy to define what is good for the infant. On this issue, the HIV pandemic stresses the discrepancy between community and health services, since the international medical culture considers the mother as the infant's sole caretaker who can make 'individual choices', and often blames her when she is the victim,[16] which is a consequence of individualising social problems (see also Chapters 2, 5 and 9 in this volume).

[16]The idiom 'blaming the victim' coined in the mid-1970s by the sociologist William Ryan was applied in the 1990s by Paul Farmer in the field of AIDS and summarises a major theoretical interpretation trend of social processes related to the AIDS pandemic (Farmer 1992).

The difficulties women face when trying to apply an alternative to breastfeeding or to limit its duration to 4–6 months reveal not only the normative strength of breastfeeding promotion and popular perceptions but also their rationales. In health services as well as in the community, biological considerations and precise categorisation have little weight compared to the social and symbolic logics in defence of breastfeeding – whatever its mode of implementation according to nutritionists' categories – when a full range of actors under various ideological or social guidance have added to its long-standing perceived benefits. This strange ambiguity turns maintaining a mode of HIV transmission into the absence of contamination and thus challenges communication about health. For this aspect, the HIV pandemic revealed, and maybe in some areas such as Burkina Faso paradoxically reinforced, the symbolic value of breastfeeding. The threat that formula feeding practices would spillover beyond HIV-positive mothers, often evoked by child specialists, never became an empirical concern since formula is a sign of mothers' HIV infection and thus a highly stigmatised behaviour.

The mothers' experiences stress the symbolic construction, perceptible in both health discourses and institutional organisation, of an opposition between breastfeeding and HIV – two heterogeneous categories. Some health workers still seem to believe, as one public health official said in the late 1990s: 'The problem is not breastfeeding, it is HIV-positive mothers'.[17] In this context, narrated experiences may be interpreted as the result of the embodiment of global categories with profound symbolic content (considering 'good' breastfeeding as opposed to 'bad' HIV) for women who may both breastfeed and be infected by HIV. As for conceptualisation of breastfeeding which, even in health settings, is still considered under a monothetic category when characterisation on a biological basis requires at least four categories,[18] this symbolic opposition, which seems hardly questioned by evidence, appears as a fundamental concept in medical culture.

The range of strategies applied by women to reduce social and biological risks for their infants and themselves is wide. For instance, they would often use several feeding options one after another when medical recommendations request that one is chosen 'for good' and applied without any variation. Women would also adapt the feeding pattern according to changing social contexts, which is not supported by PMTCT. They would set 'risk reduction' when PMTCT claims 'risk withdrawal', when they either used mixed feeding or were ready to re-start breastfeeding in case of a formula shortage. These hybrid patterns, which showed women's capacity and limits in adapting to their context, are not valued by the health system since they do not correspond to the strictly defined patterns that were validated by experimental clinical trials.[19] There, women's experiences reveal the rigidity of medical concepts, which lack the sensitivity to contexts that are empirically developed by women. Further studies in political science are necessary to understand how this lack

[17] Abidjan, personal communication, author's translation (*'Le problème c'est pas l'allaitement, c'est les femmes séropositives'.*).

[18] See footnote 4.

[19] From an epidemiological perspective, the overall reduction of milk intake should reduce HIV transmission.

of acknowledgement is, on this particular topic, related to social and gender status differences between women in Burkina Faso – who are poorly represented as a community force capable of social 'transformation' – and scientists at the international level.

Shared decision-making with fathers was advised by health workers, who acknowledge the need for fathers' psychological and material involvement to support mothers made vulnerable by the risk of HIV stigma; it may also result from defined gender roles inspired by Western-orientated patterns, which underlie UN agency recommendations for HIV counselling, implemented by health workers in PMTCT programs. Before, it was mainly women who provided care, assisted by grandmothers and elder women. Now, because they are afraid of a possible breach in confidentiality and rejection from the extended family, decision-making is increasingly limited to couples, which subsequently means greater involvement from men. This focus on the couple, which also emphasises sharing responsibilities equally between men and women and promoting rights of individuals among PLHIV whatever their gender as a means of protection against rejection, is also enhanced in some PLHIV organisations and publicly demonstrated by their leaders.

Focusing on the parental couple or nuclear family and on the mother–child interaction rather than on extended family are preventive discourses that convey social models from Western or global cultures. Whether instrumental, aimed at avoiding HIV-labelling by the extended family or intertwined with medical media and messages, these models have spread with the globalised AIDS culture conveyed particularly by NGOs and PLHIV associations. More than the 'therapeutic citizenship' that has not yet developed in Africa in the field of PMTCT (Blystad & Moland 2009), contrary to other fields (Nguyen, Ako, Niamba, Sylla, & Tiendrébéogo 2007), this individualising and nuclear pattern in family social organisation, which also corresponds to a shift in gender roles, may be the social transformation brought about by the HIV pandemic through the prevention of HIV breastfeeding transmission.

Acknowledgments We would like to thank women and caregivers that devoted time to this research. We also thank Kesho Bora Group, Centre Muraz, Association Espoir pour Demain (Bobo-Dioulasso), Centre Medical avec Antenne chirurgicale de Pissy, Vie Positive, Médecins sans Frontières (Ouagadougou), and the teams in health facilities that made this research possible.

References

Blystad, A., & Moland K. A. (2009). Technologies of hope? Motherhood, HIV and infant feeding in eastern Africa. *Anthropology and Medicine, 16*(2), 105118.

Buskens, I., Jaffe, A., & Mkhatshwa, H. (2007). Infant feeding practices: Realities and mindsets of mothers in southern Africa. *AIDS Care, 19*(9), 1101–1109.

Demographic and Health Survey Data Base, undated. *HIV/AIDS indicators country report.* Burkina Faso 1992/1993–2003. Macro Inc. Retrieved 4 January 2010, from http://www.measuredhs.com/hivdata/start.cfm

Desclaux, A. (2000). *L'épidémie invisible. Anthropologie d'un système de santé à l'épreuve du sida chez l'enfant à Bobo Dioulasso*, Burkina Faso. Lille, France: Presses Universitaires du Septentrion.

Desclaux, A., & Taverne, B. (Eds) (2000). *Allaitement et VIH en Afrique de l'ouest. De l'anthropologie à la santé publique*. Paris, France: Karthala. Retrieved 4 January 2010, from http://classiques.uqac.ca/contemporains/Desclaux_alice/allaitement_et_VIH/allaitement_et_VIH.html

Desclaux, A., & Alfieri, C. (2008). Allaitement, VIH et prévention au Burkina Faso. Les déterminants sociaux ont-ils changé? *Science et Technique, Série Sciences de la santé*, Special issue n°1, November 2008: Sida, santé publique et sciences sociales. Vingt ans d'épidémie et de recherche au Burkina Faso, 117–126.

Desclaux, A., & Alfieri, C. (2009). Counselling and choosing between infant-feeding options: Overall limits and local interpretations by health care providers and women living with HIV in resource-poor countries (Burkina Faso, Cambodia, Cameroon). *Social Science and Medicine, 69*(6), 821–829.

Desclaux, A., Crochet, S., Querre, M., & Alfieri, C. (2006). Le "choix informé" des femmes séropositives qui doivent alimenter leur enfant : interprétations locales, limites et nouvelles questions. In A. Desgrées du Lou, & B. Ferry (Eds.), *Sexualité et procréation confrontées au Sida dans les pays du Sud* (pp. 245–262). Paris, France: CEPED.

Detwyller, K. A. (1987). Breastfeeding and weaning in Mali. Cultural context and hard data. *Social Science and Medicine, 24*(8), 633–644.

Dieterlein, G. (Ed.) (1993 [1971]). *La notion de personne en Afrique noire*. Paris, France: L'Harmattan.

Farmer, P. (1992). *AIDS and accusation: Haiti and the geography of blame*. Los Angeles: University of California Press.

Hofmann, J., de Allegria, M., Sarker, M., Sanon, M., & Böhler, T. (2009). Breast milk as the "water that supports and preserves life" – Socio-cultural constructions of breastfeeding and their implications for the prevention of mother to child transmission of HIV in sub-Saharan Africa. *Health Policy, 89*, 322–323.

Leshabari, S. C., Blystad, A., & Moland, K. M. (2007). Difficult choices: Infant feeding experiences of HIV-positive mothers in northern Tanzania. *Journal of Social Aspects of HIV/AIDS, 4*(1), 544–555.

Nguyen, V. K., Ako, C. Y., Niamba, P., Sylla, A., & Tiendrébéogo, I. (2007). Adherence as therapeutic citizenship: Impact of the history of access to antiretroviral drugs on adherence to treatment. *AIDS, 21*, 31–35.

UNICEF. (2007). *The state of the world's children 2008. Child survival*. New York: UNICEF.

WHO/UNAIDS/UNICEF. (1998). *HIV and infant feeding: A guide for health care managers and supervisors*. Geneva: Suisse, WHO/FRH/NUT/CHD/98.2.

World Health Organization. (2008). *Indicators for assessing infant and young child feeding practices*. Conclusions of a consensus meeting held 6–8 November 2007 in Washington, DC, USA. Retrieved 4 January 2010, from http://whqlibdoc.who.int/publications/2008/9789241596664_eng.pdf

World Health Organization. (2009). *Rapid advice: Revised WHO principles and recommendations infant feeding in the context of HIV*. Geneva: November 2009. Retrieved 4 January 2010, from http://www.who.int/child_adolescent_health/documents/9789241598873/en/index.html

Chapter 13
Fluid Boundaries: Multiple Meanings of the Illness '*Moto*' in Northern Malawi

Laura Sikstrom, Rachel Bezner Kerr, and Laifolo Dakishoni

Contents

13.1 Introduction

The emerging social studies of childhood demonstrates that local conceptualisations of childhood influence caretaking arrangements (Weisner & Gallimore 1977; Engle & Breaux 1994; Hewlett, Lamb, Shannon, Leyendecker, & Scholmerich 1998; Matthews & Limb 1999; Gottlieb 2004; Kramer 2005; Bolin 2006), alter nutrition and feeding practices (Richards 2004[1932]; Roopnarine, Fouts, Lamb, & Lewis-Elligan 2005; Deardon et al. 2009) and health seeking practices and treatment options when a child becomes ill (Kamat 2006; Munthali 2007). In Northern Malawi, *moto*, which means 'heat' or 'fire' in the local language chiTumbuka, is a childhood illness that presents as a syndrome with common symptoms including a

L. Sikstrom (✉)
Department of Anthropology, University of Toronto, 19 Russell St., Toronto, ON, M5S-2S2, Canada
e-mail: lsikstrom@yahoo.ca

P. Liamputtong (ed.), *Infant Feeding Practices*, DOI 10.1007/978-1-4419-6873-9_13,

© Springer Science+Business Media, LLC 2011

'hot' or 'weak' body, persistent diarrhoea and fast or troubled breathing (Munthali, 2007). Often, it is an older female relative, such as the mother-in-law, who provides the final diagnosis and organises treatment. Treatment is an herbal infusion administered orally called '*mzuwula*'. However, from a public health perspective, *mzuwula* may also introduce dangerous pathogens, which could increase the chances of diarrhoeal incidence, reduce breastfeeding intensity and duration and, therefore, increase the likelihood of an early death from a preventable illness.[1] Moreover, estimates indicate that there are approximately 91,000 children, ages 0–14 year (UNAIDS, 2008) infected with HIV in Malawi, and recent studies indicate that transmission of HIV from mother to infant is significantly reduced if the mother practices exclusive breastfeeding (Coovadia et al. 2007).

The cause of *moto* is conceptualised as '*wajumpikha*' or the idea of 'crossing over' cultural taboos and expectations. The bodies of young children and elderly people are regarded as particularly vulnerable to exposure by being touched by someone engaged in 'promiscuous' sexual behaviour or by eating food from a fire shared by such an individual. Sexual promiscuity in this context is defined as sexual practices outside accepted norms, including postpartum sexual intercourse in marriage. Therefore, it has critical implications for young child care and infant feeding since the parents (and especially breastfeeding mothers) are the most likely source of infection. Many would argue that *moto* is a 'remnant cultural belief' that will disappear over time. However, in this chapter we argue that *moto* is a fluid concept that has evolved over time to provide meaning to the phenomena observed by caretakers of sick children.

This chapter will discuss these research findings in relation to Malawi's high HIV prevalence, discuss areas of further inquiry and the possible implications for public health programs focused on early child care and infant feeding. In particular, this research has implications for programs promoting exclusive breastfeeding aiming to reduce infant mortality and prevent maternal-to-child transmission of HIV (PMTCT). There are several challenges for public health programs that encounter 'culture bound syndromes' that do not fit biomedical classifications and that are fraught with multifaceted conflicts.[2] First, how do we situate our analysis of local

---

[1]Epidemiological data shows that more than 12 percent of children from rural Malawi die before their fifth birthday (MICS 2006[0]). Significantly, Malawi has the fourth[0] highest stunting rate in the world; 46 percent of under-five children are too short for their age, an indication of chronic undernutrition over an extended period of time (MICS 2006). The most common causes of death in young children are first acute respiratory infection, diarrhoea and undernutrition, malaria and HIV[0]. Some of the major immediate causes of child mortality and undernutrition include low exclusive breastfeeding rates (57 percent) and dietary deficiencies in micronutrients (Black et al. 2008a).

[2]A 'culture bound syndrome' by definition is a set of psychiatric and/or bodily symptoms that are classified as a disease in one culture but not in others. The concept first developed in psychiatry (Yap 1967) and was later used by anthropologists and sociologists the late 1970s and 1980s. Although considerable debate still exists about the term (Guarnaccia & Rogler 1999) Young's research on post-traumatic stress disorder among Vietnam war veterans demonstrates the importance of examining the social, geographical and historical context of any disease whether it is

representations of *moto* in relation to the truth claims of biomedicine, in ways that link to effective breastfeeding and complementary feeding education? In this context, these claims include, but are not limited to, the belief that the introduction of non-breast milk liquids is dangerous and potentially fatal for a child; that 'promiscuity' does not cause a child to get sick; that *mzuwula* has no medicinal benefits; that *moto* is actually a biomedical illness; and that 'traditional beliefs' are both erroneous and dangerous. Second, how can public health issues be successfully tackled when they are directly linked to the intimacy of competing gender and generational demands at the household level, while remaining respectful towards indigenous systems of healing and belief?

These issues have important repercussions for efforts to address the infant mortality and malnutrition rates in Malawi. How illnesses are treated have a very real impact on child health and mortality outcomes. Our aim is not to provide comprehensive solutions to this problem but to raise questions that will orient future research. Our discussions of *moto*, therefore, cannot and should not be separated from present day realities in Malawi. Our objectives of this study were to examine local child care practices (including feeding and care during illness), knowledge of childhood illnesses and the underlying explanatory theories that give meaning to what people do and observe when children become ill (Green, Jurg, & Djedje 1994; Yoder 1997). To this end, we conducted research in Ekwendeni region of Mzimba district, Malawi, over a 4 year period as part of the *Soils, Food and Healthy Communities Project's* (SFHC) ongoing development and research activities. The purpose of the research was to gather information that would help in developing a culturally appropriate strategy for the prevention and treatment of infant and childhood malnutrition.

13.2 Theoretical Framework

The theoretical framework for this paper, which guided the interpretation and analysis of the findings, is adapted from discussions by Good (1994, pp. 1–64) on the problem of 'belief' in medical anthropology. Good (1994) argues that there persists an empiricist tradition in medical anthropology that uncritically juxtaposes 'traditional medical beliefs' against 'biomedical knowledge'. Despite these critiques, Primary Health Care practitioners around the world, and in Malawi specifically, often implicitly or explicitly take the biomedical model as the normative framework, and try to learn about 'traditional' practices in order to design interventions to change them (Yoder 1997). More recent studies identify the ways in which dominant discourses on sexuality and morality place local, indigenous knowledge and practice as deviant and 'other' in comparison to the biomedical model (Lwanda, 2004; Adams & Pigg 2005). Our approach in this paper is to 'replace belief and

---

recognised by biomedicine or not (Young 1995, see also Lock 1995 and Kalipeni et al. 2004 for other examples).

culture as explanatory of behavior, with a theory of the relation of knowledge to practice that recognizes the situated and constructed nature' (Yoder 1997, p.141). Drawing on studies of colonial biomedical practice in Africa (Vaughan 1991), we also consider the ways in which biomedicine is a healing system with a complex set of ideas and practices that are historically situated and dynamic. We view the experience and treatment of *moto* in the contemporary period as a contested site of power and knowledge at multiple fault lines: genders, generations, classes and ethnicities (Foucault 1980). Rather than ask what *moto* is in relation to biomedical illnesses, we ask: how is *moto* interpreted in relation to current events and what are the implications for feeding and care practices?

13.3 The Study

Malawi has a population of 13 million people, most of whom are smallholder farmers, and a gross national product of $160 USD per capita (UNDP 2008). In the past decade, anywhere between 70 and 85 percent of households ran out of their own food stocks several months prior to the next harvest, creating an annual 'hungry season' (Bezner Kerr 2005; Conroy & Blackie 2005). Compounding these issues are current high rates of HIV prevalence, estimated at 11.9 percent (UNAIDS 2008), which increases household food and nutritional needs and reduces labour availability (Gillespie 2006). The dominance of HIV/AIDS in everyday life also leads to complex discourses around societal changes (Kaler 2004), which in this paper we relate to child care practices. Ekwendeni, a town of approximately 20,000 inhabitants, is in northern Malawi, in Mzimba District. Ekwendeni Hospital was founded by Scottish missionaries in the late 1800s, and is now run by the Church of Central African Presbyterian (McCracken 1977). The Primary Health Care (PHC) department has been working in the surrounding rural areas for over 20 years, with mobile maternal and child health clinics, a community grain bank and other health programs. The research was conducted as part of a participatory agriculture and nutrition project, spearheaded by Ekwendeni Hospital and described in detail elsewhere (Bezner Kerr & Chirwa 2004). All research was carried out in the Ekwendeni Hospital region of approximately 500 square kilometres with a population of approximately 70,000 people.

This research combined qualitative and quantitative research methods, with three primary types of data collection reported in this chapter: (1) semi-structured interviews; (2) focus groups; (3) participatory workshops. A survey which provides quantitative evidence of these feeding practices is described in another related paper (Bezner Kerr et al. 2007). All research activities except for the 2005 interviews are detailed in earlier papers (Bezner Kerr et al., 2007, 2008) and described briefly below.

Twenty-one semi-structured interviews on childcare and feeding practices were carried out in 2001 with a range of villagers purposefully selected based on their knowledge of child care and feeding practices (Liamputtong 2009). Two follow-up focus groups were carried out, one with a group of four older women considered to be knowledgeable about child feeding and the other with a group of eight younger women with young children. Key hospital staff informants involved in breastfeeding education and maternal and child health care were also interviewed. After further analysis of the data, the research team carried out nine follow-up interviews in 2004 on traditional herbal infusions. The second and third author contributed to the development of the interview guide. Nine informants were purposefully selected based on gender and age. Each interview took approximately one hour, and was tape-recorded. In July 2005, we conducted 38 interviews in three purposefully sampled village areas in the Ekwendeni Catchment area. Qualitative research training was conducted over three days with SFHC staff and eight Farmer Research Team (FRT) members. The interviews lasted between one and two hours and were later translated into English, and analysed by the authors for trends, differences and common themes. Following the content and thematic analysis (Liamputtong 2009), the first and third author conducted seven follow-up interviews with local female farmers and conducted two focus group discussions. In addition, the first author interviewed four staff members at Ekwendeni hospital and FRT members.

A participatory workshop was held in 2003, and participants included grandmothers, food insecure farmers, young mothers, community leaders, project participants and hospital staff with experience in breastfeeding and complementary feeding nutrition education. The workshop consisted of oral presentations, dramas and songs from the community members and researchers on the different themes, group discussions and planning for follow-up activities. The second and third author participated in these research activities, including notes and observation.

13.4 The Polluting Touch: Symptoms and Causation of *Moto*

Moto is a syndrome with a complex array of symptoms that affects children and to a lesser degree, older adults. The most common sign of *moto* is fast or troubled breathing, a persistent cough, diarrhoea, white mucus and a 'weak' child (see Table 13.1). Women described several common signs of *moto:* if a child cried when lifted, coughed a certain way, or when lifted was very light. As one young mother stated:

> The child says "ah, ah, ah" – has pains in the chest and you can hear the child breathing from far away. (the young mother points at our vehicle parked two houses away). July 2005.

A child may also be diagnosed with *moto* after death; it is suspected if white mucus comes out of the nostrils. In addition, the research identified eight types of locally defined diarrhoea, two of which are possible symptoms of *moto*. *Chikhakha* is white diarrhoea with pus that usually occurs if the mother breastfeeds while pregnant; in these cases a mother stops breastfeeding immediately. *Chingwenya* was described as the most serious type of diarrhoea since it often leads to death. A child

Table 13.1 *Moto* symptoms (August 2005 Post-Harvest Survey, N=41)

Symptom	Response
Persistent or chronic coughing	14
Diarrhoea (*Chikhakha* and *Chingwenya*)	13
Child is weak	12
Fever/High Body temperature	11
Swollen	6
Failing to breath	6
Stunted growth	5
Pale skin/hair	5
Thin/No appetite	5
Baby cries when held	4
Pneumonia	3
Ill and/or faints frequently	3
Anaemia	2
Child Looks unhealthy	1
Child Vomits	1
Malnutrition	1
Cerebral malaria	1
Child sick when mother is pregnant	1

with *Chingwenya* has chronic diarrhoea that causes wounds at the anus over time. One young mother we interviewed had a 6-month-old son who was diagnosed with *moto* by her mother-in-law. She stated that his symptoms included, anaemia, being ill frequently, a persistent cough, and he had frequent diarrhoea that sometimes had blood in it. He was treated with both traditional and Western medicines and eventually recovered.

At the heart of the cause of *moto* are ideas concerning 'promiscuity', which can take place within the household or village. Promiscuity in this case refers to several types of sexual practice: prostitution, adultery or the breaking of the 1 year postpartum sexual taboo by the husband and wife. Prostitutes (women described as 'roaming' villages looking for sex) could make a child sick if they touched or made contact (e.g. through food that they prepare and the child eats) with that child. Anyone committing adultery could make someone get *moto* within a village, and sexual intercourse between a husband and wife during the first year of the infant's life, or during the breastfeeding phase can also give *moto* to that infant, to children or the elderly:

> *Moto* is caused by '*wajumpikha*' (going across the 'boundary' or 'going out of bounds'). In this village boys and girls might have sex and when they're together their chests get warm and that heat is transferable to the child through the mother when she breastfeeds (young mother, July 2005).

Newborns less than 2 months old are considered particularly vulnerable to 'bad behaviour' of husbands (i.e. adultery or postpartum sex with the wife). In keeping with another study describing *moto* in northern Malawi (Munthali 2007), our results indicate that there are various reasons that sexual promiscuity may cause *moto*.

These findings indicate that 'crossing over' the boundaries of culturally appropriate sexual behavior is linked to *moto*. A child suffering from *moto* may have only one of the above symptoms, but more often he or she has a combination of chronic symptoms. Causation is explained with a combination of biomedical and indigenous terms such as '*wajumpikha*' 'veins' and 'blood', but is directly linked to sexual intercourse:

> If a boy or girl go out and have sex from a household, and if they cook or touch the fireplace, whatever is cooked from there will cause the child to get sick (Older woman, July 2005).

The term *moto* refers to the heat produced during sex, which is passed onto a child during breastfeeding, from the food cooked over a fire that was touched by a 'promiscuous' individual, or from direct contact with that individual. Other respondents talked about the ways in which *moto* creates 'heat' that can then be transferred to children or the elderly through breastfeeding, touch, food or through fire:

> The blood comes from the man during sex, and it's that heat or blood which is transferred to the breast of the mother and the child gets *moto* (young mother, July 2005).

Men's sperm is considered to be particularly strong and dangerous, suggesting alternative reasons (beyond HIV prevention) for the increased condom use in Malawi; national contraceptive prevalence rates have increased from 13 percent in 1992 to 26 percent in 2004 (Smith & Watkins 2005; Kalipeni & Ghosh 2006; Chimbiri 2007; Bankole, Singh, Hussain, & Oestreicher 2009).

> If the mother and father have sex when the mother is still breastfeeding the child will get *moto*. The sperm that is left in the mother is sooo strong and it affects the body of the mother. It flows to her breast in the blood, through her veins and the child will start coughing (Older woman, July 2005).

More importantly, *moto* exemplifies how particular understandings of the human body shape social interactions and bodily practice in particular places (see for example McDowell 1999; Lock & Farquhar 2007). Intimate gendered and generational social relationships (such as those between a husband and a wife, or a father and child) are regulated in this case by a specific understanding of young children's bodies. Sexually active adult bodies can pollute more vulnerable and permeable non-adult bodies (especially newborn bodies) through touch or proximity. The result is that men were rarely observed holding newborns, or feeding them and that newborns are often covered up to protect them from a man's polluting gaze.[3] 'Youth' (unmarried, post-pubescent boys and girls) are also rarely involved in child care for the same reason, unlike pre-pubescent girls, who are often left to care for younger siblings. Moreover, intergenerational conflicts between youth and elders (often elder women and their daughters-in-law) centre around accusations of carelessness, and 'bad behavior' [*Ukwenda waka* – they just wander]. These conflicts work to regulate younger women's bodies, who are blamed for children's

---

[3]In this context, two of the markers indicating a transition from 'newborn' status to 'child' is that the child develops 'curly' hair and begins to smell 'human'. This transition usually occurs at 1-2 months of age when the child's newborn (straight) hair is shaved.

illnesses, even though it is the interaction between men and women's bodies that are the polluting source. Therefore, *moto* is not merely a 'remnant cultural belief' but one aspect of a larger set of gendered and generational bodily practices that may also have health consequences for young children. See also Chapter 14 in this volume.

13.5 Permeable Bodies, Fluid Boundaries and Treatment Practice

In our findings, the most common treatment for signs of *moto* was an herbal infusion called *mzuwula*, given both as *protection* and as *treatment*. In both cases, the child is usually bathed in, and given a small handful of *mzuwula* to drink. To protect against *moto*, a child is bathed and/or given *mzuwula* at birth, before the child is touched by people from outside the household. Children's bodies are 'softer' than adults, and skin seems to be considered particularly permeable at birth, which not only allows the *mzuwula* to take effect but also makes newborns very vulnerable to polluting touches. The timing of giving *mzuwula* as protection to a newborn differs from community to community. Some communities wait until the umbilical cord falls, while others wait until the baby is taken out of the house after birth, which is usually about 1 week. Older women (especially the paternal grandmother) of that village control the practice. Men know little about the practice, and knowledge is passed onto young mothers after the birth of their first child by their mothers-in-law.

The frequency, duration and method of administering *mzuwula* differ depending on the community, the severity of the symptoms, the age of the person affected and individual discrepancy. A child might be given *mzuwula* several times a day until the sickness disappears; newborns are bathed and young children might wear amulets around their necks or beads around their waists that releases the medicines when they bath and then absorbed through the skin. One boy was given both *mzuwula* and tablets from the hospital when his diarrhoea persisted after the *mzuwula* treatment. In interviews, women would often demonstrate the method used to give children *mzuwula* by cupping their hand below their lips and tossing the pretend liquid quickly into their mouths. Elderly people are also given *mzuwula* as a treatment if they are seen to be affected with *moto*. Informants also reported that a number of different traditional herbs are also used; they were either used as a liquid to be drunk or to rub into wounds on the chest that are cut by a traditional healer. The last method is often used if the *moto* is particularly severe since it allows the medicines to enter directly into the bloodstream.

Mzuwula are species of trees that are found in the upland and river valleys. There are multiple ways that *mzuwula* is used to treat or prevent *moto*. One method involves plucking the leaves and pounding in a mortar. Some cold water is added in the mortar or as it comes out of the mortar. An axe is heated and then is held in one hand while the pounded leaves are squeezed, such that the liquid from the pounded leaves falls on the heated axe into a container. The child then drinks this liquid. In the second method, the leaves are plucked and pounded in a mortar, then water is heated and the pounded leaves are added and the child is bathed in the liquid. Another method is also to prevent *moto* from affecting the child. The *mzuwula* are dug and mixed with roots from other trees (informants would not give the names of these trees). The roots are bound together and buried at the hearth. This action prevents future *moto* occurrence within that household from happening to their children.

A common warning given by older people to the younger generation is: 'If you practice promiscuity your children will die of *moto*'. If men and women practice promiscuity, the whole village could be affected with *moto*, through the exchange of fire from one hearth to the other. Older women at the participatory workshop argued that the breaking of sexual taboos was part of a broader trend in their communities, in which young people did not respect traditional ways, leading to high rates of HIV/AIDS (Bezner Kerr et al. 2008). Survey data collected in 2002 as part of the broader research project provided strong evidence for the early introduction of herbal infusions (Bezner Kerr et al. 2007). About half of the survey respondents reported giving *mzuwula* to their infants by 1 month of age, indicating that these practices were common at the time of data collection.[4] National survey data in 1998 showed that more than 60 percent of women in the north abstained from sex for the first year of their babies' lives, compared to 20 percent in the south and central regions of Malawi (Zulu 2001). The period of postpartum abstinence has declined nationally from an average of 9 months in 1992 to 6 months in 2004 (Palamuleni 2008).

In Malawi, HIV prevention campaigns are encouraging women to resume sexual relations with their husbands early to prevent adultery (and therefore HIV). However, the period of post partum amenorrhoea has also reduced from 12.1 months in 1992 to 9 months in 2004 (NSO & ORC Macro 2005). A decline in this rate is indicative of changes in the duration and intensity of breastfeeding practices – a factor that has serious child health implications (Simondon et al. 2003). The early termination of breastfeeding puts a child at an increased risk of developing symptoms of malnutrition-related illnesses like diarrhoea (Black et al. 2008a). HIV prevention campaigns tell women to resume sex early; however, the early resumption of sexual relations may cause *moto* since the mother is still breastfeeding (the most common source of transmission) and therefore families are likely to introduce potentially diarrhoea-inducing substances like *mzuwula* to protect a child from *moto*. Mothers also reported providing their breastfeeding infant with sugar water or porridge rather than breast milk if they had recently had sex, indicating that sexual practices also alter breastfeeding practices.

---

[4]During 2008-09 fieldwork by the first author, there were persistent rumours of children being kidnapped by witches in their sleep to be tortured and/or trained to be witches. One rationale given for this increase in child kidnapping is that parents are not protecting their children with mzuwula anymore.

13.6 *Moto* in Historical and Cross-Cultural Perspective: (Dis)continuities and Flows

There are widespread pollution beliefs in sub-Saharan Africa that use 'heat' to designate a form of pollution originating from certain types of sexual intercourse, including extramarital sex and violations of the 'postpartum' abstinence period, which extends up to 2 years in many cases (van de Walle & van de Walle 1993; Green et al. 1994). For instance, the Lele of Congo identify a syndrome similar to *moto* called *hanga*, which Douglas (1992 [1966]), pp. 123, 206) translates as 'sex-pollution'. Among the Wagogo of Tanzania violations of the postpartum sex taboos by the mother and father can be the cause of the most serious cases of childhood diarrhoea (Mabilia 2005). A study of perceived barriers to exclusive breastfeeding with 320 women in Cameroon found that sexual contact is prohibited during the postpartum period, as it is thought to spoil the breast milk and harm the child (Kakute et al. 2005).

Part of the sex taboo may be connected to the 'polluting' nature that birth is ascribed; several historical studies in Malawi have noted that women underwent a period of ritual uncleanliness after the birth of a child, for about 1 month, during which time they could not cook, or eat or bathe with anyone (Read 1959; Berry & Petty 1992). Munthali (2007) has documented a period of ritual uncleanliness for women following birth in Rumphi District of northern Malawi. Our research recorded similar postpartum practices in the Ekwendeni area. Similar approaches to postpartum practices have been documented among the Wagogo of Tanzania (Mabilia 2005). Lwanda (2004, p. 30) argues that the concept of 'heat', associated with immoral acts, periods of uncleanliness (such as menstruation) or contagious diseases (such as leprosy), has long been considered taboo and part of a broader healing system practiced by all ethnic groups in Malawi. Green and colleagues (1994, p. 6) argue that 'heat' is part of a broader ethnomedical concept in sub-Saharan Africa, which is connected to states of physical health and spiritual and social relationships.

Other studies throughout sub-Saharan Africa have documented a strong belief in the importance of postpartum abstinence in order to ensure birth spacing and to protect the infant from illness (van de Walle & van de Walle 1993). There are many words in many different parts of Africa for illnesses of breastfeeding infants, caused by the mother and/or father having sexual intercourse. Infant diarrhoea is often linked to resumption of sexual intercourse (van de Walle & van de Walle 1993; Kakute et al. 2005). In Malawi, where there are common cultural continuities between different ethnic groups, there is a taboo against postpartum sexual practice and a similar illness (*tspempo* or *mdulo*) caused by promiscuity, infidelity or sexual relations at inappropriate times (Lwanda 2004; Munthali 2007).

Moto appears to be an illness that has both historical regularity within Malawi, and among Bantu speakers in sub-Saharan Africa (Munthali 2007). Missionary reports on Tumbuka theories of disease causation suggest that the concept of *moto* was a recognised illness from at least the late 19th century (Fraser 1970 [1940], pp. 144–145). Studies carried out by anthropologists in the 1930s and 1940s and by historians in the 1990s in central and northern Malawi noted that a sickly or wasted child was thought to be caused by the mother or father breaking the sexual abstinence taboo following birth, or by having an extramarital affair (Berry & Petty 1992; Soko 2002, p. 54). This suggests that the term '*moto*' is a fluid concept that emphasises causation over symptomology, which has important consequences for individual treatment choices and preventative health strategies.

13.7 What Is *Moto Really*? Biomedical Responses to Moto and Mzuwula

Throughout history, biomedical personnel have attempted to identify what *moto* 'really is'. Fraser (1970 [1940]) argued that it was 'really' a 'deadly pestilence', and in the 1950s it was considered a proxy for sickle-cell anaemia. During our research, employees working at Ekwendeni Hospital argued that *moto* is really a biomedical illness, such as pneumonia or malnutrition. As one active volunteer stated:

> There is no difference between *moto* and malnutrition only that in the past the old people said *moto* for family planning because if the mother gets pregnant while breastfeeding the [breastfeeding] child couldn't grow well because she couldn't care for him as required. But now from the Under Five [MCH] clinics and SFHC we know it is malnutrition (older woman, July 2005).

As a result, the hospital has focused their education campaigns at identifying, then eradicating, 'bad cultures' or 'traditional beliefs' that they deem harmful or irrelevant.[5] Ekwendeni Hospital, in particular, began to direct their attentions to *moto* and *mzuwula* since hospital staff argued that *mzuwula* was a dangerous 'traditional' practice that introduced liquids other than breast milk increases the child's exposure the pathogens that cause diarrhoea and other parasitic infections. As part of their efforts the hospital held of series of 're-education/behavior change/sensitization' workshop trainings with grandmothers to stop the practice. This program has increased the tensions between the hospital and the local communities, which was reflected in some informants' reluctance to speak openly about *mzuwula* and it made it impossible to determine whether villagers were stopping this practice or whether the practices had gone 'underground' (Bezner Kerr et al. 2008). Nonetheless, there is strong scientific evidence that non-exclusive breastfeeding greatly increases the risk of child mortality and morbidity (Black et al. 2008a), making the challenges for public health programs wishing to be knowledgeable and respectful of local beliefs, while recognising their dynamism and implications for child survival rates great indeed. A biomedical paradigm that reduces indigenous illness concepts to static typologies fails to pinpoint the dynamic ways in which concepts of child illness can change based on social context. While the concept of *moto* has remained constant, the symptoms and the related rationale or meaning of

[5] In an earlier paper, we reported on the disparaging attitudes that nurses and hospital staff had towards local beliefs around child feeding (Bezner Kerr et al. 2008).

moto may change over time, reflecting peoples' everyday concerns related to food security, sexuality, health and so on.

Has the concept *moto* been affected by the current social and historical context, which is characterised by high HIV infection and high malnutrition rates? Malnutrition alone has major implications for child survival. Mild to moderate child malnutrition has synergistic effects with infection (Pelletier 1994), with a recent meta-study finding that malnutrition was responsible for 2.2 million deaths annually of children under 5 years (Black et al. 2008b). Children with malnutrition develop symptoms similar to HIV such as pneumonia, progressive weight loss, chronic diarrhoea and fevers. An estimated 68,000 adults and children died from AIDS in Malawi in 2007 (UNAIDS 2008). It is a common scientific understanding that HIV contributes substantially to child mortality, but factors underlying these deaths are inadequately described in the literature (Newell et al. 2004). Early infant HIV infection and maternal death are two major risk factors for HIV-infected infants, with an estimated 50 percent dying by 2 years of age (Newell et al. 2004). One study in Zambia of children admitted for severe malnutrition found that children with HIV were lower in child growth measures and more likely to have the wasting (marasmus) type of malnutrition compared to children not infected with HIV (Amadi et al. 2001). Hospital staff at Ekwendeni Hospital started to notice the link between childhood malnutrition and pediatric HIV rates several years ago. Children are admitted to the NRU when they present with signs of malnutrition; these include kwashiorkor, marasmus and oedema. In 2005, staff started testing children at the Nutrition Rehabilitation Unit (NRU) for HIV infection because as the coordinator stated: 'Now, most of the children who die from malnutrition have HIV' (Interview, July 2005). Our point here is *not* to make a causal linkage between *moto* and a biomedical concept, be it malnutrition, diarrhoea or HIV, but rather to understand how local conditions (such as poor health care, poverty, high rates of child mortality, HIV/AIDS) recreate a fluid concept such as *moto*.

13.8 Discussion

Our data points to a persistent belief and practice in *moto, mzuwula* and related beliefs around the effects of sexual intercourse on breastfeeding and child health, despite active efforts to change these beliefs by the dominant biomedical system. In understanding the contemporary cultural and political significance, we ask why has *moto* remained despite efforts to eradicate it? Lwanda (2004) argues that the colonial and postcolonial medicine led to a governance system that pathologised, objectified and derided traditional medical beliefs in Malawi. He argues that this pathologising and objectification of indigenous beliefs, often linked to Christian discourse around immorality and ignorance, has led to a cultural duality rather than hybridity in belief systems, which was reinforced during the postcolonial period by educated, elite Malawians. Indigenous Malawian beliefs, that is, have been put 'out of the gaze', made as 'other' and dismissed as irrational, as part of a biomedical perspective that focuses on biological, individual factors that cause health problems, rather than social, political or economic dynamics (Krieger, 1994; Kalipeni, Craddock, Oppong, & Ghosh 2004).

Some respondents indicated that they combined *mzuwula* treatment with biomedical care of their sick child. In other studies, there is some evidence that Malawian families take a syncretic approach to treating child illness. One study in the northern region with the Tumbuka examined parents' ideas about child illness (Munthali 2001). Parents tried to prevent and/or treat malaria, malnutrition, measles, diarrhoea and coughs (which they attributed to be caused by parents' sexual intercourse). Preventative measures included vaccination, food taboos, isolation of sick people and observation of taboos on sexual intercourse, while treatments include the use of government health facilities, the purchase of medicines and traditional herbal remedies. Another study done in a Yao village in central Malawi examined practices and beliefs surrounding pregnancy (Helitzer-Allen, Kendall, & Wirima 1997). Pregnant women sought out advice from *nankungwi*, elderly women in the village who could no longer conceive, and whose role is passed by previous *nankungwi*. The *nankungwi* taught women about labour, delivery and caring for the baby after birth. Antenatal care at the hospital was done by the woman primarily to ensure that she did not have problems with the hospital during delivery, since she was less likely to be reprimanded for not having proof of antenatal care. Other studies in east and southern Africa have also documented this syncretic approach to treating child illness such as malaria (Haussman Muela, Muela Riberac, Mushib, & Tanner 2002; Hildenwall et al. 2007).

There is also a strong gendered element to the cause of *moto*, since prostitutes, 'loose' or 'roaming women' are often blamed for the existence of *moto*. Sexual promiscuity is often blamed on women, as part of a broader set of cultural ideas about women needing to control their sexuality. For example, in nearby Rumphi District of northern Malawi, Munthali (2007, p. 2) notes that women who have babies with *vermix caseosa* (a creamy substance which covers the newborn baby and protects the foetus) are assumed to have 'indulged' in sexual intercourse and 'laughed at' by women attending her delivery. Women who swell or have convulsions are believed to have had intercourse with many men. These ideas have historical continuity with British colonial biomedicine, which pathologised African women's sexuality and which worked in concert with African traditionalists, who tried to reinforce gender inequalities by blaming women for sexually transmitted diseases (Vaughan 1991).

In the participatory workshop this 'blaming' of women was strongly articulated by older women, who pointed to the 'weakness' of wives, or their desire to have sex, as the reason for increased rates of malnutrition. These statements are made in the context of high rates of spousal violence (Bezner Kerr 2005). According to the most recent national survey in Malawi, one in three women interviewed experienced physical violence in their lifetime, most often from their husband, and ten percent of women experienced marital rape in the last year, both acts which are likely to be underreported (NSO & ORC Macro 2005). Another study indicated that 38 percent of adolescent girls (ages 12–19 years) said their first sexual experience involved force or coercion (Moore, Awusabo-Asare, Madise, Johannes, & Kumi-Kyereme 2007).

We argue that high HIV and malnutrition rates in children must affect the ways in which people give meaning to childhood illness in Malawi. In particular, HIV is too often the 'unspoken' or 'silent' dialogue in Malawi, but its pervasive impact cannot be ignored. Part of the difficulty is that the biomedical view and the local view on HIV come from opposite ends of the spectrum. Locally, women are blamed for causing illness in their children by 'giving in' to their husbands, which leads to *moto*. Biomedically, women are blamed for causing illness in their children by not exclusively breastfeeding, leading to infection and/or HIV. What both discussions ignore, however, are the unequal power relations that make it difficult for women to act on either piece of advice. It is crucial to understand the 'micropolitics' of taking action on child illness (Kamat 2006), and how contemporary structural factors such as chronic food insecurity and HIV interact with local belief systems about health. Academic understandings of these issues are also non-existent. At the time of writing of this chapter, there was not one single publication on local theories of disease causation, or health-seeking behavior in relation to pediatric HIV, or how this might affect social relations in the communities scientists work in.

13.9 Conclusion

Chalo ni Mazgola – This World is Change

(Tumbuka Proverb)

In the past two decades, Malawi has seen consistently high rates of malnutrition among children, severe and chronic food shortages and a devastating HIV pandemic. Culture-bound illnesses such as *moto* cannot be viewed as 'traditional' throwbacks that will disappear with the corrosive authority of biomedical science. In fact, our research shows how dynamic the concept is, and how clearly it expresses parents' anxieties about their child's health, their marriage and their social relationships with in-laws, parents and neighbours. Preliminary findings indicate that HIV, malnutrition and *moto* form an inseparable complex that both reflect the present-day reality of the health and well-being of infants and young children in Malawi. *Moto*, in particular, appears to be part of a larger ethnomedical concept in sub-Saharan Africa that provides a grid through which Malawians give meaning to children's illnesses.

Similar ideas and illnesses found elsewhere in sub-Saharan Africa suggests that this may also be the case in the rest of the region. *Moto* as a syndrome that produces a complex array of symptoms is a very useful term for conceptualizing the complex relationships between poor health, behavior and poverty; how to incorporate it into public health activities is an important area of further enquiry. Exploring how HIV and chronic food insecurity are affecting, or have affected, the concept of *moto* is also an important question, both practically for infant feeding projects and for those that critically investigate public health programs. These studies should consider both cultural factors and existing structural constraints that influence the dynamics of child health care seeking and child health outcomes.

References

Adams, V., & Pigg, S. L. (eds.) (2005). *Sex in development: Science, sexuality and morality in global perspective*. Durham: Duke University Press.

Amadi, B., Kelly, P., Mwiya, M., Mulwazi, E., Sianongo, S., Changwe, F., et al. (2001). Intestinal and systemic infection, HIV, and mortality in Zambian children with persistent diarrhoea and malnutrition. *Journal of Pediatric Gastroenterology & Nutrition, 32*(5), 550–554.

Bankole, A., Singh, S., Hussain, R., & Oestreicher, G. (2009). Condom use for preventing STI/HIV and unintended pregnancy among young men in sub-Saharan Africa. *American Journal of Men's Health, 3*(1), 60–78.

Berry, V., & Petty, C. (1992). *The Nyasaland survey papers 1938–1943: Agriculture, food and health*. London: Academy Books.

Bezner Kerr, R. (2005). Food security in northern Malawi: Historical context and the significance of gender, kinship relations and entitlements. *Journal of Southern African Studies, 31*(1), 53–74.

Bezner Kerr, R., & Chirwa, M. (2004). Participatory research approaches and social dynamics that influence agricultural practices to improve child nutrition in Malawi. *Ecohealth, 1*(Suppl. 2), 109–119.

Bezner Kerr, R., Berti, P. R., & Chirwa, M. (2007). Breastfeeding and mixed feeding practices in Malawi: Timing, reasons, decision makers, and child health consequences. *Food and Nutrition Bulletin, 28*(1), 90–99.

Bezner Kerr, R., Dakishoni, L., Shumba, L., Msachi, R., & Chirwa, M. (2008). 'We grandmothers know plenty': Breastfeeding, complementary feeding and the multifaceted role of grandmothers in Malawi. *Social Science and Medicine, 66*, 1095–1105.

Black, R. E., Allen, L. H., Bhutta, Z. A., Caulfield, L. E., De Onis, M., Ezzati, M., et al. (2008a). Maternal and child undernutrition: Global and regional exposures and health consequences. *The Lancet, 371*, 243–260.

Black, R. E., Allen, L. H., Bhutta, Z. A., Caulfield, L. E., De Onis, M., Ezzati, M., et al. (2008b). Maternal and child undernutrition: Global and regional exposures and health consequences. *The Lancet, 371*, 243–260.

Bolin, I. (2006). *Growing up in a culture of respect: Child rearing in highland Peru*. Austin: University of Texas Press.

Chimbiri, A. M. (2007). The condom is an 'intruder' in marriage: Evidence from rural Malawi. *Social Science and Medicine, 64*(2007), 1102–1115.

Conroy, A., & Blackie, M. J. (2005). Introduction. In A. Conroy, & M. J. Blackie (Eds.), *Poverty, AIDS and hunger: Breaking the poverty trap in Malawi* (pp. 1–13). New York: Palgrave MacMillan.

Coovadia, H. M., Rollins, N. C., Bland, R. M., Little, K., Coutsoudis, A., Bennish, M. L., et al. (2007). Mother-to-child transmission of HIV-1 infection during exclusive breastfeeding in the first 6 months of life: An intervention cohort study. *The Lancet, 369*(9567), 1065–1066.

Deardon, K. A., Hilton, S., Bentley, M. E., Caulfield, L. E., et al. (2009) Caregiver verbal encouragement increases food acceptance among Vietnamese toddlers 1–3. *Journal of Nutrition, 139*, 1387–1392.

Douglas, M. (1992 [1966]). *Purity and danger: An analysis of concepts of pollution and taboo*. London: Routledge and Kegan Paul.

Engle, P. L., & Breaux, C. (1994). *Is there a father instinct? Fathers' responsibility for children*. New York: Population Council Series.

Foucault, M. (1980). *Power/knowledge: Selected interviews and other writings 1972–1977*. New York: Pantheon Books.

Fraser, D. (1970-originally published 1914). Winning a primitive people: Sixteen years' work among the warlike tribe of the Ngoni and the Senga and Timbuka people of Central Africa; Fraser, D.; 1914, London: Seeley Service.

Gillespie, S. (2006). AIDS, poverty and hunger: An overview. In S. Gillespie (Ed.), *AIDS, poverty and hunger: Challenges and responses* (pp. 1–32). Washington, DC: IFPRI.

Good, B. (1994). *Medicine, rationality and experience: An anthropological perspective.* Cambridge: Cambridge University Press.

Gottlieb, A. (2004). *The afterlife is where we come from: the culture of infancy in West Africa.* Chicago: University of Chicago Press.

Green, E. C., Jurg, A., & Djedje, A. (1994). The snake in the stomach: Child diarrhoea in central Mozambique. *Medical Anthropology Quarterly, 8*(1), 4–24.

Haussman Muela, S., Muela Riberac, J., Mushib, A. K., & Tanner, M. (2002). Medical syncretism with reference to malaria in a Tanzanian community. *Social Science and Medicine, 55*, 403–413.

Helitzer-Allen, D. L., Kendall, C., & Wirima, J. J. (1997). Beliefs and practices during pregnancy in a Yao community in Malawi. In E. Kalipeni, & P. Thiuri (Eds.), *Issues and perspectives on health care in contemporary Sub-Saharan Africa* (pp. 145–164). Lewiston: Edwin Mellen.

Hewlett, B. S., Lamb, M. E., Shannon, D., Leyendecker, B., & Scholmerich, A. (1998) Culture and early infancy among Central African foragers and farmers. *Developmental Psychology, 34*, 653–661.

Hildenwall, H., Rutebemberwa, E., Nsabagasani, X., Pariyo, G., Tomsona, G. O., & Peterson, S. (2007). Local illness concepts—Implications for management of childhood pneumonia in eastern Uganda. *Acta Tropica, 101*, 217–224.

Kakute, P. N., Ngum, J., Mitchell, P., Kroll, K. A., Forgwei, G. W., Ngwang, L. K., et al. (2005). Cultural barriers to exclusive breastfeeding by mothers in a rural area of Cameroon, Africa. *Journal of Midwifery and Women's Health, 50*(4), 324–328.

Kaler, A. (2004). AIDS-talk in everyday life: The presence of HIV/AIDS in men's informal conversation in Southern Malawi. *Social Science and Medicine, 59*, 285–297.

Kalipeni, E., & Ghosh, J. (2006). Concern and practice among men about HIV/AIDS in low socioeconomic income areas of Lilongwe, Malawi. *Social Science and Medicine, 64*(2007), 1116–1127.

Kalipeni, E., Craddock, S., Oppong, J. R., & Ghosh, J. (Eds.) (2004). *HIV and AIDS in Africa: Beyond epidemiology*. Malden: Blackwell.

Kamat, V. R. (2006). "I thought it was only ordinary fever!" cultural knowledge and the micropolitics of therapy seeking for childhood febrile illness in Tanzania. *Social Science and Medicine, 62*, 2945–2959.

Kramer, K. L. (2005). Children's help and the pace of reproduction: Cooperative breeding in humans. *Evolutionary Anthropology, 14*, 224–237.

Krieger, N. (1994). Epidemiology and the web of causation: Has anyone seen the spider? *Social Science and Medicine, 39*(7), 887–903.

Liamputtong, P. (2009) *Qualitative research methods* (3rd ed.). Melbourne: Oxford University Press.

Lock, M. (1995). *Encounters with aging: Mythologies of menopause in Japan and North America.* Berkeley: University of California Press.

Lock, M., & Farquhar, J. (Eds). (2007). *Beyond the body proper: Reading the anthropology of material life*. Durham: Duke University Press.

Lwanda, J. (2004). Politics, culture and medicine: An unholy trinity? Historical continuities and ruptures in the HIV/AIDS story in Malawi. In E. Kalipeni, S. Craddock, J. Oppong, & J. Ghosh (Eds.), *HIV and AIDS in Africa: Beyond epidemiology* (pp. 29–42). Hoboken: Wiley-Blackwell.

Mabilia, M. (2005). *Breastfeeding and sexuality: Behavior, beliefs and taboos among the Gogo mothers in Tanzania*. New York: Berghahn Books.

Matthews, H., & Limb, M. (1999). Defining an agenda for the geography of children: Review and prospects. *Progress in Human Geography, 23*, 61–90.

McDowell, L. (1999). *Gender, identity and place: Understanding feminist geographies.* Minneapolis: University of Minnesota Press.

McCracken, J. (1977). *Politics and Christianity in Malawi 1875–1940: The impact of the Livingstonia Mission in the Northern Province*. Cambridge: Cambridge University Press.

Moore, A. M., Awusabo-Asare, K., Madise, N., Johannes, J.-L., & Kumi-Kyereme, A. (2007). Coerced first sex among adolescent girls in Sub-Saharan Africa: Prevalence and context. *African Journal of Reproductive Health, 11*(3), 62–82.

Munthali, A. (2007). Beliefs about pregnancy, childbearing and newborn infants in a rural district in northern Malawi. In P. Liamputtong (Ed.), *Childrearing and infant care Issues: A cross-cultural perspective* (pp. 141–154). Hauppauge: Nova Science.

Munthali, A. C. (2001). Management of childhood illnesses among the Tumbuka of Rumphi District in northern Malawi. *The Society of Malawi Journal, 54*(2), 43–65.

Newell, M.-L., Coovadia, H. M., Cortina-Borja, M., Rollins, N. C., Gaillard, P., Dabis, F., et al. (2004). Mortality of infected and uninfected infants born to HIV-infected mothers in Africa: A pooled analysis *The Lancet, 365*(9441), 1236–1243.

NSO, & ORC Macro. (2005). *Malawi demographic and health survey 2004*. Zomba, Malawi and Calverton, Maryland, USA: National Statistical Office of Malawi (NSO) and ORC Macro.

Pelletier, D. (1994). The potentiating effects of malnutrition on child mortality: Epidemiology, evidence and policy implications. *Nutrition Reviews, 52*, 409–415.

Read, M. (1959). *Children of their fathers*. London: Metheun & Co.

Richards, A. I. (2004 [1932]). *Hunger and work in a savage tribe. A functional study of nutrition among the southern Bantu*. London: Routledge.

Roopnarine, J. L., Fouts, H. N., Lamb, M. E. & Lewis-Elligan, T. Y. (2005). Mothers' and fathers' behaviors toward their 3- to 4-month-old infants in lower, middle, and upper socioeconomic African American families. *Developmental Psychology, 41*, 723–732.

Simondon, K., Delaunay, V., Diallo, A., Elguero, E. & Simondon, F. (2003). Lactational amenorrhea is associated with child age at the time of introduction of complementary food: a prospective cohort study in rural Senegal, West Africa. *American Journal of Clinical Nutrition, 78*(1), 154–161.

Smith, K. P., & Watkins, S. C. (2005). Perceptions of risk and strategies for prevention: Responses to HIV/AIDS in rural Malawi. *Social Science and Medicine, 60*(3), 649–660.

Soko, B. (2002). *Nchimi chikanga: The battle against witchcraft in Malawi*. Zomba: Kachere.

UNAIDS (2008). *2008 report on the global AIDS epidemic*. Geneva: UNAIDS.

UNDP (2008). *UNDP development report 2008*. New York: Oxford University Press.

van de Walle, E., & van de Walle, F. (1993). Post-partum sexual abstinence in tropical Africa. In R. Gray, H. Leridon, & A. Spira (Eds.), *Biomedical and demographic determinants of reproduction* (pp. 446–460). Oxford: Clarendon.

Vaughan, M. (1991). *Curing their ills: Colonial power and African illness*. Stanford: Stanford University Press.

Weisner, T. S., & Gallimore, R. (1977). My brother's keeper: Child and sibling caretaking. *Current Anthropology, 18*, 169–190.

Yap, P. M (1967). Classification of the culture-bound reactive syndromes. *Australian and New Zealand Journal of Psychiatry, 1*, 172–179.

Yoder, P. S. (1997). Negotiating relevance: Belief, knowledge and practice in international health projects. *Medical Anthropology Quarterly, 11*(2), 131–146.

Young, A. (1995). *The harmony of illusions: Inventing post-traumatic stress disorder*. Princeton: Princeton University Press.

Zulu, E. M. (2001). Ethnic variations in observance and rationale for postpartum sexual abstinence in Malawi. *Demography, 38*(4), 467–479.

Part IV
Infant Feeding Beliefs and Practices Within Socio-cultural Context

Chapter 14
From Traditional to Optimal Breastfeeding Practices: Selected Cases from Central and Southern Africa

Penjani Kamudoni and Gerd Holmboe-Ottesen

Contents

14.1 Introduction

This chapter discusses the current global policy recommendation of optimal breastfeeding by illustrating the traditional norms and taboos pertaining to breastfeeding among the Yao of Malawi, Chagga, Wagogo and Haya of Tanzania. Interventions that can bridge the gap between optimal breastfeeding and traditional norms are also discussed. In conclusion, the extent to which the culture of breastfeeding can persist is discussed.

P. Kamudoni (✉)
Department of General Practice and Community Medicine, Faculty of Medicine, Institute of Health and Society, University of Oslo, P.O. Box 1130, Blindern, 0318 Oslo, Norway
e-mail: p.r.kamudoni@medisin.uio.no/penjanius@yahoo.com

P. Liamputtong (ed.), *Infant Feeding Practices*, DOI 10.1007/978-1-4419-6873-9_14,

© Springer Science+Business Media, LLC 2011

The first section presents a historical perspective of breastfeeding promotion, which gave birth to the policy recommendation of optimal breastfeeding. Thereafter, a presentation of what optimal breastfeeding entails is made. Traditional infant feeding practices from birth and interventions which can promote optimal breastfeeding are presented last.

14.2 Global Perspectives on Breastfeeding

Since the beginning of the later half of the 1950s, breastfeeding has increasingly been shown through scientific evidence to be the most effective health intervention to avert malnutrition and other childhood illnesses. It was during this time period, with the onset of the infant formula industry (Obermeyer & Castle 1996; Naylor 2001; UNICEF 2005), that declining rates in breastfeeding were experienced in Western countries. Much later, marketing of such products was followed up in developing countries, where it combined with poverty and lack of sanitary environment, had disastrous effects on infant health. This scenario prompted the global community, that is, governments and most organisations working in child health, to work towards strategies that could support mothers to breastfeed. This was significantly first noticed when UNICEF and WHO in the 1970s jointly mobilised governments and technical experts and called for the development of an international code for ethical marketing of infant formulas (Naylor 2001). The initiative led to the drafting and later to the adoption of the *International Code of Marketing of Breast milk Substitutes* by both governments and other relevant bodies (Naylor 2001; UNICEF 2005). Following these efforts, several publications and statements offering guidelines and policy changes were made, the most notable being two publications in 1989 titled: 'Protecting, Promoting and Supporting Breastfeeding: The special role of maternity services. A joint WHO/UNICEF statement' and 'Breastfeeding: Protecting a natural resource'(UNICEF 2005). These and other publications were later discussed and their contents adopted (especially the former) at a global conference co-sponsored by WHO and UNICEF among other agencies in August 1990 in Spedale degli Innocenti, Italy (Naylor 2001; UNICEF 2005). The conference, which drew together 30 governments and other key stakeholders, culminated into a globally influential declaration, which has been referred to as the *Innocenti Declaration.* The declaration served as a formalised launch of global efforts to shield mothers from emerging influences, which could deter them from breastfeeding. It regarded breastfeeding and child feeding as human rights issues for both developing and industrialised countries (UNICEF 2005). Concepts like *promotion, support* and *protection of breastfeeding* were agreed upon as universal mandates of states. Furthermore, it included practical national operational targets like appointing national breastfeeding coordinators, ensuring that maternity services were following practises to promote successful breastfeeding as recommended (UNICEF 2005). The contents of the Innocenti declaration continued to be endorsed in several global summits. With subsequent years of the declaration's implementation, the vastness of the social changes necessary to support breastfeeding and infant feeding became clear, and the need to revitalise global commitment to breastfeeding and young child nutrition was felt. In 1998, WHO and UNICEF (Innocenti) undertook consultations for a global strategy on infant feeding based on scientific and epidemiological evidence. From this initiative followed the *Global Strategy for Infant and Young Child Feeding* (GSIYF), which was fully developed by 2002. Its development was guided on scientific evidence and participation (WHO 2003). The GSIYF includes the Innocenti targets and successes, and broadens the understanding of breastfeeding and infant feeding to being a part of other global interventions. The GSIYF obligates countries to develop or reinforce comprehensive national strategies and action plans for young child feeding.

14.3 Optimal Breastfeeding

The infant feeding practices recommended by the GSIYF were termed *optimal breastfeeding practices*. These are practices that have been scientifically shown to maximise the physiological benefits to both the infant and the mother, and include the following:

- *Feeding of colostrum and early initiation of breastfeeding within the first hour after birth*: The mother's first initial breast milk has been shown to have a high concentration of antibodies, which provide the infant with natural immunity at a time when its immunity is not fully developed. Thus, initiating breastfeeding early is recommended to make it possible for the infant to suckle colostrum.
- *Exclusive breastfeeding*: This is defined as giving the infant no fluids or foods other than necessary medical prescriptions for the first 6 months of life. Breast milk is nutritionally adequate to meet the baby's needs in the first 6 months of life. In addition to containing antibodies, breast milk contains a number of components that help to protect the infant various biological mechanisms. Notably, it is rich in sugars, which are helpful in blocking the adherence of microbes to epithelial cells, which in turn prevents infections.
- *Avoidance of prelacteal feeding*: This is an important implication of the recommendation to exclusively breastfeed during the first 6 months and to feed the infant colostrum. Furthermore, avoidance of prelacteal feeding is deemed to protect the infant from contamination, which can result in enteric infections.
- *Continued breastfeeding up to 18–24 months*: After the first 6 months of birth, breast milk can still meet over a third of the infant's need. Furthermore, the protective components of breast milk are still contained in breast milk. Therefore, it is recommended that infants are to continue to be breastfed.

Breastfeeding on demand is a practice that cuts across the optimal breastfeeding practices. It entails feeding the infant as it would want to (demands to) as opposed to feeding it by schedule.

14.4 Traditional Practices and Perceptions on Breastfeeding

Although optimal breastfeeding is recommended by global and national policy making bodies as the appropriate way for mothers to feed infants, traditional institutions and communities perceive this differently. To illustrate this, perceptions and customs surrounding breastfeeding among selected tribal groups in southern Africa will be presented within the themes of the optimal breastfeeding recommendation. These cases represent the breastfeeding practices in the rural regions of the countries referred to here: Malawi, Tanzania and the Gambia.

14.4.1 Prelacteal Feeding

Feeding infants water soaked in herbs immediately after birth, before starting breastfeeding, is a custom in most traditional societies (see also Chapter 18 in this volume). In rural northern Malawi among the Tumbuka, an infusion made from crushed dried leaves of a specific tree mixed with boiled water, *mzuwala*, is the first non-breast milk substance given to infants in order to protect them against an illness called *moto*. Its signs include fast breathing, coughing, white mucus, and low weight of the child. *Moto* is believed to be caused by sexual misconduct in the child's household (Bezner, Dakishoni, Shumba, Msachi, & Chirwa 2008; Kerr, Berti, & Chirwa 2007; see also Chapter 13 in this volume). The infusion is given in varying doses usually three times a day, a spoonful each time. Some mothers would give it for 6 months while others would feed it to the child throughout the first year. Bathing the infant with some of the *Mzuwala* herbal water to further protect the child from misconduct of other people in the village is also part of the custom. Among the Haya of northern Tanzania, native beer is used as a prelacteal feed to wake the infant up from its sleep and relieve it of the exhaustion from its way out from the mother's womb into the world (Rwegelera 1963). The Yao in Malawi used to have the tradition of giving water mixed with minute quantities of maize flour to 'allow the intestines to expand' (Kamudoni 2005, p. 37). Among the Datoga, a pastoralists tribe in northern Tanzania, infants would be fed only water, in some cases diluted goat's or cow's milk prior to the first breastfeeding. In cases where labour had been particularly difficult, infants would be ritually fed a mixture of water and hot ash (Sellen 1998).

Apart from giving prelacteal feeds for diseases and conditions whose aetiology is rooted in the culture, such feeds are also customarily given for prevention of conditions which can be clearly identified in modern medicine. For instance, among the Yao in southern Malawi, infants are given a herbal infusion made from roots of a specific shrub within the first 2 weeks of birth to prevent jaundice, locally termed *mwanamphepo* (Kamudoni 2005). Among the Chagga of northern Tanzania, a herbal prelacteal feed would be given to prevent future infestation of the parasitic worms (Lema 1963).

With modern medical influence, the types of prelacteal feeds being given have changed. A notable case is the Wagogo of central Tanzania, who give a sugar or salt solution to the infant immediately after birth. However in the past, soft millet porridge with particular herbs mixed in it would be given to the infant and baby after birth as a sign of warm welcome to the baby. Recently, this porridge is to be given to only the mother instead (Mabilia 1996a, b). In relatively more urbanised communities, sugar solutions have also been reported to be given as prelacteal feeds (de Paoli, Manongi, Helsing, & Klepp 2001; Shirima, Greiner, Kylberg, & Gebre-Medhin 2001).

The traditional reasons for giving prelacteal feeds may no longer be valued where communities are becoming urbanised. However, the concept of offering other feeds to the infant before offering breast milk is still used to deal with breastfeeding challenges like lactation being delayed, or the persistent crying of the infant. In a study in central Tanzania, it was reported the use of prelacteal feeds among over a quarter of the sampled mothers who gave birth in a health facility (Agnarsson, Mpello, GunnLaugsson, Hofvander, & Greiner 2001). The feeds were given while waiting for mature milk to appear, and included plain water, sugar solution and/or plain porridge.

Although interventions to promote optimal breastfeeding are elaborated in the later part of this chapter, it is worthwhile mentioning that the use of prelacteal feeds is also tied in with other traditional beliefs, for instance, protection against illnesses as earlier highlighted. Therefore, caution is required in promoting exclusive breastfeeding especially in the early days of birth in traditional societies. One way of doing this would be to assure mothers that vaccine antigens given to mothers at birth are adequate to protect babies from any childhood illnesses. As such, babies would not require to have drinks or feeds to prevent illnesses.

14.4.2 Discarding of Colostrum

Traditions surrounding the feeding of colostrum vary. Among the Chagga of northern Tanzania, colostrum is believed to be good for the infant, and is hence fed to it. In the same regard, animal colostrum from their livestock is drunk only by children (Lema 1963). Likewise, the Wagogo of central of Tanzania would feed their babies colostrum (Mabilia 1996a, b). The mothers in this tribe believe that every child has specifically tailored for their own child, although they do not associate it with nutritional benefits. It is fed to the infant with the belief that ‘it is necessary to suck it to allow the true milk to come’. Also among the Tumbuka in northern Malawi, colostrum is being perceived as being good for infants. Among the Datoga of Tanzania, there is no taboo against feeding of colostrum; however, most mothers among those sampled in a study by Sellen (1998) reported discarding colostrum. They discard colostrum based on thinking that it will give the infant digestive problems because it is thought to be ‘too heavy’ for the infant’s stomach. Others associate the look of colostrums with ‘being bad’ and think that it will make the child sick. The notion of the mother’s milk being bad will be elaborated when discussing breastfeeding taboos later in the chapter. Mixed practices towards feeding of colostrum have also been reported in more recent studies. Agnarsson et al.

(2001), in a study in central Tanzania in a community of a modern hospital, reported that some mothers had no opinion on colostrum while some mothers discarded it, and washed the breast with traditional medicine. Similarly, mothers' reasons for discarding colostrum were related to the notion that it was 'bad milk'; and hence could harm the baby and cause digestive problems. Discarding of colostrum, although not as a universal practice, has also been reported in less traditional communities (de Paoli et al. 2001;Shirima et al. 2001; see also Chapters 1 and 18 in this volume).

It is interesting to note that traditional norms against the feeding of colostrum have not been widely reported in literature, although the practice of discarding colostrum is still prevalent. On the other hand, the fear of colostrum being harmful reported by mothers in traditional societies is rational, given the unusual colouring and consistency it has, compared to mature milk. Adequate communication to mothers could easily help address their fears and clarify that colostrums is 'the best milk', hence its stronger colouration than that of the 'good milk'. Analogies of baby livestock which do feed on their mother's colostrums could also be utilised (Semega-Janneh, Bohler, Holm, Matheson, & Holmboe-Ottesen 2001).

14.4.3 Exclusive Breastfeeding and Introduction of Complementary Feeding

Once lactation is established, breastfeeding is carried out on demand – without any schedule – in all the tribal groups mentioned earlier here. Crying is perceived as a sign of the baby being hungry, and therefore, it would need to be breastfed. Such that among the Wagogo, if a mother is far from her infant and her milk pours out spontaneously at the place where she is, it means that her infant is crying, and is 'calling' for its milk. The relationship between crying and breastfeeding is so strongly established in the mothers' mind, such that a baby is not offered the breast if it is not crying even if several hours have passed since the last breastfeeding (Mabilia 1996a, b). There are no traditional customs specifying the time at which supplementary fluids should be introduced in the tribal groups in question.

Supplementary foods are introduced based on the mother's own understanding of when her breast milk *quantity* is not adequate to satisfy the baby (Mabilia 1996a, b). Among the Wagogo, developmental milestones, such as the time when the baby begins to sit up on its own, would be associated with the need to introduce such foods. Among Chagga mothers, appearance of new teeth would be used as a sign that the baby can start new foods (Lema 1963). However, even before such a developmental milestone is observed, Chagga mothers would make the baby taste and familiarise itself with the food it would be eating in the future (Lema 1963). Such that as early as 3 weeks before birth, small quantities of foods such as cream from cow's milk or bananas would be introduced to the baby.

Supplementary foods can also be given to the infant when the *quality* of the mother's breast milk is perceived to turn bad, implying that the baby cannot feed on 'bad' milk. This would be effectuated regardless of the developmental milestones being reached or not. Circumstances under which the mother's milk can turn 'bad' are specific and are in most cases related to the taboos surrounding breastfeeding. Among the Wagogo, mother's ill health especially when she would have either of the following signs, fever, an abscess, a sore on a breast, would make her milk from either both or one breast bad (Mabilia 1996a, b). When milk has stayed too long in the breasts, it will also be considered 'bad', and therefore, discarded. Becoming pregnant is also perceived to alter the mother's body, making her milk indigestible and liable to cause diarrhoea. Sexual relations of either parent outside marriage can also make the mother's breast milk impure and cause sickness to the infant. Pregnancy, in essence, will imply that the mother has to totally stop breastfeeding. Similar taboos have also been reported among the Tumbuka and Datoga (Sellen 1998; Bezner et al. 2008; see also Chapters 13 and 18 in this volume).

The types of supplementary foods are dependent on the adults' diets. Pastoralist tribes like the Datoga would largely give cow's milk as a supplementary food, while agrarian tribes like the Wagogo, Tumbuka, would give cereal gruel.

It is interesting to note that although there are many customs surrounding breastfeeding, stopping exclusive breastfeeding is at the mother's discretion. Furthermore, mothers would associate the infant's increase in physical growth with its diminishing satisfaction from breast milk. This phenomenon of associating increase in physical growth with sufficiency of breast milk is very logical and scientifically valid although it is a gradual process that does not occur until after 6 months. This instinctive way of thinking by mothers could explain the perception of insufficient milk syndrome, which is commonly reported from both traditional and modernised societies as the reason why mothers stop exclusive breastfeeding before 6 months (see also Chapters 9, 18, 20, and 21 in this volume). It is challenging for a mother to still perceive her breast milk as being enough, when the infant is physically increasing in size, and hence, that could be why in later infancy any infant crying is perceived as the infant being unsatisfied. This could further explain why mothers who exclusively breastfeed for 6 months are those who are highly motivated and/or well informed about exclusive breastfeeding and/or have a supportive social network around. Therefore, these mothers can easily deal with the psychological pressure of handling the growing infant when it is agitated. In this regard, exclusive breastfeeding has been consistently reported to be practised by indeed a minority of mothers in both traditional and modernised societies (Kamudoni 2005). This emphasises why intervening is required to enable mothers to exclusively breastfeed for 6 months.

14.4.4 Breastfeeding Cessation

In all tribal groups, breast milk is perceived as being good for the infant. After the first 6 months and before children are weaned, breast milk will still constitute a major part of their diet. Supplementary foods are not given as frequently as the number of adult meals. In some tribal groups like among the Datoga, semi-solid foods would only be introduced after weaning – the supplementary foods are non-human milks and gruels.

Breastfeeding is stopped by mothers as either a natural weaning process or in response to taboos as earlier mentioned (for instance, pregnancy). Children are completely stopped from breastfeeding usually around 24 or 30 months. However, age is not the basis for the weaning, but rather developmental milestones such as child being able to walk quickly. Prolonged breastfeeding is perceived as spoiling the child, and interfering with marital relations. Hence, when the children have reached specified development milestone, they must be weaned according to tradition. After weaning, mothers in some tribes, like the Wagogo, will feed the children extra meals in addition to or to replace the adult monotonous diet (Mabilia 1996a, b). For this reason, women would choose to stop breastfeeding during the rainy season, as there is more food than at any other period of the year. However, among other tribes, like the Haya, no special foods are prepared for the children; they would eat the food served to the rest of the family (Rwegelera 1963). See also Chapter 18 in this volume.

14.4.5 Other Breastfeeding Practices

14.4.5.1 Unilateral Breastfeeding

Twins are breastfed exceptionally with each twin feeding from the same breast all the time, that is, one breast for each twin, especially among the Haya, the Wagogo (Mabilia 1996a, b; Rwegelera 1963). In the event of death of one of the twins, mothers will feed the surviving twin from only one breast. Although instances where a death of a twin has occurred are rare events, such practice can greatly reduce the mother's breast milk output. Interventions, which are tailor-made for particular cultural contexts, can best deal with such kind of practices. Not much has been written over current breastfeeding practices of multiple birth infants. These are usually excluded from most studies on infant practices, as they represent only a small fraction of infants.

14.4.5.2 Wetnursing

In the event of death of a mother before the child is properly weaned or before the mothers even begins breastfeeding the child, one of the female relatives (either paternal or maternal) who is not breastfeeding but is most likely to re-lactate would be requested to take over breastfeeding of the child. If a mother falls pregnant at a time when it will be considered undesirable for the child to stop receiving breast milk, a wetnurse will take over the breastfeeding of the child (Rwegelera 1963). Utilisation of wetnurses is a possibility that has also been promoted as a safe breastfeeding method in preventing mother-to-child-transmission of HIV for HIV-infected mothers in low-income settings. However, it has not been successfully adopted given that it makes the mothers likely to have their status known by their community, even when they have not been ready to disclose their status. Studies indicate that HIV-infected mothers face negative community reactions and are stigmatised. Therefore, some mothers may opt not to disclose their status (Chinkonde, Sundby, & Martinson 2009). See also Chapters 12 and 13 in this volume.

14.4.5.3 Special Feeding for Pregnant and Lactating Mothers

Unlike in other tribal groups in Africa, among the Chagga, mothers are provided with a wider variety of foods and allowed to eat more during both pregnancy and lactation. The mothers are encouraged to eat more and gain weight. Furthermore, in the first 3 months of life, mothers are excused from regular work like agricultural-related work. However, this is not common in other tribal groups in Africa. A similar strategy of giving mothers a leave from agricultural work has been utilised by the Baby Friendly Community Initiative, to be described in more detail later, has proven to be successful.

14.5 Transitioning from Traditional to Optimal Breastfeeding Practices

The above traditional practices illustrate the strong values with which breastfeeding is perceived in most cultures. Furthermore, they also indicate the challenges that are bound to be faced in promoting a new culture of breastfeeding as given by the optimal breastfeeding recommendations. Nevertheless, as rural communities are eventually becoming modernised and access and use of modern health care services are increasing, the influences of the culture of optimal breastfeeding are inevitable. Furthermore, with urbanisation, the traditional support systems may be eroded or changed and mothers may be exposed to mass media (Omer-Salim, Persson, & Olsson 2007). This scenario makes it possible for modern health care-based concepts and information like optimal breastfeeding to be assimilated. This explains to a greater extent the trends of relatively higher rates of optimal breastfeeding practices in semi-urban areas (Kamudoni, Maleta, Shi, & Holmboe-Ottesen 2007).

Our observation in Malawi is that while semi-urban residence is associated with optimal breastfeeding practices, rural habitation is related to a lower proportion of mothers practising optimal breastfeeding. However, it seems that residence in fully urbanised locations unlike (in semi-urbanised locations) in most low-income countries, including countries mentioned in this chapter, is associated with low levels of exclusive breastfeeding and shorter duration of breastfeeding in general. This is likely to be the result of women undertaking formal employment, and hence having limited time to spend directly with the child. In these settings, also high education is likely to be associated with low exclusive breastfeeding rates. The influences that have resulted in the penetration of optimal breastfeeding practices have come as a result of interventional programs, which have been carried out both by governments and non-governmental agencies intervening both at policy level and at community level (as vertical parallel programs). These interventions have been carried out based on a number of models and which will be discussed below.

14.5.1 The Baby Friendly Hospital Initiative (BFHI)

14.5.1.1 Background

The BFHI is a global initiative which was pioneered by the World Health Organisation (WHO) and United Nations International Children's Fund (UNICEF) in 1992 (see also Chapter 4 in this volume). The background to this initiative can be traced back as far as the 1980s when UNICEF and WHO published the joint statement in 1989 titled 'Protecting, Promoting and Supporting Breastfeeding: The special role of maternity services', one of the publications central to the Innocenti meeting. The publication argued that in order to reverse the declining breastfeeding rates during this time, maternity policies and procedures needed to be adjusted to favour the lactation and physiological needs of mothers and infants. Influences on successful breastfeeding were also discussed (Naylor 2001). These were summarised as a set of ten action statements entitled 'The Ten Steps to successful Breastfeeding'. The idea of giving recognition to the hospitals who adopted and adhered to these ten steps was conceived at one of the meetings in the following months after the Innocenti declaration. The BFHI was, therefore, launched to recognise the facilities that had adopted and were implementing 'The ten steps'. To date, more than 15 000 hospitals in 134 countries (including all the countries in southern Africa) have been awarded the 'Baby friendly' status. In most of the countries of southern Africa as elsewhere, the BFHI was adopted in the 1990s soon after its global launching by Ministries of Health as a policy strategy for healthcare in these countries. As such, the process of accreditation of the hospitals is embedded within the Ministries of Health and UNICEF. This is unlike in most countries in the West where implementation of the BFHI has been implemented largely by other agencies outside Ministries of Health.

14.5.1.2 Ten Steps to Successful Breastfeeding Promotion

The ten steps can be described as mainly focusing on two things: educating healthcare staff on breastfeeding and management of problems related to it; and supporting the mothers to successfully breastfeed (Table 14.1). The first component is covered in the first two steps, which are centred on universally informing and training all staff in health facilities on breastfeeding. This is built on the understanding that health workers' attitudes are influential in the mothers' choice to either optimally breastfeed or not. Hence, unless they perceive optimal breastfeeding as the way to feed infants, the health workers are less likely to promote it. In the same regard, in the face of divergent opinions on infant feeding among health workers, a clearly defined policy act would still ensure promotion of breastfeeding.

Table 14.1 The ten steps to successful breastfeeding

Step 1. Have a written breastfeeding policy that is routinely communicated to all health care staff
Step 2. Train all healthcare staff in the skills necessary to implement this policy
Step 3. Inform all women about the benefits and management of breastfeeding
Step 4. Help mothers initiate breastfeeding within half an hour of delivery
Step 5. Show mothers how to breastfeed and how to maintain lactation (by expressing milk) even if they should be separated from their infants
Step 6. Give newborn infants no food or drink unless medically indicated. No promotion of formula milks
Step 7. Practise 'rooming-in'. Allow mothers and infants to stay together 24 hours a day
Step 8. Encourage breastfeeding on demand
Step 9. Give no artificial teats or pacifiers/dummies to breastfeeding babies
Step 10. Foster the establishment of breastfeeding support groups and refer mothers to them on discharge from the hospital or clinic

The third to the ninth step focus on direct support to the mother to enable her to breastfeed. The initial step of these entails informing the mother about the benefits and management of breastfeeding to enable her to make an informed choice about breastfeeding. This is based on the understanding that decisions regarding infant feeding are to be freely made by the mother and cannot be imposed by others. The subsequent steps are concerned with the actual help to the mother to initiate and maintain optimal breastfeeding during her hospital stay. Common practices that could hinder breastfeeding are to be replaced with evidence-based practices proven to promote breastfeeding. For instance, dummies or any objects simulating the breast which infants can suckle are not to be given. In addition, mothers are supposed to remain together with their infants for all the twenty-four hours of the day, and offering the breast whenever the baby would like to suckle it. The last of the ten steps focuses on linking the mother to community-based groups to support her to continue breastfeeding after leaving the hospital. Another aspect of the BFHI which is not covered in the 10 steps, sometimes referred to as the eleventh step, is that a 'Baby-friendly' hospital follows the International Code of Marketing of Breast milk Substitutes, which requires that all infant formula should be paid for by current market prices and should not be received as a donation or gift (Naylor 2001; see also Chapters 10 and 19 in this volume).

14.5.1.3 Impact of the BFHI

Abundant evidence has shown that the BFHI has had impact on breastfeeding practices in places where it is implemented (Philipp & Merewood 2004; Philipp & Radford 2006; Saadeh & Akre 1996). Longer exclusive breastfeeding durations and earlier initiation of breastfeeding has been found in randomised controlled trials evaluating the impact of the BFHI. Similarly, recent national Demographic and Health Surveys (DHS) in Tanzania, Malawi and South Africa have also documented an increase in the same outcomes during the period over which the BFHI has been implemented in these countries (Shirima et al. 2001; Hussein 2005).

14.5.1.4 Limitations of the BFHI

The impact of the BFHI has mostly been limited to mothers who opt to give birth in health facilities, which happen to be baby friendly (Bhandari, Kabir, & Salam 2008). In community-based studies in Malawi and Tanzania, breastfeeding practices were assessed in rural and semi-urban settings. Residents in the rural setting were being served by baby-friendly certified facilities, unlike in the semi-urban setting. Exclusive breastfeeding was almost non-existent in the rural communities unlike in the more urbanised ones (Vaahtera et al. 2001; Kamudoni et al. 2007). Furthermore, home births still constitute the majority of the births, raising a need to adapt the BFHI to include other influential people like traditional midwives when conducting training on optimal breastfeeding for health workers, if its impact is to be increased. Even for mothers who give birth in baby-friendly facilities, breastfeeding support is limited to the hospital premises, given the logistical challenges of linking up with mothers outside the hospital setting. High health staffs turn over in low-income settings also implies that staff training has to be ongoing in order to sustain baby-friendly services, which is costly and may make it difficult for facilities to sustain a good standard of the baby-friendly services. In spite of these limitations, the BFHI has been one of the most successful programs in impacting the way mothers breastfeed.

14.5.2 Community-Based Breastfeeding Interventions (CBBI)

While BFHI has promoted breastfeeding through focusing on policy and changing maternity services, evidence has shown that achieving optimal infant child feeding practices requires an integrated, comprehensive strategy that also includes community-based interventions. It has been realised that use of community-based approaches in breastfeeding promotion is an important model. The Global Strategy for Infant and Young Child Feeding of 2003 has included CBBIs as a new operational target (WHO 2003). CBBI are based on the understanding that optimal breastfeeding requires maternal choice combined with the ability to implement that choice, which is in turn affected by social, physical, and logistical factors that are immediate to the mother's experiences. Communication is a core aspect of CBBI. Strategies used in this regard seek to address not only individual beliefs of the mother but also the beliefs of those who influence her within her community, as for instance family members and elders. Targeting community influential individuals provides a mechanism for shifting cultural knowledge, norms and expectations. Unlike the BFHI, CBBIs have been mostly carried out on a relatively smaller scale, for instance, within selected areas in districts and in rare circumstances conducted as national projects. Some examples of CBBIs are discussed below.

14.5.2.1 The Baby Friendly Community Initiative (BFCI)

The BFCI is an adaptation of the BFHI, which focuses on making community changes instead of maternity health services changes to promote breastfeeding. It has been implemented on national scale in the Gambia and at a smaller scale with different emphasis in other parts of the world. Although not documented to have been implemented in countries in southern Africa, there is growing recognition of this model, indicated from anecdotal reports and in publications. In the Gambian model, '10 steps to successful infant feeding' were developed, which included both breastfeeding and other issues to protect maternal and child health (Semega-Janneh et al. 2001). These steps are promotional messages, which are based on integrating the traditional knowledge and practices within local communities with optimal breastfeeding and modern infant care practices. Village support groups are created comprising three to five women and three men, and these support groups are given training on the ten steps, which they then pass along to pregnant and lactating women, their spouses and extended family. The idea is to elicit all practices within the family to favour optimal breastfeeding. For instance, the family would provide maternity leave from farm work to the breastfeeding mother; or men in particular would construct shelters in the farms to enable mothers to breastfeed. The village support groups integrate the awareness campaigns into the ordinary village events like drama, traditional festivals and so on. To become baby-friendly, a community must select the village support group and have its members receive the training. Community health nurses provide supervision to the village support groups. The approach has been effective at among other things creating a culture of optimal breastfeeding, and has the unique feature of involving men, which has contributed to the acceptability of its promotional messages (Semega-Janneh et al. 2001).

14.5.2.2 Peer Support-Based Interventions

In peer support (also referred to as peer counselling) interventions, mothers who have previous breastfeeding experience are trained on optimal breastfeeding practices and follow-up of their fellow mothers to give them home-based support on breastfeeding. The number of visits may vary considerably depending on the availability of the peer counsellors and other factors. Most commonly, a total of 6–15 visits would be made to the mother. These would be from the last month of pregnancy until the sixth month or earlier after the infant's birth. The spacing of the visits may vary. However, it is very usual to have more visits made within the first week of birth, for instance, a visit within 2 days after birth, followed by one at the 5th day and another during the 10th day. Subsequent visits would then be more spaced, for instance, being made biweekly or monthly or longer depending on resources. In general, more visits are made within the first month to ensure that the mother is adequately assisted to establish breastfeeding. During the visits, peer counsellors would provide needed information pertaining to optimal breastfeeding practices at that particular stage. Of all CBBIs, this model is seemingly the most resource-intensive, given the time required by the peer counsellors in making the home visits. According to our knowledge, there is no documentation indicating that this model of intervention has been implemented on large national scale.

14.5.2.3 Mother Support Groups

In mother support groups, mothers periodically meet to share their breastfeeding experiences. In so doing, they both seek to learn from others ways to address the breastfeeding challenges they may be encountering and at the same time offer their own experiences as a learning ground for others. Occasionally, a professional in healthcare would visit them to address any questions, which are beyond their common experiences. In terms of use of resources, this is least resource-intensive.

14.5.2.4 Impact and Limitations of CBBI

CBBIs are mostly associated with greater impact compared to the BFHI on both duration of exclusive breastfeeding and breastfeeding in general, although their impact on the latter has been reported to be much more. In comparison with the BFHI, CBBIs have been reported to have greater impact. The limitation of CBBIs is that they are dependent on volunteerism, which may be difficult to sustain in the long run.

14.5.3 Sustaining the Optimal Breastfeeding Culture

Our discussion in this chapter raises the question on whether the optimal breastfeeding culture can be sustained or not. The traditional breastfeeding practices represent the most common way of infant feeding in most communities in southern Africa, including Malawi and Tanzania as mentioned earlier. Nevertheless, these communities are also not spared from the promotion of the culture of optimal breastfeeding, which come along with modern health care. However, awareness campaigns which most communities are exposed to are not adequate to ensure that mothers exclusively breastfeed, although such campaigns are an important step in initiating behavioural change. Mothers require both a supportive environment and personal skills to be able to exclusively breastfeed.

A supportive environment can be achieved by undertaking deliberate measures within the different sectors of communities to make breastfeeding easier. For instance, this would entail providing adequate maternity leave to allow mothers to spend ample time with the infants at least during the first 6 months where they are to breastfeed exclusively (see Chapter 8 in this volume). In scenarios where long maternity leaves may not be feasible, mothers may be provided with breastfeeding rooms and breaks during working hours to enable them to breastfeed from the workplace. In farming communities, households and/or the community could arrange to take up most of the farm work for mothers who are lactating. In addition, breastfeeding shelters could be constructed to allow mothers to breastfeed while working on the farms. The BFCI in the Gambia is a good example where these measures have been taken. The personal skills which mothers require to breastfeed optimally are additional child care skills. Such skills would enable the mother to deal with a crying infant in the middle of the night and to deal with the fear of their breast milk being insufficient. Mothers can get this support through counselling from health personnel or people in their social network who have successfully breastfed.

The fact that additional support is required for mothers to optimally breastfeed highlights the implication that in the absence of any intervention, exclusive breastfeeding will hardly be practised. Therefore, the extent to which optimal breastfeeding promotion interventions are scaled up and the extent of the permanence of the measures they take will likewise define the extent to which optimal breastfeeding culture is adopted and sustained. Most interventions, as earlier elaborated, have focused on providing mothers with child care skills and have given minimal emphasis to providing a supportive environment. The provision of child care skills is in itself an undertaking which requires a lot of human and financial resources. Community measures to adapt community structures to support breastfeeding are cost-effective in the long run. Nevertheless, resources are still required to initiate such community changes. Unless if governments and non-governmental organisations would make even much more stronger commitment and set aside more resources for breastfeeding, mothers may never have the possibility to embrace the new culture of optimal breastfeeding.

14.6 Conclusion

Global infant feeding policies uphold optimal breastfeeding as the strategy for infant feeding. However, the practises of optimal breastfeeding are unusual in traditional customs in most parts of central and southern Africa.

Intervening in infant feeding practices through providing additional child care skills and a supportive environment seems to provide a bridge for transitioning from traditional infant feeding practices to optimal breastfeeding practices. The extent to which interventions take into account traditional beliefs of the communities which they target is important for the success of the interventions. Further to this, interventions which provide both child care skills and an enabling environment to breastfeed are bound to make a greater impact in effecting change for optimal breastfeeding than those where a single focus is made. Community-based breastfeeding interventions such as the Baby Friendly Community Initiative have been associated with making a greater impact on mothers to optimally breastfeed than those which are health facility-based like the Baby Friendly Hospital Initiative. The fact that intervening requires both human and financial resources is crucial in the sustenance of the culture of optimal breastfeeding. The sustenance of the culture of breastfeeding is dependent on the permanence of the measures brought about by interventions, and more so, on the availability of resources to scale up such interventions.

References

Agnarsson, I., Mpello, A., GunnLaugsson, G., Hofvander, Y., & Greiner, T. (2001). Infant feeding practices during the first six months of life in a rural area in Tanzania. *East African Medical Journal, 78*(1), 9–13.

Bezner, K. R., Dakishoni, L., Shumba, L., Msachi, R., & Chirwa, M. (2008). "We grandmothers know plenty": Breastfeeding, complementary feeding and the multifaceted role of grandmothers in Malawi. *Social Science and Medicine, 66*(5), 1095–1105.

Bhandari, N., Kabir, A. K., & Salam, M. A. (2008). Mainstreaming nutrition into maternal and child health programmes: Scaling up of exclusive breastfeeding. *Maternal and Child Nutrition, 4*(Suppl 1), 5–23.

Chinkonde, J. R., Sundby, J., & Martinson, F. (2009). The prevention of mother-to-child HIV transmission programme in Lilongwe, Malawi: Why do so many women drop out. *ReproductiveHealth Matters, 17*(33), 143–151.

de Paoli, M., Manongi, R., Helsing, E., & Klepp, K. I. (2001). Exclusive breastfeeding in the era of AIDS. *Journal of HumanLactation, 17*(4), 313–320.

Hussein, A. K. (2005). Breastfeeding and complementary feeding practices in Tanzania. *East African Journal of Public Health, 2*(1), 27–31.

Kamudoni, P., Maleta, K., Shi, Z., & Holmboe-Ottesen, G. (2007). Infant feeding practices in the first 6 months and associated factors in a rural and semiurban community in Mangochi District, Malawi. *Journal of Human Lactation, 23*(4), 325–332.

Kerr, R. B., Berti, P. R., & Chirwa, M. (2007). Breastfeeding and mixed feeding practices in Malawi: Timing, reasons, decision makers, and child health consequences. *Food Nutrition Bulletin, 28*(1), 90–99.

Lema, N. T. (1963). Tribal customs in infant feeding. II. Among the Chagga. *East AfricanMedical Journal, 40*, 370–375.

Mabilia, M. (1996a). Beliefs and practices in infant feeding among the Wagogo of Chigongwe (Dodoma rural district), Tanzania. I. Breastfeeding. *Ecology and Food Nutriton, 35*(3), 195–207.

Mabilia, M. (1996b). Beliefs and practices in infant feeding among the Wagogo of Chigongwe (Dodoma rural district), Tanzania. II. Weaning. *Ecology and Food Nutriton, 35*(3), 209–217.

Naylor, A. J. (2001). Baby-Friendly Hospital Initiative. Protecting, promoting, and supporting breastfeeding in the twenty-first century. *Pediatic Clinical of North America, 48*(2), 475–483.

Obermeyer, C. M., & Castle, S. (1996). Back to nature? Historical and cross-cultural perspectives on barriers to optimal breastfeeding. *MedicalAnthropology, 17*(1), 39–63.

Omer-Salim, A., Persson, L. A., & Olsson, P. (2007). Whom can I rely on? Mothers' approaches to support for feeding: An interview study in suburban Dar es Salaam, Tanzania. *Midwifery, 23*(2), 172–183.

Kamudoni, P. (2005). *Infant feeding practices and perceptions*. Unpublished Master thesis in International Community Health, University of Oslo.

Philipp, B. L., & Merewood, A. (2004). The Baby-Friendly way: The best breastfeeding start. *Pediatic Clinics of North America, 51*(3), 761–83.

Philipp, B. L., & Radford, A. (2006). Baby-Friendly: snappy slogan or standard of care? *Archives of Dissertation of Child Fetal Neonatal Education, 91*(2), F145–F149.

Rwegelera, G. G. (1963). Tribal customs in infant feeding 1. Among the Haya. *East Africal Medical Journal, 40*, 366–369.

Saadeh, R., & Akre, J. (1996). Ten steps to successful breastfeeding: a summary of the rationale and scientific evidence. *Birth, 23*(3), 154–160.

Sellen, D. W. (1998). Infant and young child feeding practices among African pastoralists: The Datoga of Tanzania. *Journal of Biosocial Science, 30*(4), 481–499.

Semega-Janneh, I. J., Bohler, E., Holm, H., Matheson, I., & Holmboe-Ottesen, G. (2001). Promoting breastfeeding in rural Gambia: Combining traditional and modern knowledge. *Health Policy Plan, 16*(2), 199–205.

Shirima, R., Greiner, T., Kylberg, E., & Gebre-Medhin, M. (2001). Exclusive breast-feeding is rarely practised in rural and urban Morogoro, Tanzania. *Public Health Nutrition, 4*(2), 147–154.

UNICEF. (2005). *Celebrating the Innocenti Declaration on the protection, promotion and support of breatsfeeding, 1990–2005*. UNICEF, Innocenti Research Centre.

Vaahtera, M., Kulmala, T., Hietanen, A., Ndekha, M., Cullinan, T., Salin, M. L., et al. (2001). Breastfeeding and complementary feeding practices in rural Malawi. *Acta Paediatrics, 90*(3), 328–332.

World Health Organization (2003). *Global strategy for infant and young child feeding*. Geneva: World Health Organization.

Chapter 15
Hoki Ki Te Ukaipo: Reinstating Māori Infant Care Practices to Increase Breastfeeding Rates

Marewa Glover and Chris Cunningham

Contents

15.1 Introduction

He aroha whaereere, he potiki piripoho.
A mother's love, a breast-clinging child.

There are marked cultural differences in infant care practices (Panaretto, Muller, Patole, Watson, & Whitehall 2002) and the meanings attached to these practices. In New Zealand, infant care practices are associated with differences in outcomes for

M. Glover (✉)
Social & Community Health, School of Public Health, University of Auckland, Private Bag 92019, Auckland, New Zealand
e-mail: m.glover@auckland.ac.nz

P. Liamputtong (ed.), *Infant Feeding Practices*, DOI 10.1007/978-1-4419-6873-9_15,

© Springer Science+Business Media, LLC 2011

both mother and child. Sources of support and advice for the mother, infant feeding, infant sleeping and traditional 'cultural' practices were examined for a range of New Zealand mothers to illuminate inter- and intra-ethnic differences with Māori found to exhibit the broadest range of practices seen in New Zealand populations (Abel, Park, Tipene-Leach, Finau, & Lennan 2001).

Traditional Māori infant care practices have been systematically, although unevenly, lost as the 'benefits' of Western and modern practices have been sold to new Māori mothers. Associated with this change in behaviour are infant care outcomes, which are poorer for Māori than for other ethnic groups in New Zealand. Sudden Infant Death Syndrome (SIDS) rates are higher and have been known to be higher for some decades (Scragg & Mitchell 1998). Breastfeeding rates are lower, bedsharing and its attendant risks are more frequently seen for Māori, yet the knowledge and practice of Māori traditions by contemporary Māori mothers is poor.

In this chapter, we will discuss several issues relevant to Māori infant feeding practices. In particular, we will focus on pre-European Māori infant care, newcomers (Pākehā) and the colonisation of New Zealand, the introduction of foreign infant care practices, the growth of the artificial baby milk industry, the destruction of Māori infant feeding traditions, Māori mothers and breastfeeding among Māori today, influences that divert Māori women from breastfeeding, and tobacco smoking as a significant barrier to breastfeeding for Māori women. We conclude our chapter by discussing some opportunities for intervention.

15.2 Pre-European Māori Infant Care

Māori migrated from Eastern Polynesia and, according to the archaeological record, settled in New Zealand around AD 1000 or 1100. Ancient Māori society was essentially tribal, with each *iwi* (tribe) being a nation unto itself (Te Awekotuku 1991), holding political authority as *tangata whenua* (people of the land) in their region. Each tribe, or even *hapū* (sub-tribe), formulated and followed distinct sets of *tikanga* (protocols, lore) governing daily life and interaction within the *whānau* (immediate and customary extended family), and *hapū/iwi* and interaction with other *iwi*. Many *tikanga* were concerned with tribal survival (Glover, McKree, & Dyall 2007), for example, *whakapapa* (geneaology, particularly the tracking of biological and non-biological family relationships and the continuance of family bloodlines) was a significant *tikanga* for Māori (Glover & Rousseau 2007). Flowing from this central and all important necessity – to survive as a unique people and culture – fertility and the continuance of *whakapapa* were governed by elaborate and varied *tikanga*. There were *tikanga* guiding the forming of partnerships to have offspring; *tikanga* establishing what was appropriate behaviour for women, respect towards women and care of women. *Tikanga* were practiced especially for pregnant women, and there were many *tikanga* guiding birthing practice and infant care (Palmer 2002; Glover 2007).

The *whakatauki* (proverb) at the opening of this chapter refers to the mother's provision of infant care practices. One interpretation gives the meaning as: 'A mother would rather suffer than to see her child in any form of misfortune' (Te Whare Wānanga o Awanuiārangi no date). The *whakatauki* comes from a time when Māori language was largely oral and speech, chants, *karakia* (prayer) and songs were more rhetorical, relying on the invoking of visual images through the use of metaphor. Though the *whakatauki* refers specifically to breastfeeding, breastfeeding itself is used as a metaphor to convey the essence of the love and care required when raising a child. The child's well-being is central. The *whakatauki* also comes from a time before artificial alternatives to breast milk were available to Māori. Breastfeeding was not separated from the essential practices of infant care – it was assumed and it was natural.

The historical record supports that Māori infants were always breastfed before colonisation (Papakura, cited in Ellis-Loschmann 1997). Best (1929) recorded that infants were fed for varying lengths of time, for example, until they could turn over without assistance, until teeth appeared, or for as long as the child chose to breastfeed. Papakura (cited in Ellis-Loschmann, 1997) reported that breastfeeding was usually continued until the child was walking. When the biological mother for whatever reason could not breastfeed or was temporarily unavailable for breastfeeding, the baby would have been breastfed by another woman in the *whānau*. Māori lived in extended communal *whānau* groupings and childrearing was to a certain extent shared. For instance, the Māori word for mother – *whaea*, was used by children when referring to all women of their mother's generation. Similarly, children were collectively called son and daughter. Even in modern times, some Māori report that breastfeeding anothers' baby is normal (Glover, Manaena-Biddle, Waldon, Cunningham 2008; McLeod 2008). One study on traditional Māori food sources reports the use of a freshwater mussel (*kakahi*) for mixing up an alternative food when a wetnurse could not be found, as follows:

> To any one who enjoys the shell-fish of the salt water the kakahi is very tasteless and insipid. In olden days, however, the kakahi was very important. It was used in the feeding of motherless infants where a wet-nurse could not be secured. The kakahi was cooked and the child fed with the soft paru, or visceral mass, which, further softened with the water retained in the shell, could be sucked like milk. Three or four kakahi formed a meal. Hence the Māori said, Ko te kakahi te whaea o te tamaiti (The kakahi is the mother of the child). Ka whakangotea ki te wai o te kakahi (It was suckled on the juice of the takahi), (Hiroa 1921, p. 450).

15.3 New-Comers (Pākehā) and the Colonisation of New Zealand

Māori were exposed to European ideals and technologies occasionally during the seventeenth and eighteenth century as explorers, whalers and sealers, and missionaries driven by European capitalism continued the search for new environmental and human resources to exploit. Māori and their land were discovered relatively late in the process of European colonisation, and by the 19th century, two-thirds of the world was colonised by European nations (see Glover, Dudgeon, & Huygens 2004 for a fuller discussion of the colonisation of Australia and New Zealand and the effects on the Indigenous peoples). Colonisation of New Zealand did not begin in earnest until the early 1800s, when in 1840 the Treaty of Waitangi was signed by over 500 tribal leaders and a representative of the British Crown. The Treaty allowed for the establishment of a settler government, guaranteed that *iwi* would maintain their *tino rangatiratanga* (sovereignty) and guaranteed protection over property rights and *taonga* (cultural and social properties) (Durie 2003). The Treaty promised that Māori would have equal citizenship rights to settlers, implying equal opportunity and access as well as spiritual and cultural freedom.

European colonisation followed familiar processes whereby control over spirituality, land, law, language and education, health and family structures and finally culture itself passed from the Indigenous people to the colonisers (Nairn 1990). Thus, in New Zealand it was mainly English worldviews that were introduced and enshrined in the new institutions established by the settlers and their government. Racism, particularly a belief in the superiority of the European colonisers and conversely the belief in the inferiority of the *natives,* was integral to the colonising processes that led to Māori worldviews and ways of life being systematically replaced. In contravention of the Treaty, European settlers established a national government excluding Māori and used the British army to force land sales and seize land. Overt legislation and policy destroyed the economic base and undermined the Māori spirit and culture. For example, the Tohunga Suppression Act of 1907 forbade the role of *tohunga* (people with superior knowledge in a particular area/Indigenous healers) and enabled Christianity to supplant the ancestral gods or spiritual guardians (Roberts, Norman, Minhinnick, Wihongi, & Kirkwood 1995).

15.4 The Introduction of Foreign Infant Care Practices

Māori would have observed and been subjected to 'lessons' in infant care from early on as a focus on health and well-being followed a period where introduced diseases had decimated the Māori population. Some practices, however, would not have been unusual. For example, the foreign practice of 'wetnursing' could have been seen to be similar to pre-existing Māori practice. The commercialisation of wetnursing as a profession and the use of strangers, however, may have been a new concept, although captives from other *iwi* could have been put to use as wetnurses by Māori in ancient times.

European ideas about the unsuitability or inadequacy of breast milk and the concocting of alternative 'milk' or cereals to feed infants, which date back centuries (Davidson 1953) before Māori exposure to them, would have been looked upon with curiosity, yet Māori were keen to benefit from their encounters with foreigners and were quick to adopt practices and technologies. Some Māori women would have been early-adopters of such practices.

15.5 Bonnie Babies for a Strong Nation

Improving the health of mothers and thereby their babies grew out of turn of the century (1900) national British security concerns to build a stronger and healthier next generation of fighters and workers (Bryder 2008). A number of male physicians and paediatricians supported the idea that a child's first few years determined later physical and intellectual capacity. In New Zealand, they were at the forefront of the response to high infant mortality and illness. In 1907, the Society for Promoting the Health of Women and Children, later to become the Royal New Zealand Plunket Society (Plunket), was established. The Society was set up to apply scientific principles to nutrition of babies, and was strongly rooted in eugenics and patriotism (Stace 1997). Its 1917 'Save the Babies' Week had the slogan 'The Race marches forward on the feet of Little Children'. Plunket was largely a women's movement, run by volunteers, sometimes with Government support. Clinics were established and nurses were employed to educate and support mothers who 'were ignorant of the correct methods of child-rearing and needed to be educated' (Bryder 2003, p. ix).

Among the male physicians working for improved infant health and heavily involved with Plunket was Truby King, who in 1904 was medical superindendent of Seacliff Lunatic Asylum near Dunedin, New Zealand. His role involved running the attached 900 acre farm. The high rate of mortality from scouring among the calves on the farm led him to studying the tracts on the artificial feeding systems. At the urging of his wife, he turned his scientific study from improving the artificial feeding systems for the calves to trying to develop a more nutritionally adequate artificial milk for their adopted daughter who was not thriving on the mixture of cow's milk and cane sugar that she had been having. Though he never wavered in his belief that breast milk was best, King developed and went on to promote 'a healthy system of artificial feeding', which he passed on to others who in turn set about teaching nurses and mothers and the newly formed Plunket volunteers (Bryder 2003).

King and his medical contemporaries believed a germ-free environment was necessary for disease prevention. Plunket's 1912 book *The Feeding and Care of Baby* promoted a by-the-clock routine of feeding, bathing and sleep. As Bryder (2003, p. 75) explains, 'this approach was believed to produce a well-balanced adult, who could exercise self-control and cope with deferred gratification. In the less child-centred world before the Second World War, it was also regarded as convenient for the parents'. This philosophy and the practices consistent with it would have contradicted *whānau*-centred Māori values of *aroha* (love) and infant care *tikanga* epitomised in the contemporary saying 'baby's the *rangatira*' (Glover et al. 2008, p. 57); that is the baby is the chief and she/he sets the pace: they feed when they are hungry and they sleep when they are tired. Some of the ancient practice of the *wharemoe* (sleeping house, typically a *raupo* hut the whole *whānau* slept in) has been retained. Particularly, it has remained common for mothers to sleep their babies next to them (Escot et al. 2009). This has become a major topic of contention between Māori and Pākehā (non-Māori) SIDS prevention workers and epidemiologists over the past 15 years (Thompson, Thach, Becroft, Mitchell, & the New Zealand Cot Death Study Group 2006).

15.6 The Growth of the Artificial Baby Milk Industry

Although King emphasised the preference of breastfeeding for infants, he was concerned about 'progressive nutritional failure from generation to generation' and argued for the very best artificial feeding in these cases (Bryder, 2009, p. 56). Māori women would likely have been exposed to and influenced by artificial baby milk marketing in New Zealand and given poorer Māori health, artificial feeding was seen as beneficial. Certainly, by 1955 Māori mothers were being encouraged to re-adopt breastfeeding of babies as the norm (Keritapu, 1955), clearly in response to a reduction of the practice of breastfeeding.

'King's particular contribution to the New Zealand infant welfare movement', writes Bryder (2003, p. 14), 'was the introduction of American formulae for infant feeding'. He devised two artificial baby food products: Kariol (New Zealand Cream or New Zealand Emulsion) and Karilac (also called Plunket Emulsion). Karilac consisted of vegetable oil, cod liver oil and dextrose and Karilac was a mixture of lactose, dextrose and gelatine, which was dissolved in water and added to cow's milk. King established a factory for their production, which in 1927 was taken over and established as the Karitane Products Society (KPS), whose profits were used to fund the Plunket Society. Plunket's artificial feeding practices relied on KPS products and indeed for a time was limited to them, as Plunket nurses were not permitted to prescribe patent medicines or promote commercial products, other than KPS products (Bryder 2003).

King was not alone in New Zealand in his establishment of a commercial artificial baby milk factory. In 1904, a dried-milk factory was built in a small rural town in New Zealand. This was the beginning of Glaxo, which became a major producer and exporter of 'baby formula', powdered milk and toddler cereals. Glaxo was marketed in England using the slogan 'Glaxo builds bonnie babies' (McCloy 2008). It was also used by soldiers in the First World War, ensconcing it almost as an institution in itself.

The marketing of artificial baby milk and infant foods continued unrestricted in New Zealand until the 1980s when The International Code of Marketing of Breastmilk Substitutes was formulated to protect infants from 'inappropriate feeding practices (including the unnecessary and improper use of breastmilk substitutes)' (Smith 2004, p. 371). The uncanny similarities between the history of and harmful, and addictive, nature of artificial baby milk products and tobacco products are only just beginning to be discussed (Smith 2004). The parallels include that: prior to marketing restrictions these industries falsely promote their products to be beneficial while omitting information on the significant health risks; the decision to use artificial baby milk, like the loss of autonomy that occurs for smokers even after one cigarette (Scragg, Wellman, Laugesen, & DiFranza 2008), is often irreversible for that child and the social and economic costs are also huge. Smith (2004, p. 377) reminds us that 'artificial feeding is the tobacco of the twenty-first century'.

15.7 The Destruction of Māori Infant Feeding Traditions

The following poem captures the feeling and concerns overheard at a Māori Sudden Infant Death Syndrome *hui* (meeting run in accordance with Māori protocols) in the early 1990s. It conveys the widely held belief that a law was passed in 1909 forbidding Māori women to breastfeed, at least in public. The stories told by Māori participants in the *hui* also implied that Māori women were encouraged to sleep babies face-down, that they sensed or were told that their infant care practices were unhygienic and their milk was inadequate and or inferior to introduced alternatives. Flour and water, referred to in the poem, was a commonly used and promoted European preparation called Pap, which dates back to 1465 (Davidson 1953). Further, the poem captures how the introduced foreign ways are adopted as the new norm to be passed on inter-generationally.

15.7.1 Apnoea

Don't look at me in that punishing way
and say I'm a bad parent
because I sleep my baby on its stomach
and don't breastfeed it.
It was your idea after all – remember?
Remember, back in 1909
you used to say our lives were full of germs
the very air in our homes was infested
and you said it was healthier for baby
to sleep on its tummy so as not to ingest it
and you passed a law – remember?
Your Native Affairs Amendment Act
forbidding our babies their mother's milk
a milk you thought inferior
and for fear of losing our babies altogether
for that was your threat and your practice
some mothers mixed up what looked like milk
but was only flour and water
and some babies died as the imitation milk
gummed up their interior.
Even so, it was your ways that were passed down

from Māori mother to Māori mother.
So, don't look at me and say I'm a bad parent
when my child becomes another
Māori-cot-death-statistic.
You've got to take some credit for it. Remember
(Glover 2001, p. 24).

The law referred to above does not exist, but the myth conveys the depth of censure Māori women used to experience when breastfeeding (Ellis-Loschmann 1997). Ellis-Loschmann (1997) surmises that a number of factors could have contributed to the creation and maintenance of this 'urban-myth'. Firstly, Victorian era class systems and strictures around modesty/decency would have deemed public displays of the breast, even in the act of breastfeeding, offensive. Secondly, the pre-existing Māori public health system rapidly deteriorated, with for example the Midwives Registration Act of 1904 restricting the role of lay midwives; the Tohunga Suppression Act 1907 and other laws aimed at destroying Māori culture, such as the Native Schools Act 1867 forbidding Māori language to be spoken in schools.

In 1909, the Department of Health recruited District nurses (non-Māori) to work with Māori, though their focus at first was typhoid fever and other acute illnesses. Some of the Health Department's District Health Nurses, however, also undertook Karitane Nurse training exposing them to Plunket philosophies. Plunket primarily worked only with Pākehā women.

During the 1924 Campaign for Safe Maternity, legislation was introduced to completely eliminate untrained midwives (Donley 1986 cited in Palmer 2002). The cumulative effect was that by the 1930s, birthing among Māori women increasingly shifted to hospitals. Palmer (2002) concludes that Māori participation in the national maternity system was encouraged by, Government policy, for example, the 1937 Committee of Inquiry into Maternity Services supported hospitalised childbirth attended by doctors and obstetric nurses; financial incentives, for example, the 1924 ten pound maternity subsidy to help cover doctors fees; and endorsement within Māoridom, for example, the Māori Members of Parliament Apirana Ngata, Maui Pomare and Peter Buck, fiercely advocated complete acceptance of Pākehā knowledge in hygiene, sanitation and medicine.

By the 1950s, Plunket was advocating breastfeeding for 6–9 months, although breastfeeding for 9 months was 'becoming exceptional' (Bryder 2003, p. 121). This was because the use of alternative baby milk was so popular and the prevalence of breastfeeding had reduced so much, though prevalence was still mainly based upon Pākehā women's experiences.

Following the Second World War, New Zealand experienced rapid economic growth. There was a shortage and thus high demand for labour which attracted many Māori to live in the cities. To encourage Māori assimilation, tribal structures were discouraged. By 1961, approximately forty percent of the Māori population lived in urban areas, and by 1963, ninety-five percent of all Māori births were taking place in hospital (Palmer 2002). Plunket did not begin to deliver to Māori women until the late 1960s and in limited urban areas. In 1977, Plunket was finally funded to take total responsibility for health surveillance of all babies and pre-school infants in the 'special needs' areas of south Auckland where a third of the population were Māori or Pacific Islanders (Bryder 2008).

15.8 Māori Mothers and Breastfeeding Among Māori Today

While some Māori still practice traditional maternity and infant care practices, such as the ritual disposal of the placenta and use of traditional processes for naming their children, breastfeeding as the norm did not survive the introduction of European models of care (Abel et al. 2001).

For Māori, the fertility rate has fallen dramatically from historical rates of over 6 per woman in the 1960s to a rate of 2.7 per woman in 2008 (Statistics New Zealand 2009) with the median age of Māori mothers being 25 years. These data compare with a fertility rate of 1.96 and median age of 29 years for all NZ women (Statistics New Zealand 2009). The major change in Māori fertility is that fewer older Māori women are having babies, while first time Māori mothers are significantly younger than non-Māori mothers. This relatively youthful profile for Māori mothers means that the types of support services and advice needed is markedly different than for older, non-Māori mothers.

Breastfeeding rates in New Zealand, and for Māori particularly, are difficult to measure due to inconsistencies in the way breastfeeding has been measured over time (Thornley, Waa, & Ball. 2007). In 2002, Māori breastfeeding rates were reported to be consistently lower than overall New Zealand rates, with only 13–14 percent of Māori babies vs. 19–21 percent of European and other babies fully[1] breastfed at 6 months (Thornley et al. 2007). Plunket breastfeeding data for 2006 (Table 15.1) shows how exclusive and full breastfeeding reduces down to 25 percent by 4–8 months.

Table 15.1 Percentage of Plunket babies exclusively and fully fed in 2006

Age of infant	Māori	Pacific	Asian	European/other	All
2–6 weeks	58	56	55	71	66
10–16 weeks	45	48	52	59	55
4–8 months	17	19	25	29	25

Source: Royal New Zealand Plunket Society (2006), in Glover et al. (2007)

15.9 Influences That Divert Māori Women from Breastfeeding

A study of Māori women's infant feeding practices (Glover et al. 2009) proposed that for Māori women, breastfeeding is the *tika* (culturally right) way to feed baby. For some mothers, breastfeeding is still the norm and they and their *whānau* assume

[1]Fully breastfed: the infant has taken breastmilk only, and no other liquids or solids except a minimal amount of water or prescribed medicines, in the past 48 hours (Ministry of Health 2002a)

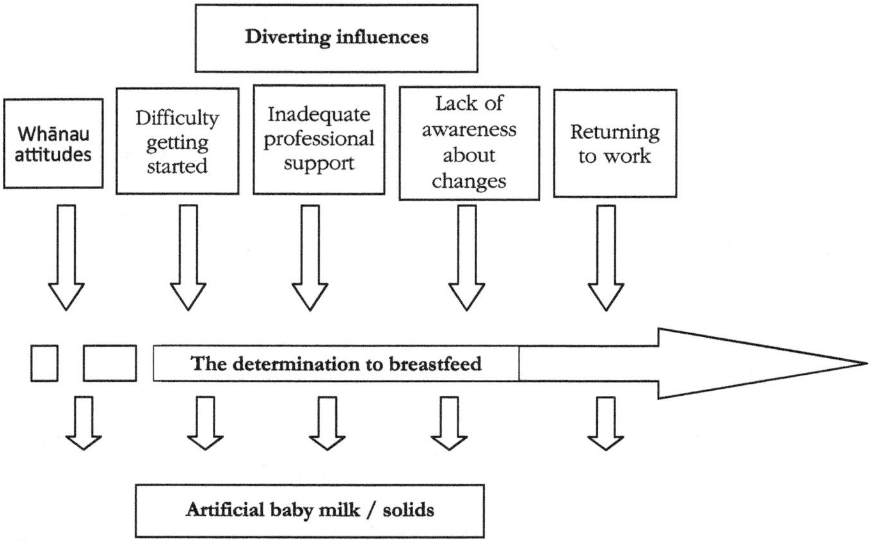

Fig. 15.1 *Te Reo o te Aratika.* Source: Glover et al. (2007)

that they will breastfeed. However, for some new mothers artificial feeding or switching baby to artificial baby milk and solids early occurred as a result of influences that diverted women from the preferred pathway of breastfeeding. The model, *Te Reo o te Aratika* (Fig. 15.1), shows the five diversionary influences that were identified:

- breakdown in the breastfeeding norm within the *whānau*;
- early interruptions to or difficulties establishing breastfeeding;
- negative or insufficient maternity support for breastfeeding;
- lack of knowledge about how breastfeeding changes over time, and
- returning to work.

The first diverting influence is the contemporary infant feeding norm within the *whānau*, including how babies have been fed within the *whānau* in the past and *whānau* attitudes towards breastfeeding and historically high levels of using artificial milk. The inter-generational differences that emerged during Glover et al.'s (2007) research supported the findings of other researchers that beliefs and practices introduced to Māori by European/Pākehā immigrants to New Zealand have supplanted Māori infant feeding practices (Abel et al. 2001). Thus, in some Māori *whānau*, bottle-feeding, or breastfeeding for a few weeks only, has become the norm and new mothers within these *whānau* feel that they are breaking the cycle if they choose to breastfeed exclusively. They may experience less support to breastfeed and/or active discouragement from advisors who are not aware of cultural infant care values and practices and support mechanisms unique to Māori. This negative environment can start to occur during pregnancy, soon after birth and as long as the mother continues to breastfeed. How women have fed their previous babies can also determine intent to breastfeed new babies.

The second diverting influence occurs within the first 6 weeks of baby's birth. This is when physiological, social and cultural factors influence the mother–infant dynamic and undermine the maintenance of breastfeeding or hinder its establishment. Physiological barriers to breastfeeding, for example, inverted nipples or prematurity of the baby, can make it more difficult to establish exclusive breastfeeding from birth. Given that each mother–infant dyad is unique, the baby's inclination to suckle and the strength of the mother's determination to breastfeed and her self-efficacy, for instance, combine in a dynamic way to influence the ease with which breastfeeding is established. Interruptions to immediate establishment of exclusive breastfeeding and difficulties, such as, painful cracked nipples can put women off breastfeeding.

The third diverting influence occurs when women's experience of maternity services they receive is negative or insufficient. The absence of effective antenatal education – targeted to the specific needs of a younger, culturally diverse population – can leave a bottle-feeding status quo unchallenged. Insufficient postnatal instruction and support to breastfeed can leave a woman having difficulties establishing breastfeeding with no choice but to turn to artificial baby milk. Culturally insensitive behaviour and/or conflicting advice can cause women to distrust the health professionals, effectively cutting them off from professional support. Feeling pressured to breastfeed and/or pressured to breastfeed a particular way can be disempowering and can undermine a woman's confidence in her ability to breastfeed her child.

An extension of this influence is the sometimes conflicting health promotion messages which new mothers receive. Māori mothers sometimes cited a return to tobacco smoking as a reason for stopping breastfeeding so as to not expose the infant to tobacco smoke. They understood the negative influences of environmental tobacco smoke, but were confused about the possible transmission of nicotine (or other chemicals) through breast milk. A second negative influence was messages the mothers had heard about bedsharing and sudden infant death. Bedsharing promoted breastfeeding, but a desire to 'keep babies safe' led to separate sleeping arrangements and a reduced convenience of breastfeeding, which in turn led to bottle-feeding.

The fourth diverting influence occurs at about 4 months. At the time of Glover et al.'s (2007) research, postnatal midwifery care in New Zealand usually had ended pending transition to a well child care service, which scheduled early childcare checks to occur around 5 months of age. If mothers have not been adequately educated as to the natural growth spurts and resulting physiological changes that occur in the breasts, they may conclude that their milk is insufficient. The participants in Heath, Tuttle, Cleghorn, and Parnell's study (2000) similarly appeared to know little about breastfeeding. For instance, only 17 percent were aware that frequent breastfeeding was an effective way of increasing breast milk supply.

The fifth main factor that diverts a woman from breastfeeding is the need to return to work. Māori *whānau* are more economically deprived, and therefore, women are under pressure to return to work for financial reasons (cf Chapters 7, 8, and 9 in this volume). In New Zealand, some women qualify for paid parental leave, which allows them to take 3 months off work. Thus, Government policy in a de facto manner withdraws support for women who wish to breastfeed for more than 3 months. Paid parental leave, therefore, provides for some babies to be exclusively breastfed for the first 3 months, which is inconsistent with international expert opinion to feed babies breast milk exclusively for 6 months.

Social discouragement of breastfeeding in public compounds the difficulties women can encounter if they try to persist with breastfeeding upon their return to work. Most of the participants in Heath et al.'s (2000) study reported that it was embarrassing to breastfeed in public. Heath et al. (2000) also heard anecdotal reports of mothers being asked not to breastfeed in restaurants, shops and shopping malls (see also Chapters 3 and 4 in this volume). Only a few (12 percent) of the mothers in Heath et al.'s (2000) study recalled being encouraged to breastfeed. Heath and colleagues (2000) conclude that social change is necessary to enable more women to continue on with breastfeeding past 3 weeks (when many of their participants stopped).

15.10 Tobacco Smoking: A Significant Barrier to Breastfeeding for Māori Women

Unlike most women of the world, Māori women rapidly took up smoking tobacco upon its introduction to New Zealand in the 1800s. This historical anomaly resulted in Māori women having the highest rate of smoking and smoking-related lung cancer in the world (Doll 1978). Māori women have almost twice the incidence of cervical cancer than non-Māori women (Ministry of Health 2005). Despite a falling smoking prevalence rate for most groups in New Zealand, Māori women still have the highest rates at 45 percent (vs. 19 percent non-Māori non-Pacific women (Ministry of Health 2009). Tobacco smoking is the biggest killer of Māori (Laugesen & Clements 1998). Exposure to second-hand smoke in utero harms the health of the unborn child and is associated with increased ectopic pregnancies, spontaneous abortions, still births, neonatal and perinatal deaths. At first visit with a midwife for pregnancy, in 2007, 42.9 percent of Māori women smoked. This reduced to 34.1 percent at the 4–6 weeks postpartum visit (New Zealand College of Midwives 2008). These excessively high rates of smoking during pregnancy are significantly associated with the disproportionately high rates of Sudden Unexpected Deaths in Infancy (SUDI) for Māori. More than 60 percent of New Zealand infants dying of SUDI were Māori in 2003–2007 (Child and Youth Mortality Review Committee 2009). Smoking is associated with both premature birth and intrauterine growth retardation, and so with lower birth weight, all factors that undermine successful initiation and continuation of breastfeeding.

Health promotion efforts to reduce people's exposure to second-hand smoke and that warn of the risks to health from smoking have been very effective in New

Zealand. A 2006/2007 New Zealand health survey found that just 4.8 percent of children under 2 years of age are exposed to environmental tobacco smoke in the home. However, significant inequalities persist. Māori children were at twice the risk (Ministry of Health 2008). Māori women have the highest smoking prevalence rates in New Zealand, with 52.5 percent of women of childbearing age smoking (The Quit Group & the Ministry of Health 2009).

One of the unintended negative impacts of the successful social marketing campaigns to increase smoke-free environments and reduce harm from exposure to second-hand smoke could be that women who are unable to stop smoking during pregnancy, or who relapse to smoking soon after pregnancy, believe that the health risk from their smoking outweighs the benefits of breastfeeding and they choose to stop breastfeeding. Whilst stopping smoking remains one of the most important changes a person can make to improve their health, advice to breastfeeding mothers who smoke should be that it is best to continue breastfeeding despite their smoking status.

15.11 Opportunities for Intervention: Conclusion

Breastfeeding Māori infants has the potential to yield a greater health benefit for Māori due to the higher prevalence rates for a number of conditions that can be moderated by having been breastfed (Heath et al. 2000). The risks of SUDI, persistent otitis media and the resulting hearing loss, and juvenile diabetes are all lessened for infants who are breastfed. Between 2003 and 2005, the leading cause of admission to a public hospital among 1–4 years old was respiratory disease (Robson & Harris 2007). Exclusive breastfeeding is also associated with a significant reduction in the incidence of lower respiratory problems (Wright, Holberg, Martinez, Morgan, & Taussig 1989).

The diversionary influences and barriers to breastfeeding outlined in this chapter highlight critical foci and times for intervening. Māori women share many of the challenges to breastfeeding experienced by other women. What is unique to Māori is that foreign infant care practices have displaced pre-European Māori infant feeding practices to such a degree that Māori women now have the lowest rates of exclusive or full breastfeeding in New Zealand. Promotion of breastfeeding to Māori should focus on re-establishing breastfeeding as a *tikanga* (right cultural practice) rather than a perceived lifestyle choice (Glover et al. 2007). Public health policies are needed to support breastfeeding from birth, throughout infancy and beyond. Currently, in New Zealand paid parental leave supports exclusive breastfeeding for only the first 3 months for some babies. This provision should be extended to benefit all babies of mothers who were working pre-pregnancy, and to provide for a longer period of time off work.

Not only is social change needed to create more supportive environments for breastfeeding, Tipene-Leach, Abel, Park, Finau, and Lennan (2000) argue for structural change to reduce 'non-modifiable' risk factors, such as reducing the economic inequality between Māori and Pākehā/European. The public health approach in New Zealand relies heavily on motivating individual change. This is not consistent with the more holistic understanding of health, as conveyed in contemporary Māori health models such as *Te Whare Tapa Wha* (the four-sided house). The four sides of the house, which are interdependent and must be maintained in balance to enjoy stability are: *te taha wairua* (the spiritual realm), *te taha whānau* (the family and wider community of support); *te taha tinana* (the physical body); and *te taha hinengaro* (the psychological world) (Durie 1994). Te ao tūroa (the long-standing world) has been proposed as an additional realm to cover the broader political and environmental impacts on health (Glover 2005). A more holistic approach would situate breastfeeding, which is one modifiable behaviour, within a programme focused on the re-establishment of a range of Māori infant care *tikanga*. For example, providing *whānau*, especially those who have been disconnected from family/ancestral sources of the knowledge, with information on Māori *tikanga* concerning traditional disposal of the *whenua* (placenta) and *pito* (navel), *karakia* (chants), naming practices, safe sleeping practices and how to protect baby from toxins such as environmental tobacco smoke.

Recognising the *whānau* as the foundation of Māori society is central to Government policy. One of the key threads through *He Korowai Oranga*, one of the Governments' key Māori health policy strategies (Ministry of Health 2006), is *tino rangatiratanga*, the capacity for *whānau* to make informed decisions about health and to apply these decisions positively. Supporting *whānau* to implement effective breastfeeding practices is directly relevant to *He Korowai Oranga*: 'development of *whānau*, *hapū*, *iwi* and Māori communities'. *He Korowai Oranga* acknowledges 'the need to foster conditions that build on strengths and assets of *whānau* and encourage their health and well-being'. Also, it is stated that: 'services should be organised around the needs of *whānau* and not the needs of providers'. For Māori, this means health providers need to deliver in to environments where Māori *whānau* gather (the home, marae, sports events) at times that are convenient to *whānau*. This would require a radical restructuring of the way the health system operates and is currently the subject of a major review being promoted by the coalition government (the Whānau Ora Task Force, http://www.msd.govt.nz/about-msd-and-our-work/work-programmes/initiatives/whanau-ora/index.html).

In the interim, decolonisation principles need to inform the design of *whānau ora* policies and intervention programmes. In relation to the re-establishment of breastfeeding, the process of conscientisation (Freire 1972) suggests that it is useful to encourage critical reflection upon the history outlined in this chapter, the foreign beliefs and practices that were introduced and how legislation and institutions were used to systematically displace Māori beliefs and practices. It would be useful to raise Māori awareness of and facilitate a critical analysis of the role of the multinational artificial baby milk and infant food industry and their marketing tactics and develop a Māori appropriate counter-industry strategy. This would assist in affirming the legitimacy of Māori knowledge and encourage cultural renewal (Dudgeon & Williams 2000).

References

Abel, S., Park, J., Tipene-Leach, D., Finau, S., & Lennan, M. (2001). Infant care practices in New Zealand: A cross-cultural qualitative study. *Social Science and Medicine, 53*, 1135–1148.

Best, E. (1929 reprinted 2005). *The whare kohanga (The "Nest House") and its lore.* Wellington: Te Papa.

Bryder, L. (2003). *A voice for mothers: The Plunket Society and infant welfare, 1907–2000.* Auckland: Auckland University Press.

Bryder, L. (2008). The Plunket Society: Part of the New Zealand way of life? *Australian Historical Studies, 39*(2), 183–198.

Bryder, L. (2009). From breast to bottle: A history of modern infant feeding. *Endeavour, 33*(2), 54–59.

Child and Youth Mortality Review Committee, Te Rōpū Arotake Auau Mate o te Hunga Tamariki, Taiohi. (2009). *Fifth Report to the Minister of Health: Reporting mortality 2002–2008.* Wellington: Child and Youth Mortality Review Committee.

Davidson, W. D. (1953). A brief history of infant feeding. *The Journal of Pediatrics, 43*(1), 74–87.

Doll, R. (1978). Atmospheric pollution and lung cancer. *Environmental Health Perspectives, 22*, 23–31.

Dudgeon, P., & Williams, R. (2000). Culturally appropriate therapies, models and services. In P. Dudgeon, D. Garvey, & H. Pickett (Eds.), *Working with Indigenous Australians: A handbook for psychologists* (pp. 389–394). Perth: Gunada.

Durie, M. (1994). Whaiora : Maori health development. Auckland: Oxford University Press.

Durie, M. (2003). Providing health services to indigenous peoples. *British Medical Journal, 327*, 408–409.

Ellis-Loschmann, L. (1997). *Maori women's experience of breastfeeding.* Wellington: Victoria University, unpublished Master's thesis.

Escott, A., Elder, D. E., & Zuccollo, J. M. (2009). Sudden unexpected infant death and bedsharing: referrals to the Wellington Coroner 1997–2006. *N Z Med J*, 122(1298), 59–68.

Freire, P. (1972). *Pedagogy of the oppressed.* New York: Herder and Herder.

Glover, M. (2001). *Hui.* Auckland: Glover.

Glover, M. (2005). Analysing smoking using Te Whare Tapa Wha. *New Zealand Journal of Psychology, 34*(1), 13–19.

Glover, M. (2007). How researching breastfeeding helped my own breastfeeding experience. *Breastfeeding Communique, 18*, 19–23.

Glover, M., & Rousseau, B. (2007). "Your child is your whakapapa": Māori considerations of assisted human reproduction and relatedness. *Sites: New Series, 4*(2), 117–136.

Glover, M., Dudgeon, P., & Huygens, I. (2004). Colonisation and racism. In I. Prilleltensky, & G. Nelson (Eds.), *Community psychology: Wellness & liberation* (pp. 330–344). New York: Palgrave MacMillan.

Glover, M., Manaena-Biddle, H., & Waldon, J. (2007). Influences that affect Māori women breastfeeding. *Breastfeeding Review, 15*(2), 5–14.

Glover, M., McKree, A., & Dyall, L. (2007c). *Māori attitudes to assisted human reproduction: An exploratory study. Summary report.* Auckland: Social & Community Health, School of Population Health, University of Auckland, p. 36.

Glover, M., Manaena-Biddle, H., Waldon, J., Cunningham, C. (2008). *Te Whaangai UU – Te Reo o Aratika: Māori Women and Breastfeeding.* Auckland: University of Auckland, Social and Community Health.

Glover, M., Waldon, J., Manaena-Biddle, H., Holdaway, M., & Cunningham, C. (2009). Barriers to best outcomes in breastfeeding for Māori: Mothers' Perceptions, Whānau Perceptions, and Services. *Journal of Human Lactation Online*. First published on March 13, 2009 as doi:10.1177/0890334409332436.

Heath, A. M., Tuttle, C. R., Cleghorn, C. L., & Parnell, W. R. (2000). A survey of knowledge, attitudes and practices associated with infant feeding in a New Zealand Māori population. *Journal of the New Zealand Dietetic Association, 54*(2), 94–98.

Hiroa, T. R. (1921). Maori food supplies of Lake Rotorua, with methods of obtaining them, and usages and customs pertaining thereto. *Transactions and Proceedings of the New Zealand Institute,* 53, 433–451.

Keritapu. (1955). Mothercraft: The Maori mother and her child. *Te Ao Hou. The New World,* No.10, April, 62–64. Downloaded 22 November 2009, from http://teaohou.natlib.govt.nz/journals/teaohou/issue/Mao10TeA/c53.html

Laugesen, M., & Clements, M. (1998) *Cigarette smoking mortality among Maori 1954–2028.* Wellington: Te Puni Kokiri (Ministry of Maori Development).

McCloy, N. (2008). *Made in New Zealand.* Auckland: Random House New Zealand.

McLeod, M. (2008). *Breastfeeding support in the Tairawhiti region: A formative evaluation.* Gisborne, New Zealand: Tairawhiti District Health Board.

Ministry of Health. (2005). *Cervical screening in New Zealand: A brief statistical review of the first decade.* Wellington: Ministry of Health.

Ministry of Health. (2006). *Whakatataka Tuarua: Maori Health Action Plan 2006–2011:* Wellington: Ministry of Health.

Ministry of Health. (2008). *Health behaviours and risk factors. A portrait of health – Key results of the New Zealand Health Survey.* Wellington: Ministry of Health.

Nairn, M. (1990). *Understanding colonization.* Auckland: Workshop material distributed by CCANZ Programme on Racism.

New Zealand College of Midwives, & The Midwifery and Maternity Providers Organisation. (2008). *Smoke free outcomes with midwife lead maternity carers: An analysis of smoking during pregnancy from the New Zealand College of Midwives midwifery database information 2004–2007.* Wellington: New Zealand College of Midwives & The Midwifery and Maternity Providers Organisation.

Palmer, S. K. (2002). *Hei oranga mo ngā wāhine hapū (o Hauraki) i roto i te whare ora.* Unpublished PhD thesis, Department of Psychology, University of Waikato, Hamilton, New Zealand.

Panaretto, K. S., Muller, R., Patole, S., Watson, D., & Whitehall, J. S. (2002). Is being Aboriginal or Torres Strait Islander a risk factor for poor neonatal outcome in a tertiary referral unit in north Queensland? *Journal of Paediatric Child Health, 38,* 16–22.

Roberts, M., Norman, W., Minhinnick, N., Wihongi, D., & Kirkwood, C. (1995). Kaitiakitanga: Maori perspectives on conservation. *Pacific Conservation Biology, 2,* 7–20.

Robson, B, & Harris, R. (Eds). (2007). *Hauora: Māori Standards of Health IV. A study of the years 2000–2005.* Wellington: Te Rōpū Rangahau Hauora a Eru Pōmare.

Scragg, R. K. R., & Mitchell, E. A. (1998). Side sleeping position and bed sharing in the sudden infant death syndrome. *Annals of Medicine, 30*(4), 345–349.

Scragg, R. K. R., Wellman, R. J., Laugesen, M., & DiFranza, J. R. (2008). Diminished autonomy over tobacco can appear with the first cigarettes. *Addictive Behaviors,* 33, 689–698.

Smith, J. (2004). Mothers' milk and markets. *Australian Feminist Studies, 19*(45), 369–379.

Stace, H. (1997). *Gene dreaming: New Zealanders and eugenics.* Professional Historians' Association of New Zealand/Aotearoa. Retrieved 22 November 2009, from http://www.phanza.org.nz/content/gene-dreaming-new-zealanders-and-eugenics

Statistics New Zealand (2009). *Fertility rates: Māori and total mothers.* Retrieved 12 December 2009, from www.stats.govt.nz

Te Awekotuku, N. (1991). *He tikanga whakaaro: Research ethics in the Maori community.* Wellington: Manatu Maori (Ministry of Maori Affairs).

Te Whare Wananga o Awanuiarangi. (n.d.) Te Hiringa i te Mahara: Whakatauki. Retrieved 26 August 2009, from http://s3.amazonaws.com/THM/resources/curriculum/maori_language/Fun_Task_4.pdf

The Quit Group and the Ministry of Health. (2009). *Maori smoking and tobacco use 2009.* Wellington: Ministry of Health.

Thompson, J. M. D., Thach, B. T., Becroft, D. M. O., Mitchell, E. A., & the New Zealand Cot Death Study Group. (2006). Sudden infant death syndrome: Risk factors for infants found face down differ from other SIDS cases. *Journal of Pediatrics, 149*(5), 630–633.

Thornley L, Waa, A., & Ball, J. (2007). *Comprehensive plan to inform the design of a national breastfeeding promotion campaign.* Wellington: Quigley & Watts.

Tipene-Leach, D., Abel, S., Park, J., Finau, S., & Lennan, M. (2000). Māori infant care practices: Implications for health messages, infant care services and SIDS prevention in Māori communities. *Pacific Health Dialog, 7*(1), 29–37.

Wright, A. L., Holberg, C. J., Martinez, F. D., Morgan, W. J., & Taussig, L. M. (1989). Breast feeding and lower respiratory tract illness in the first year of life. Group Health Medical Associates. *British Medical Journal, 299*, 946–949.

Chapter 16
Infant Feeding in Indigenous Australian Communities

Jane A. Scott and Colin W. Binns

Contents

16.1 Introduction

Prior to European invasion, the Australian Aboriginal people had followed a hunter-gatherer existence for at least tens of thousands of years, and possibly for as long as 100,000 years (Gracey 2000a). They had successfully adapted to life in a variety of diverse terrains, which included 'coastal areas, riverine areas, tropical forests, savannah woodlands, temperate timbered and grassed areas in the south and on the east coast, and harsh, hot and extremely dry deserts in central Australia' (Gracey 2000a, p. 1362S). The population density was greater in the more environmentally hospitable and fertile coastal and river areas and sparse in the central desert regions (Saggers & Gray 1991). As pre-agriculturalists, they did not plant crops or raise domesticated animals and their diet was limited to the naturally occurring plants and animals available in the areas that they inhabited. While the Australian Aborigines were adept at catching fish, birds and reptiles and hunting small to large mammals such as possums and kangaroos, according to Saggers and Gray (1991, p. 26), their diet was primarily vegetarian 'with meat making up a minor, but qualitatively important part of the diet'. Saggers and Gray (1991) describe a nomadic

J.A. Scott (✉)
School of Medicine, Flinders University, Adelaide, South Australia, Australia 5042
e-mail: jane.scott@flinders.edu.au

P. Liamputtong (ed.), *Infant Feeding Practices*, DOI 10.1007/978-1-4419-6873-9_16,
© Springer Science+Business Media, LLC 2011

lifestyle dictated by the need to take advantage of the seasonally available plant life and to find reliable water sources. Most environments, particularly the harsh desert areas, could only support small groups of people. For most of the year, they roamed in widely dispersed, small bands of ten to thirty related people (Saggers & Gray 1991), but also gathered 'regularly for games, fights, corroborees (ceremonial dances), initiations and exchange of news' (Gracey 2000a, p. 1362S).

In traditional societies, such as that of the early Australian Aborigine, for which food supplies were scarce and infant mortality was high, breastfeeding was a biological imperative and provided an irreplaceable source of optimal nutrition and immuno-protective factors (Cuthbertson 1999). This chapter primarily describes the infant feeding patterns of Indigenous Australians;[1] however, the infant feeding traditions and contemporary feeding behaviours of Indigenous Australians share many similarities with those of other Indigenous populations.

16.2 Traditional Infant Feeding Practices

Prior to European contact, breastfeeding amongst Australian Aboriginal women was universal, with mothers carrying and feeding their children while they collected food (Hitchcock 1989b). Lactational failure or maternal death, in the absence of domesticated animals which could be milked, meant certain death for an infant unless there was another woman who could feed the infant. While the use of wetnurses has been reported among traditional Aboriginal women (Hitchcock 1989b), it may have been unlikely in small bands with a limited number of childbearing-aged kinswomen (Cuthbertson 1999).

Mothers breastfed their infants frequently and exclusively for 6 months or more and prolonged breastfeeding was the norm with children reportedly being breastfed for up to 4 years and sometimes longer (Mathews 1960). This practice of prolonged breastfeeding has been offered as one possible explanation for the reportedly low birth rate in traditional Aboriginal society (Saggers & Gray 1991; see also Chapter 15 in this volume). Breastfeeding through hormonal mechanisms exerts a natural contraceptive effect, and exclusive and prolonged breastfeeding increases the interval between births. This has a direct effect on infant mortality, as a short birth interval carries an increased risk of undernutrition and death for subsequent siblings (Rutstein 2005). The age at which solids were introduced can only be speculated; however, it is likely that Aboriginal infants were weaned onto traditional bush foods such as '*damper* (a bread made from ground grass seeds), honey, wild fruit and vegetables, tubers, birds and their eggs, kangaroo meat, lizard, fish, turtles and other aquatic foods' (Gracey 2000b, p. 1276). Mouth-to-mouth feeding, whereby the mother pre-masticated the food, was probably the only way to feed weaning foods to infants (Cuthbertson 1999).

[1]The Indigenous Australian population includes Aboriginal and Torres Strait Islander peoples. In this chapter, both the terms Indigenous and Aboriginal are used according to their original use in the references cited.

16.3 Contemporary Infant Feeding Practices

Increasing urbanisation and Western influence has had a negative impact on the breastfeeding practices of Indigenous Australian and other indigenous populations (Gracey 2002). These days, with the exception of those living in remote areas, Indigenous Australians have lower breastfeeding initiation rates than non-Indigenous people (Australian Bureau of Statistics 2006). This is also the case in other Indigenous populations such as the Mãori in New Zealand (Ministry of Health 2002; see also Chapter 15 in this volume) and the First Nations, Inuit and Métis peoples in Canada (McShane, Smylie, & Adomako 2009).

While there is relatively limited data on breastfeeding practices among Indigenous Australians, there is evidence that breastfeeding practices reflect the degree of urbanisation of the community studied. An anthropometric study of Aboriginal children conducted in Western Australia in 1981 (Gracey, Murray, Hitchcock, Owles, & Murphy 1983) revealed that mothers in remote communities practiced traditional feeding behaviours with all mothers initiating breastfeeding and 90 percent continuing to breastfeed beyond 2 years. In contrast, only 71 percent of mothers living in or outside big country towns were breastfeeding at 3 months and less than half at 2 years. Among mothers living in the rural closely settled south-west of Western Australia, less than half were still breastfeeding at 6 months and none at 2 years. Another study of Aboriginal women living in Perth conducted contemporaneously in the early 1980s (Phillips & Dibley 1983) revealed that while 82 percent of mothers initiated breastfeeding, only 50 percent were still breastfeeding at 3 months.

Twenty years later, this negative association with urbanisation was still apparent in the Western Australian Aboriginal Child Health Survey, which reported that the proportion of Aboriginal children who had ever been breastfed increased steadily with isolation from 81.5 percent for children in Perth to 96.3 percent of children in the most remote areas (Zubrick et al. 2004) (see Fig. 16.1).

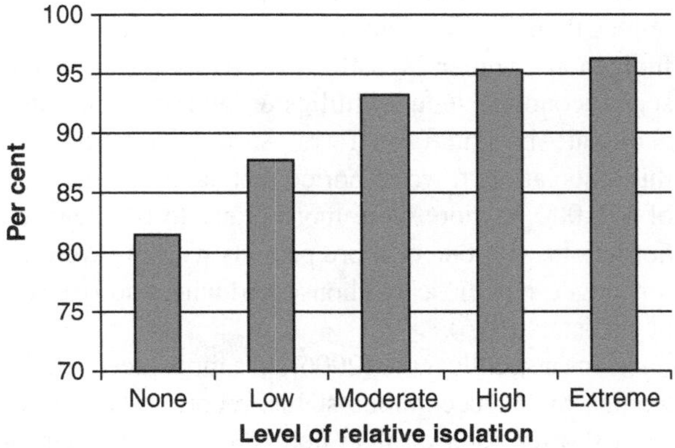

Fig. 16.1 Proportion of Aboriginal children aged 0–17 years (Children whose mother is also their primary care giver) ever breastfed by level of relative isolation. Source: Zubrick et al. (2004) The Western Australian Aboriginal Child Health Survey: The Health of Aboriginal Children and Young People

A decline in breastfeeding among non-Indigenous Australian women was observed from the mid-1950s until the early 1970s (Hitchcock 1989a), after which time breastfeeding initiation and duration increased steadily until the early 1990s when they appeared to plateau with roughly 90 percent of non-Indigenous women initiating breastfeeding and 50 percent of women stopping before their infants reach 6 months of age (Donath & Amir 2005; Graham, Scott, Binns, & Oddy 2005). This decline in breastfeeding among non-Indigenous women paralleled, and probably pre-empted, a decline in breastfeeding experienced by Indigenous women, as demonstrated in data from an isolated Queensland Aboriginal community collected over a 20 year period. Dugdale (1980) reported the prevalence of breastfeeding at 1 month of age among this community had declined from 77 percent in 1953 to a low of 51 percent in 1963 before rising again to 66 percent in 1972.

Evidence of a resurgence in breastfeeding among urban Indigenous women is provided by a number of contemporary studies. Holmes, Phillips, and Thorpe (1997a) reported that 84.5 percent of a group of Aboriginal new-mothers living in Melbourne in 1991 had initiated breastfeeding, which was higher than the initiation rate of 75.6 percent for Victorian women in general. However, the prevalence of breastfeeding declined more rapidly among Aboriginal women and only 50 percent of Aboriginal babies were still being breastfed at 3 months and 32 percent at 6 months compared with 57.7 percent and 43.5 percent of non-Indigenous babies, at 3 and 6 months respectively. A high initiation rate of 89 percent was reported in the mid-1990s for Aboriginal mothers living in the Perth metropolitan region (Eades, Read, & Bibbulung Gnarneep Team 1999). Similarly, Binns and colleagues (2006), in a longitudinal study of Aboriginal women giving birth in Perth in 2001/02, reported that 89.4 percent of mothers were discharged from hospital breastfeeding, declining to 58.8 percent at 6 months. The breastfeeding initiation and prevalence at 6 months was higher among Aboriginal mothers than among non-Aboriginal breastfeeding women (89.4 percent compared to 83.8 percent and 58.8 percent compared to 49.9 percent, respectively).

The initiation and duration of breastfeeding is influenced by a complex variety of socio-demographic, biomedical and psycho-social factors. Socio-economic status has been found consistently to be a strong predictor of breastfeeding outcome (Scott & Binns 1998). The breastfeeding rates of urban Indigenous women reflect their socio-economic status, and several studies have reported that urban Indigenous women breastfeed for as long as non-Indigenous women of the same socio-economic status (Phillips & Dibley 1983; Hitchock & Coy 1989). The 1994 National Aboriginal and Torres Strait Islander Survey provided further evidence of this association. It was reported that babies from households with an annual income of $25,000 or more were more likely to be breastfed and Indigenous babies in a household with one or more persons working were more likely to be breastfed and for longer than those in a household where no-one was working (Australian Bureau of Statistics 1996).

Binns and colleagues (2006), in a more recent study that stratified non-Aboriginal women by socioeconomic status, reported that while Aboriginal women breastfed for a shorter duration than non-Aboriginal women of the highest socio-economic

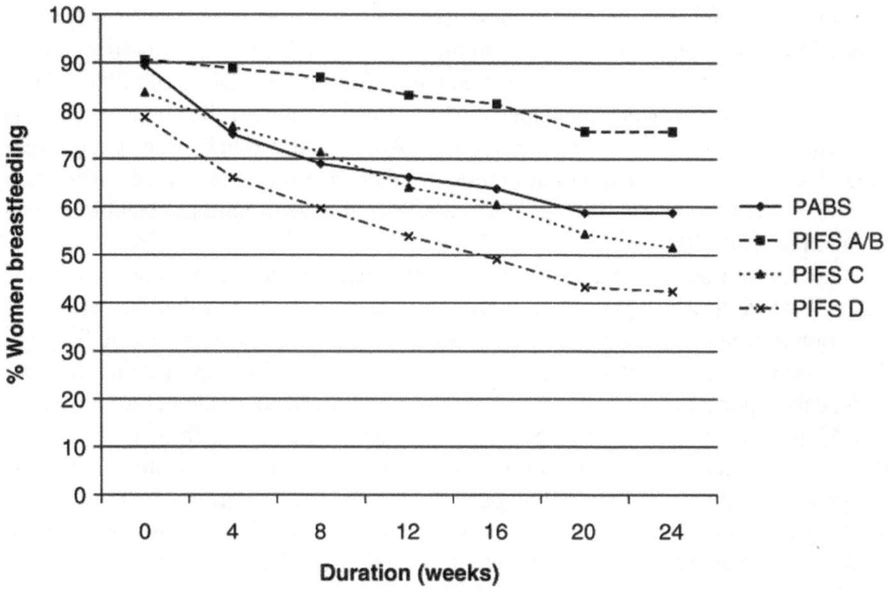

Fig. 16.2 Prevalence of breastfeeding among Aboriginal women compared with non-Aboriginal women, according to social rank (Based on Congalton scale using partner's occupation as a measure of social status, where the highest rank (group A) is assigned to professionals and academic occupations and the lowest rank (group D) is assigned to unskilled occupations. PABS, Perth Aboriginal Breastfeeding Study; PIFS, Perth Infant Feeding Study.). Source: Binns et al. (2006)

status, they breastfed for significantly longer than non-Aboriginal women of the lowest socio-economic status (see Fig. 16.2).

The most recent national survey of Indigenous women indicates that breastfeeding initiation rates remain higher among remote Indigenous women than non-remote Indigenous women. According to the 2004–2005 National Aboriginal and Torres Strait Islander Health Survey (NATSIHS), 92 percent of Indigenous mothers aged 18–64 years living in remote areas reported having ever breastfed their babies, compared with 81 percent of those living in non-remote areas. Information about recent breastfeeding is limited to women living in non-remote areas participating in the 2004–05 NATSIHS who had a child aged 0–3 years. This survey indicated that, overall, fewer Indigenous children than non-Indigenous children had ever been breastfed (79 percent compared to 88 percent) and this finding was consistent across all states of Australia (Australian Institute of Health and Welfare 2007).

Data from the Western Australian Aboriginal Child Health Survey (Zubrick et al. 2004) provide evidence that Indigenous mothers breastfeed longer than non-Indigenous women, a practice reported also for Indigenous populations in Canada (McShane et al. 2009). Just over one-quarter (26.8 percent) of Aboriginal women living in the Perth metropolitan region had breastfed for 12 months or more (Zubrick et al. 2004) compared with 19.2 percent of non-Aboriginal women (Scott, Binns, Oddy, & Graham 2006). There was also a negative effect of urbanisation on duration among Aboriginal women with almost half (48.7 percent) of Aboriginal children living in areas of extreme isolation having been breastfed for 12 months or more. Evidence from the Perth Aboriginal Feeding Survey (Binns et al. 2006) indicates that Indigenous women exclusively breastfeed for longer than non-Indigenous women. They reported that 31.5 percent of Aboriginal mothers were exclusively breastfeeding at 6 months, which is much higher than the 18.4 percent of women who reported fully breastfeeding[2] to 25 weeks in the 2001 National Health Survey (Donath & Amir 2005).

There is limited information on the age at which Indigenous mothers introduce solids. The Perth Aboriginal Study (Binns et al. 2006) reported that 50 percent of Aboriginal women in Perth had introduced solids before 4 months (median age 3.9 months). A recent study from Victoria of Aboriginal children under the age of 5 years reported that 35 percent of children had received solids before 4 months and 42 percent between 4 and 6 months (Adams 2006). Data from the 2004–05 NATSIHS indicated that the early introduction of solids was more common amongst Indigenous mothers and that Indigenous infants aged 0–3 months were almost twice as likely to be given solid foods as non-Indigenous infants (18 percent compared to 10 percent) (Australian Institute of Health and Welfare 2007).

The Western Australian Aboriginal Child Health Survey (Zubrick et al. 2004) provides evidence of an association between age of introduction and level of urbanisation. In general, children living in the least remote areas received solids at an earlier age than those living in areas of extreme isolation (see Fig. 16.3).

A traditional practice among Aboriginals is to wait until a child demands food before breastfeeding or giving other foods (Harrison 1986 as cited in National Health and Medical Research Council 2000, p. 106). This tradition will not adversely affect a well-nourished child. However, lack of hunger and apathy are

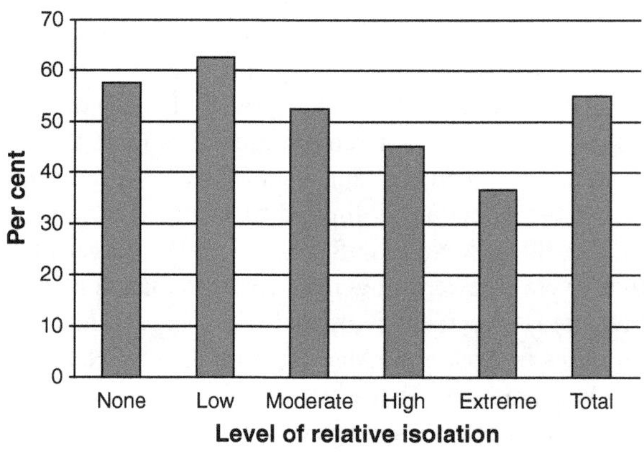

Fig. 16.3 Proportion of Aboriginal children aged 0–17 years (Children whose mother is also their primary care giver) who received solids at or before 4 months of age. Source: Zubrick et al. (2004) The Western Australian Aboriginal Child Health Survey: The Health of Aboriginal Children and Young People

[2]Infants classified as 'fully' breastfeeding may be consuming juice, water, etc, and therefore are not directly comparable to the WHO definition of 'exclusive' breastfeeding, which means that no other food or drink, not even water, is given to the infant.

commonly seen in mild malnutrition (Waterlow 1994), and a child with mild growth failure may fail to show an active interest in food at an appropriate time. Adherence to this traditional practice may disadvantage infants if their mothers wait for signs of hunger before feeding them and Indigenous mothers should be encouraged to introduce solids by 6 months of age. In addition to the *timely* introduction of weaning foods, it is also important that weaning foods be *adequate*, in as much that they provide sufficient energy, protein and micronutrients, and *safe*, that is hygienically stored and prepared and fed with clean hands (WHO/UNICEF 2003). Many Aboriginal mothers, especially those in remote communities, do not have the chance to learn about appropriate Western weaning foods and live in environments that are not conducive to the hygienic preparation and storage of weaning foods, thus placing Aboriginal children, particularly those between the ages of 6 months and 2 years, at risk of malnutrition and infectious diarrhoea (Mathews 1998).

16.4 Factors Influencing Breastfeeding in Indigenous Populations

Few longitudinal infant feeding studies among Indigenous Australian women have been conducted, primarily due to logistical problems associated with following a population with high residential mobility. Hence, there is limited quantitative data to provide insight into factors associated with breastfeeding outcome among this group. The Perth Aboriginal Breastfeeding Study (PABS) conducted by Binns, Gilchrist, Gracey, Zhang, Scott, and Lee (2004) reported that breastfeeding initiation was positively associated with perceived paternal support and maternal age and negatively associated with parity, all factors previously identified as being associated with breastfeeding among a group of non-Aboriginal Perth women (Scott, Binns, & Aroni 1997).

A small number of qualitative studies of Indigenous women provide a richer insight into factors that influence the decision of Indigenous women to breastfeed. Unlike non-Aboriginal Australian women who appear to make an informed choice to breastfeed on the basis of benefits to the infant, cost and convenience (Binns & Scott 2002), Holmes, Thorpe, and Phillips (1997b) reported that Aboriginal women simply assumed that they would breastfeed and were not aware of having made an active choice. Their findings suggest that ‘there was a strong sense among both men and women that breastfeeding is natural, accepted and a traditional practice – that Aboriginal women *ought* to breastfeed’ (Holmes et al. 1997b, p. 505). The belief that breastfeeding is ‘normal’ was also prevalent among Māori women (Glover, Manaena-Biddle, & Waldon 2007), who indicated that breastfeeding is the *tika* (right) way to feed an infant and that they and their *whanau* (partner and extended family) assumed that they would breastfeed (see also Chapter 15 in this volume).

Holmes and colleagues (1997b) reported that some Aboriginal women expressed a sense of shame and embarrassment associated with breastfeeding, a sentiment seldom reported by non-Aboriginal women (Binns & Scott 2002). They contend that ‘this attitude may have been instilled in mission days and reinforced by the dominant colonial culture's emphasis on the breast as an object of sexual desire' (Holmes et al. 1997b, p. 505). Similarly, some Māori women believed that breastfeeding in public was unacceptable, a belief that Glover and colleagues (2007) suggest was fuelled by a reportedly widely, but mistakenly, held belief among Māori women that a law was passed in the early 1900s forbidding Māori women to breastfeed, at least in public (see also Chapter 15).

While breastfeeding is generally perceived by Aboriginal women to be the accepted and traditional practice, some older women have little or no breastfeeding experience. With the advent of artificial feeding technology, infant feeding began to be viewed as a science (Mulford 1995) and in the 1940s, 1950s and 1960s, artificial feeding was often presented as a superior way to feed an infant (Hitchcock 1989a; see Chapters 2, 3 and 5 in this volume). According to Jelliffe (1976, p. 1227), 'infant feeding came to be considered almost as an engineering exercise, with the child refuelled with mathematically calculated amounts of known nutrients delivered mechanically from a feeding bottle'. Holmes and colleagues (1997b, p. 505) too argue that 'pressures to feed artificially during these decades when Aboriginal women lived on missions, can also be viewed as part of the policy of assimilation actively pursued at that time'.

16.5 Smoking and Alcohol Intake and Breastfeeding

Smoking, both maternal (Amir & Donath 2002) and paternal (Xu, Binns, Zhang, Yang, & Zhao 2010), has been negatively associated with breastfeeding outcomes. Although Gilchrist, Binns, Scott, Gracey, and Smith (2004) failed to find an association between smoking and breastfeeding duration in the Perth Aboriginal Breastfeeding Study, probably due to a relatively small sample size, smoking has been linked consistently to shorter breastfeeding duration in most other studies (Amir & Donath 2002). Smoking is common among Indigenous mothers, with 54 percent of Indigenous women aged 25–44 years admitting to smoking daily compared with 23 percent of non-Indigenous women (Australian Institute of Health and Welfare 2007). Similarly, smoking is also more prevalent among Indigenous fathers and the majority of Indigenous infants are likely to be exposed to tobacco smoke (Eades et al. 1999) and the associated health risks. While Indigenous mothers (and fathers) should be encouraged and supported to give up smoking for their own health and that of their infant, Indigenous mothers who smoke should still be encouraged to breastfeed as breastfeeding offers protection to the infant against the detrimental health effects of exposure to environmental smoke (Dorea, 2007). See also Chapter 15 in this volume.

Alcohol has been shown also to have a detrimental affect on lactation performance by blocking the release of oxytocin and the degree of inhibition is dose-dependent (Giglia & Binns 2006). Consumption of two standard drinks or more has been associated with earlier cessation of breastfeeding, deficits in infant psychomotor development and disrupted infant sleep–wake behavioural patterns (Giglia & Binns 2006). Alcohol drinking at risky or high risk levels is more prevalent among Indigenous women of childbearing age than non-Indigenous women (15 percent compared to 4 percent) (Australian Institute of Health and Welfare 2007). The National Health and Medical Council (2009) recommends for breastfeeding women that:

- Not drinking alcohol is the safest option.
- Women should avoid alcohol in the first month after delivery until breastfeeding is well established.
- After that:
  - alcohol intake should be limited to no more than two standard drinks a day
  - women should avoid drinking immediately before breastfeeding
  - women who wish to drink alcohol could consider expressing milk in advance (NHMRC 2009, p. 81)

16.6 The Importance of Breastfeeding Among Indigenous Populations

Indigenous children have higher hospital admission rates for gastroenteritis (Gracey, Lee, & Yau 2004) and respiratory infections (Moore et al. 2007) than non-Indigenous children. Up to 95 percent of Aboriginal infants experience chronic suppurative otitis media, a severe form of middle ear infection, during the first 3 months of life. In some communities, recurrent otitis media leads to hearing impairment in up to 50 percent of children (Armstrong, Laing, Wilkes, & Laing 2008), which can lead to learning difficulties – perpetuating a cycle of disadvantage. The immuno-protective benefits of breastfeeding are well recognised (Chirico, Marzollo, Cortinovis, Fonte, & Gasparoni 2008). There is convincing evidence that breastfeeding, particularly exclusive breastfeeding for 3 months or more, provides protection against otitis media (Ip et al. 2007) and breastfeeding for at least 3 months has been shown to be associated with lower rates of chest infections among Aboriginal children (Oddy et al. 2008).

Chronic diseases such as type 2 diabetes and cardiovascular disease, and their associated lifestyle risk factors, are highly prevalent amongst Indigenous adults (Trewin & Madden 2005). The high prevalence of these diseases and associated premature mortality contribute in part to a life expectancy among both female and male Indigenous Australians that is approximately 17 years shorter than their non-Indigenous counterparts (Trewin & Madden 2005). In the past decade or so, research attention has focussed on the long-term health outcomes associated with breastfeeding. A number of systematic reviews have been conducted which have demonstrated a small protective effect of breastfeeding on obesity, blood pressure, total serum cholesterol and type 2 diabetes (Horta, Bahl, Martines, & Victora 2007; Ip et al. 2007). The promotion of the traditional feeding practice of exclusive and prolonged breastfeeding may be an important strategy in the battle to reduce the inequitable prevalence of chronic disease amongst Indigenous Australians.

16.7 Conclusion

Traditionally, breastfeeding was universal and prolonged amongst Indigenous mothers. While European settlement and urbanisation has had a negative impact on the breastfeeding practices of Indigenous women, those living in remote communities generally continue to adhere to traditional feeding practices and are just as likely as non-Indigenous mothers to initiate breastfeeding and more likely to breastfeed for 12 months or longer. The Statement of Intent between the Government of Australia and the Aboriginal and Torres Strait Islander Peoples of Australia, released following the *Close the Gap* Indigenous Health Equality Summit held in Canberra in March 2008, identified a shared determination to close the fundamental divide between the health outcomes and life expectancy of the Aboriginal and Torres Strait Islander peoples of Australia and non-Indigenous Australians (Indigenous Health Equality Summit March 2008). Breastfeeding is one way to ensure that short- and long-term health benefits are passed onto Indigenous children and should be actively promoted and supported as a means of *closing the gap* between the health outcomes of Indigenous and non-Indigenous children and adults.

References

Adams, K. (2006). *Koori kids' ears and health: A community report from Onemda VicHealth Koori Health Unit.* Melbourne: Centre for Health and Society, School of Population Health, The University of Melbourne.

Amir, L., & Donath, S. (2002). Does maternal smoking have a negative physiological effect on breastfeeding? The epidemiological evidence. *Birth, 29*, 112–123.

Armstrong, J. E., Laing, D. G., Wilkes, F. J., & Laing, O. N. (2008). Olfactory function in Australian Aboriginal children and chronic otitis media. *Chemical Senses, 33*(6), 503–507.

Australian Bureau of Statistics (1996). *National Aboriginal and Torres Strait Islander survey 1994: Health of Indigenous Australians. ABS Cat. No. 4395.0.* Canberra: Australian Bureau of Statistics.

Australian Bureau of Statistics (2006). *National Aboriginal and Torres Strait Islander health survey: Australia, 2004–05.* Canberra: Australian Bureau of Statistics

Australian Institute of Health and Welfare (2007). *Aboriginal and Torres Strait Islander health performance framework, 2006 report: Detailed analysis. AIHW Cat. No. IHW 20.* Canberra: Australian Institute of Health and Welfare.

Binns, C., & Scott, J. (2002). Breastfeeding: Reasons for starting, reasons for stopping and problems along the way. *Breastfeeding Review, 10*, 13–19.

Binns, C., Gilchrist, D., Gracey, M., Zhang, M., Scott, J., & Lee, A. (2004). Factors associated with the initiation of breast-feeding by Aboriginal mothers in Perth. *Public Health Nutrition, 7*(7), 857–861.

Binns, C. W., Gilchrist, D., Woods, B., Gracey, M., Scott, J., Smith, H., et al. (2006). Breastfeeding by Aboriginal women in Perth. *Nutrition and Dietetics, 63*, 8–14.

Chirico, G., Marzollo, R., Cortinovis, S., Fonte, C., & Gasparoni, A. (2008). Antiinfective properties of human milk. *Journal of Nutrition, 138*(9), 1801S–1806S.

Cuthbertson, W. F. J. (1999). Evolution of infant nutrition. *British Journal of Nutrition, 81*, 359–371.

Donath, S. M., & Amir, L. H. (2005). Breastfeeding and the introduction of solids in Australian infants: Data from the 2001 National Health Survey. *Australian & New Zealand Journal of Public Health, 29*(2), 171–175.

Dorea, J. (2007). Maternal smoking and infant feeding: Breastfeeding is better and safer. *Maternal and Child Health Journal, 11*(3), 287–291.

Dugdale, A. E. (1980). Infant feeding, growth and mortality: A 20-year study of an Australian Aboriginal community. *The Medical Journal of Australia, 2*, 380–385.

Eades, S. J., Read, A. W., & Bibbulung Gnarneep Team (1999). Infant care practices in a metropolitan Aboriginal population. *Journal of Paediatrics and Child Health, 35*, 541–544.

Giglia, R., & Binns, C. (2006). Alcohol and lactation: A systematic review. *Nutrition and Dietetics, 62*(2), 103–116.

Gilchrist, D., Binns, C., Scott, J., Gracey, M., & Smith, H. (2004). Aboriginal mothers, breastfeeding and smoking. *Australian and New Zealand Journal of Public Health, 28*, 225–228.

Glover, M., Manaena-Biddle, H., & Waldon, J. (2007). Influences that affect Maori women breastfeeding. *Breastfeeding Review, 15*(2), 5–14.

Gracey, M. (2000a). Historical, cultural, political, and social influences on dietary patterns and nutrition in Australian Aboriginal children. *American Journal of Clinical Nutrition, 72*(Suppl), 1361S–1367S.

Gracey, M. (2000b). Infant feeding and weaning practices in an urbanizing traditional, hunter-gatherer society. *Pediatrics, 106*(Suppl 5), 1276–1277.

Gracey, M. (2002). Child health in an urbanizing world. *Acta Paediatrica, 91*, 1–8.

Gracey, M., Murray, H., Hitchcock, N. E., Owles, E. N., & Murphy, B. P. (1983). The nutrition of Australian Aboriginal infants and young children. *Nutrition Research, 3*, 133–147.

Gracey, M., Lee, A. H., & Yau, K. K. W. (2004). Hospitalisation for gastroenteritis in Western Australia. *Archives of Disease in Childhood, 89*(8), 768–772.

Graham, K. I., Scott, J. A., Binns, C. W., & Oddy, W. H. (2005). National targets for breastfeeding at hospital discharge have been achieved in Perth. *Acta Paediatrica, 94*, 352–356.

Hitchcock, N. E. (1989a). Infant feeding in Australia: An historical perspective. Part 2: 1900–1988. *Australian Journal of Nutrition and Dietetics, 46*(4), 102–108.

Hitchcock, N. E. (1989b). Infant feeding in Australia: An historical perspective. Part 3: Australian aborigines and recent migrants. *Australian Journal of Nutrition and Dietetics, 46*(4), 108–111.

Hitchock, N. E., & Coy, J. F. (1989). The growth of healthy Australian infants in relations to infant feeding and social group. *Medical Journal of Australia, 150*, 306–311.

Holmes, W., Phillips, J., & Thorpe, L. (1997a). Initiation rate and duration of breast-feeding in the Melbourne Aboriginal community. *Australian & New Zealand Journal of Public Health, 21*(5), 500–503.

Holmes, W., Thorpe, L., & Phillips, J. (1997b). Influences on infant-feeding beliefs and practices in an urban Aboriginal community. *Australian & New Zealand Journal of Public Health, 21*(5), 504–510.

Horta, B. L., Bahl, R., Martines, J. C. & Victora, C. G. (2007). *Evidence on the long-term effects of breastfeeding. Systematic reviews and meta-analysis.* Geneva: World Health Organization.

Indigenous Health Equality Summit (2008). Close the gap: Statement of intent. Retrieved 10 September 2009, from http://www.hreoc.gov.au/Social_Justice/health/statement_intent.pdf

Ip, S., Chung, M., Raman, G., Chew, P., Magila, N., DeVine, D., et al. (2007). *Breastfeeding and maternal and child health outcomes in developed countries.* Rockville: Agency for Healthcare Research and Quality.

Jelliffe, D. B. (1976). World trends in infant feeding. *American Journal of Clinical Nutrition, 29*(11), 1227–1237.

Mathews, J. (1998). The crisis in Aboriginal health: The generation gap. *Australasian Science, October*, 41–45.

Mathews, M. (1960). Food consumption and dietary levels of groups of Aborigines living on naturally occurring foods. In C. P. Mountford (Ed.), *Records of the American-Australia scientific expedition to Arnhem Land, 1948*. Melbourne: Melbourne University Press.

McShane, K., Smylie, J., & Adomako, P. (2009). Health of First Nations, Inuit, and Métis children in Canada. In J. Smylie, & P. Adomako (Eds.), *Indigenous children's health report: Health assessment in action*. Toronto: Keenan Research Centre.

Ministry of Health. (2002). *New Zealand's breastfeeding rates – Statistics from breast-feeding: A guide to action.* Auckland: Ministry of Health.

Moore, H., Burgner, D., Carville, K., Jacoby, P., Richmond, P., & Lehmann, D. (2007). Diverging trends for lower respiratory infections in non-Aboriginal and Aboriginal children. *Journal of Paediatrics and Child Health, 43*(6), 451–457.

Mulford, C. (1995). Swimming upstream: Breastfeeding care in a nonbreastfeeding culture. *Journal of Obstetrics, Gynaecology and Neonatal Nursing, 24*(5), 464–474.

National Health and Medical Research Council. (2000). *Nutrition in Aboriginal and Torres Strait Islander peoples: An information paper.* Canberra: National Health and Medical Research Council.

National Health and Medical Research Council. (2009). *Australian guidelines to reduce health risks from drinking alcohol.* Canberra: National Health and Medical Research Council.

Oddy, W. H., Kickett-Tucker, C., De Maio, J., Lawrence, D., Silburn, S. R., Stanley, F. J., et al. (2008). The association of infant feeding with parent-reported infections and hospitalisations in the West Australian Aboriginal Child Health Survey. *Australian & New Zealand Journal of Public Health, 32*, 207–215.

Phillips, F. E., & Dibley, M. J. (1983). A longitudinal study of feeding patterns of Aboriginal infants living in Perth 1980–82. *Proceedings of the Nutrition Society of Australia, 8*, 130–133.

Rutstein, S. (2005). Effects of preceding birth intervals on neonatal infant and under-five years mortality and nutritional status in developing countries: Evidence from the demographic and health surveys. *International Journal of Gynecology and Obstetrics, 89*(Suppl 1), S7–S24.

Saggers, S., & Gray, D. (1991). *Aboriginal health and society.* St Leonards: Allen and Unwin.

Scott, J., & Binns, C. (1998). Factors associated with the initiation and duration of breastfeeding: A review of the literature. *Australian Journal of Nutrition and Dietetics, 55*, 51–61.

Scott, J., Binns, C., & Aroni, R. (1997). The influence of reported paternal attitudes on the decision to breast-feed. *Journal of Paediatrics and Child Health, 33*, 305–307.

Scott, J. A., Binns, C. W., Oddy, W. H., & Graham, K. I. (2006). Predictors of breastfeeding duration: Evidence from a cohort study. *Pediatrics, 17*, e646–e655.

Trewin, D., & Madden, R. (2005). *The health and welfare of Australia's Aboriginal and Torres Strait Islander Peoples 2005. ABS Catalogue No. 4704.0.* Canberra: Australian Bureau of Statistics and Australian Institute of Health and Welfare.

Waterlow, J. (1994). Relationship of gain in height to gain in weight. *European Journal of Clinical Nutrition, 48*(Suppl. 1), S72–S73.

WHO/UNICEF. (2003). *Global strategy for infant and young child feeding.* Geneva: World Health Organization.

Xu, F., Binns, C., Zhang, H., Yang, G., & Zhao, Y. (2010). Paternal smoking and breastfeeding in Xinjiang, PR China. *Journal of Human Lactation*, published online 23 June 2010, DOI: 10.1177/0890334410369480.

Zubrick, S. R., Lawrence, D. M., Silburn, S. R., Blair, E., Milroy, H., Wilkes, T., et al. (2004). *The Western Australian Aboriginal Child Health Survey: The health of Aboriginal children and young people.* Perth: Telethon Institute for Child Health Research.

Chapter 17
Breastfeeding, Vertical Disease Transmission and the Volition of Medicines in Malawi

Robert Pool, Christopher Pell, Blessings Nyasilia Kaunda, Don Mathanga, and Marjolein Gysels

Contents

17.1 Background

The data on which this paper is based were collected as part of a multi-country anthropological study of the acceptability of intermittent preventing treatment of malaria in infants (IPTi) (Gysels et al. 2009). Intermittent preventive treatment (IPT) of malaria involves the administration of treatment doses of an anti-malarial drug at predetermined intervals, regardless of parasitaemia or symptoms. Compared to continuous chemoprophylaxis, IPT reduces the number of times an individual has to be given the antimalarial, and can avoid the problem of delivery if it is given at routine health visits: IPT during pregnancy (IPTp) is linked to ongoing routine antenatal care, and IPT for infants (IPTi) is delivered through the expanded programme of immunisation (EPI) (Egan, Crawley, & Schellenberg 2005). At the time of the acceptability study, IPTi with sulfadoxine-pyrimethamine (SP) was being implemented in two districts in central Malawi (Lilongwe and Salima). The SP

R. Pool (✉)
CRESIB (Barcelona Centre for International Health Research), Hospital Clinic – University of Barcelona, Rosselló 132, sobreático 1a., 08036, Barcelona, Spain; Centre for Global Health and Inequality, University of Amsterdam, Spui 21, 1012WX Amsterdam, The Netherlands
e-mail: robert.pool@cresib.cat

P. Liamputtong (ed.), *Infant Feeding Practices*, DOI 10.1007/978-1-4419-6873-9_17,
© Springer Science+Business Media, LLC 2011

was administered at the time of DPT2 (10 weeks), DPT3 (14 weeks) and measles vaccinations (9 months).

During interviews and focus group discussions for the acceptability study, there was evidence that some women thought that malaria could be transmitted from mother to child through breastfeeding. Given the attention devoted to preventing the vertical transmission of HIV during health education given to breastfeeding women everywhere, and given reports in the literature of beliefs about breast milk's capacity to transmit other diseases (Mull 1992; Nielsen, Konradsen, Mudasser, & van der Hoek 2001; Hofmann, De Allegri, Sarker, Sanon, & Bohler 2009), it did not seem surprising that mothers should believe that they could transmit various diseases to their infant through breastfeeding. However, we had not encountered the notion of vertical transmission of malaria before, either during our own research on socio-cultural issues relating to malaria or in the literature, and we considered that it warranted further investigation, particularly because such beliefs could have implications for malaria prevention.

Related to this, we were also interested in finding out whether women thought that malaria medication taken by a mother could be passed on to her infant through breastfeeding and have an effect on the infant's illness, and whether this might influence their attitudes towards malaria prevention interventions aimed at infants. In order to investigate these questions, eight supplementary focus group discussions (FGDs) were carried out in Malawi, one of the five research sites.

17.2 The Study

The study was carried out in Lilongwe and Salima districts in central Malawi. Malawi is one of the world's poorest countries, with a Human Development Index that places it 162 out of 179 countries (United Nations Development Programme 2008). Malawi's infant mortality rate is high at 76 per 1000 live births and around half of Malawian children are chronically malnourished (National Statistical Office (NSO) [Malawi] & ORC Macro 2005). Infant feeding typically involves short periods of exclusive breastfeeding (around two months) and extended complementary breastfeeding (over 23 months). It is estimated that HIV prevalence in Malawi has stabilised at between 16 and 17 percent (Joint United Nations Programme on HIV/AIDS (UNAIDS) & World Health Organization (WHO) 2008). Although malaria transmission in Malawi varies locally, in Lilongwe it is described as endemic, perennial, and in Salima endemic-prone seasonal (www.mara.org.za).

The initial data on malaria and breastfeeding were gleaned from 57 in-depth interviews, 137 questionnaires and 18 focus group discussions (FDGs) with women participating in the IPTi acceptability study in Malawi. These were part of the main data set which also included interviews and FGDs with men, opinion leaders, health workers and traditional healers (Gysels et al. 2009). Women were not asked specifically about breastfeeding in these interviews, but the topic did arise spontaneously during discussions about malaria prevention, transmission and diagnosis. The data presented below, which are more focused on women's views on the vertical transmission of malaria and the effects of malaria medication taken by the mother on her infant, were taken from both the main study and the eight supplementary FGDs carried out after the end of the main data collection phase. These FGDs were held in the villages surrounding the health centres (Mitundu and Mchoka) and outreach clinic (Chimoga) where the main study had been carried out.

During the supplementary FGDs, women were asked about their views on the role of breastfeeding in infant health and how it affected the infant's susceptibility to illness in general and malaria in particular. Ethical clearance for the study was obtained from the ethics committees of the Malawi College of Medicine, Blantyre, and the Hospital Clinic of the University of Barcelona.

17.3 Breastfeeding and Health

With the single exception of one woman, who said that she thought bottle-fed babies were healthier, the women who participated in the supplementary FGDs were unanimous that breastfed babies were healthier and less susceptible to disease: 'Giving breast milk helps the baby to fight off many diseases' was a common comment. This view of the importance of breastfeeding was based partly on their own experience (they claimed they could easily see the difference between breastfed and bottle-fed babies) and on the fact that this was what they were repeatedly told to do at the clinic. Related to the latter, a few women said that they breastfed longer to please clinic staff who had told them to do so. In both the supplementary FGDs and in the main data where breastfeeding was discussed, women all claimed that they breastfed for at least two years.

Although they all agreed that breastfeeding was 'good', the women did not think that it prevented disease, because disease was something that was unavoidable – infants get sick whatever mothers do to prevent it – but that it reduced the chance of them getting sick and it reduced the severity when they did fall ill. These views were repeated in the context of discussions specifically about malaria. Women knew that malaria was transmitted by mosquitoes and that the best protection was to avoid being bitten, by sleeping under bednets for example; but if the child did get bitten, the illness would be less severe if they were breastfeeding.

R3: The one who gets malaria frequently is the one who is not breastfed. The baby becomes very weak in the knees because of lack of breast milk, and becomes susceptible to malaria, while the one breastfeeding has all the energies from the milk, from the first time, that they start taking the yellowish milk, and that milk energises the knees.

R4: A child who is not breastfed is a weakling and will get more severe malaria, and suffer from malaria more often, while the breastfed do not get malaria that often.

This protection was sometimes linked to 'vitamins':

The ones who are not breastfed get more malaria, since they do not have any vitamins in their body, there is no prevention in the body, and thus they suffer from more malaria.

These views were very similar to those about the way in which both childhood vaccination and intermittent preventive treatment of malaria worked; it did not prevent disease – i.e. stop its occurrence entirely – but rather reduced its incidence and attenuated its severity.

Women agreed that the longer they breastfed, the longer their infant was protected. Some women also linked longer breastfeeding to their own health; because it entailed longer sexual abstinence and greater birth spacing, it reduced the negative impact on women's bodies of giving birth. One woman expressed this clearly by arguing that it was obvious from the physical difference between urban women who practice family planning and rural women with many children. Another one said:

> If you are on family planning, your body gets stronger, you look more beautiful and you gain more strength as compared to a woman who gives birth year after year. That woman who gives birth year after year does not look good, and the other child does not get enough breast milk and the father too is never there to help with the babies and that causes you to overwork, some fathers are only available when they want to make you pregnant again.

Women sometimes linked birth spacing back again to infant health. For example, in a FGD in the main dataset, one woman argued that:

> Another advantage is that the children grow up healthy because you don't have other young ones to breastfeed or look after…and if you have a few children, you have more time to take good care of them…not bearing children like *sasakawa* [referring to a method of maize planting where by one seed is planted per hole but the holes are close together].

17.4 Disease Transmission Through Breastfeeding

All the women in the supplementary FGDs said that diseases could be transmitted to their infants through breastfeeding, and that they would not allow other women to breastfeed their infants for this reason.

> R8: There are some who do breastfeed for other women.
> R6: Yes there are, such as a mother and a daughter breastfeeding for each other, but it is not allowed.
> R7: It is because of the blood, some diseases are transmitted through the blood and that is dangerous for the baby. Nowadays there are diseases out there, AIDS, and for someone to just breastfeed your child is not good.

They all knew that HIV could be transmitted through breastfeeding, though various other diseases were also spontaneously mentioned, including TB, flu, asthma, tetanus and cholera.

Almost all the women were also aware of the need to breastfeed exclusively, and in one FGD they protested loudly when one woman said that she gave her newborn baby some water.

> R: When a baby is born, I take water on a spoon and give a few drops to the baby, because my breasts are still dry and the milk is not coming out.
> R2: No, no, no, a baby is not supposed to be given any water, just the breast milk [unanimous response].

However, in the main dataset, mention was often made of older relatives (in particular mothers-in-law) who were keen to give the infant water and other foods.

Also, when the discussion was not explicitly about exclusive breastfeeding, some women did mention giving water when the infant refused to take the breast or there was insufficient milk.

Malaria was not mentioned spontaneously in connection with the vertical transmission of disease, but when asked, women tended to have mixed views about this. In two FGDs, women were unanimous that only mosquitoes transmitted malaria. However, in two FGDs they were unanimous that malaria could be transmitted through breast milk. And in the remaining four, there were mixed views. In the mixed opinion FGDs, there was lively discussion:

R2: Yes, because the malaria stays in the blood, and when my baby is breastfeeding, the milk is coming from my body, thus through my blood, the baby can get malaria from my breast.
R3: No, it cannot happen, the baby cannot get my malaria like that...
R5: I got really sick with malaria, but my baby has not been sick, so my baby can't get my malaria.
R6: The baby can get my malaria; it depends on how serious it is. The more severe malaria will attack the baby... that's what I think...
R7: I don't think the malaria can be passed from mother to baby because malaria is not passed from one person to the other through blood.

Women were aware that malaria is 'in the blood' and those who claimed that it could be transmitted through breastfeeding thought that the mechanism of transmission was the blood circulating in the breasts rather than the breast milk as such:

The baby can get the malaria from the mother, through the blood, since breast milk comes from the body whose blood is circulating with malaria, and so the baby can get the malaria too.

They were unable to articulate the precise mechanism, however.

17.5 The Quality of Breast Milk

All the women agreed that disease (particularly HIV) could be transmitted from mother to infant through breastfeeding, and some thought that malaria could also be transmitted in this way. They mostly thought that this transmission occurred through the blood of the mother circulating in the breasts rather than through the milk itself and that the actual quality of the breast milk would not be affected by the mother's illness. This was expressed in terms of it having been 'made by God'. The women did think that the amount of milk could be reduced as a result of the mother's lack of appetite during illness. However, 'when women have malaria, they do not eat much and that causes the milk not come out'. However, there was a parallel and somewhat contradictory discourse in which they talked about breast milk becoming 'bad' due to various factors. First, breast milk can turn bad as a result of the mother being ill.

When I am sick, my whole body is affected, thus the milk too will be infected, the milk too has a disease, and that is why children become malnourished because they have drunk milk that is infected from their mother. That means as a mother I have a bad body, a sick body, that causes my child to be malnourished.

When I have malaria, the milk becomes bad, the milk becomes hot because of the fever that I have and becomes bad for the child to suck, and thus I wait for my body to cool down so that the milk can cool down too for the baby.

Second, breast milk can become bad if the woman becomes pregnant again while still breastfeeding. Some mothers, however, contested the belief that breast milk becomes tainted during pregnancy and contrasted it with what they are taught at the clinic:

R4: Some babies, when they drink the milk from their pregnant mother, they get diarrhoea and the mother has to stop breastfeeding.
R5: Yes, but from what we have learnt from the clinic…even if a woman finds herself pregnant, she should not stop breastfeeding, because when she stops, the baby will lose the protection from the breast milk.

Third, breast milk could become bad if one of the parents had an extramarital affair while the mother was breastfeeding. Women said that the locally defined disease *kusempha* was caused by the infidelity committed by one of the parents and passed to the child through breastfeeding:

When the mother or the father goes and sleeps with another person and the mother breastfeeds the child, or the father carries the child, the child reacts by becoming ill.

Hence, while women claimed that a mother's illness would not generally affect the quality of her breast milk, they did think that some illness could affect the child through breastfeeding, and that breast milk could become 'bad' as a result of the breastfeeding mother becoming pregnant or one of the parents committing adultery.

17.6 Medication and Breastfeeding

Women, being aware of the possibility of vertical HIV transmission, talked about the role of blood circulation through the breasts enabling HIV transmission. We wanted to know whether they thought that medication that they had taken for malaria could be transmitted to their infant through their breast milk, and whether they thought that this medication would have an effect on their infant's illness. Their views on this varied: in two of the supplementary FGDs women were unanimous that this happened; in three of the FGDs they were unanimous that it was not possible; and in the remaining three there were mixed views.

Women who thought that the vertical transmission of medication was possible used the same reasoning they had used for the vertical transmission of illness:

The baby gets the medication from the mother's breast because of the blood that passes through the breast, and when the baby sucks from the breast, the medication too gets sucked in the process.

It can happen, because these things are interconnected, when a woman eats more food, she has more milk, and if she takes medicine into her body, then the medicine can also be found in her breast and her milk.

The women who disagreed with this seemed to think that there was some sort of barrier that prevented medication travelling from their body to that of their infant.

R1: No, the baby cannot get my medication, because I am the one who has taken the drugs, they cannot be passed to the baby.
R7: But the food that you eat is turned into milk, so cannot the medication also be passed from the breast milk to the baby?
R3: Oh no, food is one thing and medication is another. Medication meant for me works in my body and nowhere else. For my baby I have to get her own medication.
R4: My baby cannot get any of the medication I take. For example if I take Fansidar [sulfadoxine-pyrimethamine – an anti-malarial], it just works on the parasites that are in my body, and when it gets to the breast, it kills the parasites that cause malaria only, it does not influence my breast milk nor the baby.

After further discussion, however, it turned out that the reasons that medication taken by the mother did not affect the breastfeeding infant; it was not so much because the breast prevented the transmission of the medication to the infant in some way, but because of characteristics of the medicine itself; medicine that is meant for the mother only has an effect on the mother, whether or not it is passed on to the infant.

The medication I take is for me and me alone, not for my baby, so I don't think it passes through my breasts.

I think that, when I take drugs that are meant for me, they are only for me. If my baby is ill, I have to go to the clinic and get medicine for his illness. There is no way that my medication can pass through my breast to work in my child's body. It [medicine] can be passed, but it only affects the milk itself [not the infant's illness].

Drugs do not pass through the breast milk because my baby's body is a different body; the child needs its own medication for it to be well.

The baby cannot get my medication. If I take Panadol, it is for my body and mine alone.

This was also clear in the wider dataset, where people spoke about medicines, vaccination and IPTi as though they were active agents. They worked because they 'received', 'liked' or 'accepted' the child. Similarly, the drug could also 'reject' the child, and following perceived side effects of IPTi, mothers talked about the drug 'refusing' the child. It was, therefore, the drug that either accepted or rejected the child, not the other way round.

17.7 Conclusion

Women were generally knowledgeable about the benefits of breastfeeding and aware of the importance of long-term breastfeeding and of exclusive breastfeeding during the first months. They thought, as do women in most societies, that breast milk is the most valuable food for newborn infants (Liamputtong 2007; see also other Chapters in this volume). They all claimed to breastfeed for at least two years with some claiming that they did this exclusively for the first six months. However, this might have been subject to desirability bias due to the clinic setting of the study. Indeed, Bezner Kerr, Dakishoni, Shumba, Msachi, and Chirwa (2008) report, in northern Malawi, that mothers fear health workers' disapproval if they discover that they have not exclusively breastfed (see also Chapter 13 in this volume). Moreover, the frequent mention of older relatives giving infants water during the first months suggests that this was more frequent than the women cared to admit. Furthermore, elsewhere in Malawi (Bezner Kerr et al. 2008; see also Chapters 14 and 13 in this volume) and more widely in sub-Saharan Africa, older relatives play an important role in breastfeeding decision-making and tend to discourage exclusive breastfeeding (Leshabari, Koniz-Booher, Astrom, de Paoli, & Moland 2006; De Allegri, Sarker, Hofmann, Sanon, & Bohler 2007; Fjeld et al. 2008). And breastfeeding practices of Malawian mothers have been described as 'far from optimal' (Piwoz et al. 2006).

Women generally associated breastfeeding with health. It had a positive effect on themselves as well as on their infants, reducing the incidence and severity of illness in their infants and enabling birth spacing that enhanced their own health, which also indirectly benefited the health of their children. But, they also talked about it in terms of danger. They were aware of the risk of vertical transmission of HIV and, similarly to what has been reported in the wider literature (Mull 1992; Hofmann et al. 2009), they thought that other diseases could be passed to infants through breastfeeding. However, they seemed to keep these two aspects separate and formulate them as two distinct discourses: a positive one in which their own breastfeeding practices were good and a negative one, which they did not see as applying to themselves but to 'other' women who might be HIV-positive or have other illnesses, and who were seen as a potential threat to their own infants through shared breastfeeding. However, there was some ambiguity here, as the general claim that they were committed to exclusive breastfeeding (whatever they 'really' did in practice) suggests that at some level they were well aware of the possibility that they themselves might be a potential source of HIV infection for their own infants.

The women did not spontaneously mention malaria when we asked about the vertical transmission of disease, and when we asked them explicitly about this, their views were very mixed, giving the impression that it was something that they had not really thought about. This is surprising, as we had expected them to be more unanimous about the possibility of vertical transmission of malaria given that they generally thought that various diseases could be transmitted in this way, that they saw this transmission as taking place through the 'blood' rather than through breast milk[1], that they were knowledgeable about malaria parasites being in the blood, and given that the focus of the project was malaria. Perhaps it was because they were so knowledgeable about malaria that so many of them did not associate malaria with vertical transmission. Data from the main study show that although some women thought that malaria could be caused by hard work in the hot sun or exposure to cold winds, most knew that it was transmitted by mosquitoes, and some even named the anopheles vector. There is not much literature on this, and we have only found an odd reference to the belief that malaria could be transmitted through breastfeeding (in Yemen) (Al-Taiar, Jaffar et al. 2008; Al-Taiar, Chandler, Al Eryani, & Whitty 2009).

Women saw the vertical transmission of disease as occurring through the 'blood' in the breasts rather than breast milk, thus suggesting that they thought that the

[1] In Burkina Faso, women thought that disease was transmitted through breast milk, which was seen as having 'the same potential as blood to transmit disease' (Hofmann et al. 2009)

milk itself is always 'good'. This is not the case, however, and there was also much ambiguity relating to the perceived quality of breast milk. On one hand, participants argued that a mother's illness would not generally affect the quality of her breast milk, which was 'God given' and, therefore, good by definition. But on the other hand, they claimed that breast milk could become 'bad' for various reasons: if the mother is sick, then this can make her milk 'bad', which in turn causes illness in the child (i.e. rather than her simply passing on the disease through her breast), and if she becomes pregnant and continues breastfeeding or if either of the parents commit adultery. This is very similar to what has been reported in the vast literature on 'bad' breast milk from all over the world, where it is also often related to the mother's own ill health or bodily constitution (Mull 1992; Fjeld et al. 2008), to witchcraft or other supernatural causes (Mull 1992; Pool 1994; Mabilia 2005;) or, most commonly, to the behaviour of the parents: either the mother getting pregnant again while she is still breastfeeding or to adultery by one of the parents (Fernandez & Guthrie 1984; Mull 1992; Vong-Ek 1993; Liamputtong-Rice 2000; Nielsen et al. 2001; Mabilia 2005; Fjeld et al. 2008).

Given women's awareness of the possibility of vertical HIV transmission, how they talked about the role of blood circulation through the breasts enabling HIV transmission, and their statements on how food eaten by the mother is transformed into breast milk, one might assume that they would also accept that medication consumed by the mother would be passed to the infant in a similar way. Their views on this were mixed: about half of the women in the supplementary FGDs thought that this was possible, while the other half insisted that this was not possible.[2] However, all the women, including those who thought that medication could be passed to the infant, agreed that medication taken by the mother and intended to treat illness in the mother would have no effect on illness in the infant. Women were adamant that if they and their infant both had malaria, then the infant would need its own medicine in order to be cured.

The underlying assumption here seems to be that medicines are not just chemical substances that act equally on all human bodies and that those bodies react in a uniform way, however, the medication was introduced. It is as though medicines have volition – the power to choose, to exercise will; as though they act on an individual level and 'know' which individual body, they are supposed to have an effect on. Perhaps this idea has been stimulated by the distinction between adult and infant doses as prescribed in clinics (and in this particular setting perhaps also by the presence of intermittent preventive treatment for pregnant women (IPTp) and for infants (IPTi), both using the same drug). Whether or not this is the case, the notion of medicine being the active agent, of having volition, clearly resonates with the broad concept of 'medicine' in traditional African aetiology and cosmology as 'substances with the power to influence people, events and outcomes' – i.e. as substances with volition (Pool 1994).

---

[2]Nichter and Nichter (1996) have reported women deliberately consuming medicines intended for their babies as a means of transferring the qualities of the medicine to their baby.

The points above all have implications for health-seeking behaviour for infants.

First, the distancing of vertical transmission of disease to more distant others could lead to women underestimating the chances of themselves being HIV-positive and, thus, delay their seeking voluntary counselling and testing (VCT).

Second, the idea that malaria can be transmitted vertically is clearly present; and, even though this is a relatively small and perhaps not widely representative group, it does suggest that this belief may be more widespread. As a result, women may tend to be fatalistic about the use of malaria prevention interventions such as IPT and the use of bednets, thinking that their infants are still likely to get malaria anyway through breastfeeding, which women admit they cannot avoid.

Third, the notion of the volition of medicines, while potentially detrimental to health interventions, could be adapted and used to support messages relating to the proper use of medication, thus ensuring better adherence. For example, IPTi with drugs requiring multiple doses (as opposed to the single dose of SP administered in the clinic in the study reported above) would have to be partly administered at home. Given that the infants getting this treatment are not actually sick, parents may be tempted to use the additional doses for themselves or sell them on to neighbours (and indeed there is evidence of this from our data in other countries using a three-dose regimen – see Pool et al. 2008 and Gysels et al. 2009). Emphasising that the drugs are for 'that child only' will resonate with existing beliefs, thus enhancing adherence.

Acknowledgments The authors would like to thank the mothers and other community members who gave up their time to participate in this study. The project was funded by a grant from the Bill and Melinda Gates Foundation through the IPTi Consortium.

References

Al-Taiar, A., Jaffar, S., Assabri, A., Al-Habori, M., Azazy, A., Al-Gabri, A., et al. (2008). Who develops severe malaria? Impact of access to healthcare, socio-economic and environmental factors on children in Yemen: A case-control study. *Tropical Medicine and International Health, 13*(6), 762–770.

Al-Taiar, A., Chandler, C., Al Eryani, S., & Whitty, C. J. (2009). Knowledge and practices for preventing severe malaria in Yemen: The importance of gender in planning policy. *Health Policy Plan* [Advance Access published online on September 2, 2009].

Bezner Kerr, R., Dakishoni, L., Shumba, L., Msachi, R., & Chirwa, M. (2008). "We grandmothers know plenty": Breastfeeding, complementary feeding and the multifaceted role of grandmothers in Malawi. *Social Science and Medicine, 66*(5), 1095–1105.

De Allegri, M., Sarker, M., Hofmann, J., Sanon, M., & Bohler, T. (2007). A qualitative investigation into knowledge, beliefs, and practices surrounding mastitis in sub-Saharan Africa: What implications for vertical transmission of HIV? *BMC Public Health, 7*, 22. Retrieved 6 July 2009, from http://www.biomedcentral.com/1471-2458/7/22

Egan, A., Crawley, J., & Schellenberg, D. (2005). Intermittent preventive treatment for malaria control in infants: Moving towards evidence-based policy and public health action. *Tropical Medicine and International Health, 10*(9), 815–817.

Fernandez, E. L., & Guthrie, G. M. (1984). Belief systems and breast feeding among Filipino urban poor. *Social Science and Medicine, 19*(9), 991–995.

Fjeld, E., Siziya, S., Katepa-Bwalya, M., Kankasa, C., Moland, K. M., & Tylleskar, T. (2008). 'No sister, the breast alone is not enough for my baby' a qualitative assessment of potentials and barriers in the promotion of exclusive breastfeeding in southern Zambia. *International Breastfeeding Journal, 3*, 26. Retrieved 6 July 2009, from http://www.internationalbreastfeedingjournal.com/content/3/1/26

Gysels, M., Pell, C., Mathanga, D. P., Adongo, P., Odhiambo, F., Gosling, R., et al. (2009). Community response to intermittent preventive treatment of malaria in infants (IPTi) delivered through the expanded programme of immunization in five African settings. *Malaria Journal, 8*, 191.

Hofmann, J., De Allegri, M., Sarker, M., Sanon, M., & Bohler, T. (2009). Breast milk as the "water that supports and preserves life" – socio-cultural constructions of breastfeeding and their implications for the prevention of mother to child transmission of HIV in sub-Saharan Africa. *Health Policy, 89*(3), 322–328.

Joint United Nations Programme on HIV/AIDS (UNAIDS), & World Health Organization (WHO) (2008). *Sub-Saharan Africa AIDS epidemic update regional summary* (UNAIDS/08.08E/JC1526E) Geneva: Joint United Nations Programme on HIV/AIDS (UNAIDS) and World Health Organization (WHO). Retrieved 6 July 2009, from http://data.unaids.org/pub/Report/2008/JC1526_epibriefs_subsaharanafrica_en.pdf

Leshabari, S. C., Koniz-Booher, P., Astrom, A. N., de Paoli, M. M., & Moland, K. M. (2006). Translating global recommendations on HIV and infant feeding to the local context: The development of culturally sensitive counselling tools in the Kilimanjaro Region, Tanzania. *Implement Science, 1*, 22.

Liamputtong, P. (2007). On childrearing and infant care: A cross-cultural perspective. In P. Liamputtong (Ed.), *Childrearing and infant care issues: A cross-cultural perspective* (pp. 3–29). New York: Nova Science.

Liamputtong-Rice, P. (2000). *Hmong women and reproduction*. Westport, CT: Bergin and Garvey.

Mabilia, M. (2005). *Breast feeding and sexuality: Behaviour, beliefs and taboos among the Gogo mothers in Tanzania*. New York: Berghahn Books.

Mull, D. S. (1992). Mother's milk and pseudoscientific breastmilk testing in Pakistan. *Social Science and Medicine, 34*(11), 1277–1290.

National Statistical Office (NSO) [Malawi], & ORC Macro (2005). *Malawi demographic and health survey 2004*. Calverton: National Statistical Office (NSO) [Malawi] and ORC Macro.

Nichter, M., & Nichter, M. (1996). *Anthropology and international health: Asian case studies*. Amsterdam: Gordon and Breach.

Nielsen M. H. A., Konradsen, F., Mudasser, M., & van der Hoek, W. (2001). *Childhood diarrhea and hygiene: Mother's perceptions and practices in the Punjab, Pakistan*. IWMI Working Paper 25. Colombo, Sri Lanka: International Water Management Institute (IWMI).

Piwoz, E. G., Ferguson, Y. O., Bentley, M. E., Corneli, A. L., Moses, A., Nkhoma, J., et al. (2006). Differences between international recommendations on breastfeeding in the presence of HIV and the attitudes and counselling messages of health workers in Lilongwe, Malawi. *Internatinal Breastfeeding Journal, 1*(1), 2. Retrieved 6 July 2009, from http://www.internationalbreastfeedingjournal.com/content/1/1/2

Pool, R. (1994). Dialogue and the interpretation of illness: Conversations in a Cameroon village. Oxford: Berg.

Pool, R., Mushi, A., Schellenberg, J. A., Mrisho, M., Alonso, P., Montgomery, C., et al. (2008). The acceptability of intermittent preventive treatment of malaria in infants (IPTi) delivered through the expanded programme of immunization in southern Tanzania. *Malaria Journal, 7*, 213.

United Nations Development Programme (2008). *Human Development Reports: Malawi. 2008 Statistical Update*. Retrieved 6 July 2009, from http://hdrstats.undp.org/en/2008/countries/country_fact_sheets/cty_fs_MWI.html

Vong-Ek, P. (1993). How popular beliefs influence breastfeeding practices in northeast and central Thailand. *Journal of Primary Health Care and Development, 6*, 61–76.

Chapter 18
Infant Feeding Beliefs and Practices in Islamic Societies: Focusing on Rural Turkey

Meliksah Ertem

Contents

18.1 Introduction

The World Health Organization (WHO) has established recommendations for infant feeding that advocate exclusive breastfeeding up to 6 months postpartum and prolonged breastfeeding well into the second year of life (WHO, 2002). Despite biomedical recommendations for infant feeding, mothers have varied practices, for example, they introduce foods other than breast milk before 6 months of age. These practices are based on cultural norms or folk traditions. Cultural factors, taboos, local ecology, socio-economic factors have a powerful influence on behaviours like infant feeding practices and eating patterns. It is worth understanding people's behaviour before making any judgment on it. There are many differences between communities regarding infant feeding. In Islamic communities, mothers tend to breastfeed their infants. However, there are also some practices that do not fulfil the recommendations of the World Health Organization (Kramer, & Kakuma 2002). In Western Europe, the barriers to breastfeeding are lack of motivation of mothers to breastfeed, embarrassment, lack of social support, early return to full-time

M. Ertem (✉)
Department of Public Health, Faculty of Medicine, Dicle University, Diyarbakir, Turkey
e-mail: mertem@dicle.edu.tr; mertem85@hotmail.com

P. Liamputtong (ed.), *Infant Feeding Practices*, DOI 10.1007/978-1-4419-6873-9_18,
© Springer Science+Business Media, LLC 2011

employment and so on (Libbus, Bush, & Hockman 1997; Stewart-Knox, Gardiner, & Wright 2003). The main barriers are somewhat different in Islamic or Eastern communities. In Islamic countries most of the mothers are fully motivated to breastfeed, and they have no shame or embarrassment while breastfeeding (Shaikh, & Ahmed, 2006).

In Turkey, 99.8 percent of the people are Muslims belonging to the Sunni denomination although there are religious minorities including Jews and Christians. Approximately, 10 million of the people in Turkey are ethnic Kurds who live primarily in the east of the country. Syrian Christians (*Suryani*) and Arabs are other minorities living in southeastern region. Although Turkey is an Islamic country, it incorporates both Eastern and Western cultural values and it is referred to as a country in transition. For example, according to Islamic law, women could not be in decision-making position, but since 1927 Turkey has begun to see more female lawyers, judges, and diplomats. In contrast to many Islamic countries, the population growth rate is falling in Turkey, but it remains higher than EU countries. The geographical distribution of population has shifted over the past 80 years, from being three-quarters rural in 1927 to being two-thirds in urban at present. Between 1998 and 2003, the under-five mortality rate dropped from 52 to 37 percent live births and the infant mortality rate dropped from 43 to 29 percent live births (Turkish National Health Survey (TNSA) 2003). Turkey is a country that displays stark regional differences in socio-economic conditions. While most of the populations in the eastern region live under poor socio-economic conditions in rural areas, the western region consumes most of the public and private sector resources and is highly urbanised. Although Turkish laws may be considered relatively liberal with respect to gender equality, patriarchal ideology impacts strongly on everyday social life and this is more stark in the eastern part of Turkey. The ethnic, linguistic, and religious structure of Turkish society is relatively complex. Muslims form the majority of the population, but there are also Christian, Jewish and other minorities. The Kurds and Arabs form the major ethnic groups, specifically in the east and southeastern of Turkey. About 4% of the women living in the Southeastern region of Turkey cannot speak the official language of Turkey. This suggests that Kurdish women have fewer opportunities for self-development than their Turkish counterparts. Although having children and bringing them up is accepted as women's duty and these are seen as important responsibilities of women and a reason for societal existence in southeastern rural areas of Turkey, in western region of Turkey more than 20 percent of women work outside of home to earn money.

In Turkey, nearly 1.5 million new births take place each year and 95% of newborns are breastfed (Tuncbilek, Kurtulus, E., & Hancioglu 1999). The southeastern region of Turkey is the least developed where people have more Eastern or Islamic cultural values. In the region, the vast majority of mothers are illiterate or with only a little formal education. Several mothers in this region belong to an ethnic minority, and speak Kurdish as their mother tongue. Problems in regard to infant feeding include giving sugar water to newborn babies before colostrum, late start of breastfeeding, too early or too late weaning and negative effects of pacifiers (Saka, Ertem, Musayeva, Ceylan, & Kocturk 2005). The aim of this chapter is to make sense of mothers' disparate and often complex practices and illustrate the biocultural nature of the infant feeding processes in southeastern Turkey. These are based on my research conducted in the southeastern region of Turkey. The data were collected using both qualitative and quantitative methods in 2005.

18.2 Breastfeeding Behaviour and Perception in Rural Turkey

Breastfeeding in Turkey is fully endorsed and accepted as a natural and necessary way to nurture infants. Almost all mothers breastfeed their infants at least for a short period (Unsal, Atlıhan, Ozkan, Targon, & Hassoy 2005; Akyuz, Kaya, & Senel 2007). With a multicultural structure, Turkish mothers have positive opinions on breast milk. They consider human milk as the best nutrient for good child growth, development and health of infants. Breast milk is also regarded as having a preventative effect on childhood diseases, and mothers' opinions of breast milk include vitamins (Samli et al. 2006). Positive feelings on breastfeeding are also apparent amongst women in the southeastern region (Saka et al. 2005).

In the region, breastfeeding on demand is practised through the day and night whenever baby wants. In many families, babies sleep with their mothers and it is easy to breastfeed during the night. Mothers breastfeed infants more than ten times during a 24 hour period. Breastfeeding is accepted as a natural way of life and there is no shame in showing the breast while breastfeeding. Mothers breastfeed their infants in the fields where they work, in health centres or outside her homes, near to their doorways when socialising with their friends. In the southeastern region of Turkey, the breastfeeding takes place freely everywhere, mothers may put a piece of thin white cloth on their breast, sit at a corner and breastfeed their infants. Although the breast is perceived as a sexual object, this perception changes by the time mothers start breastfeeding in Turkey. In some rural areas of southeastern Turkey, it is forbidden for men to even touch the breasts of breastfeeding mothers. Breasts are considered as the right of infants. According to the views of the participants in my research, infants have priority in the parents' lives and breasts should be saved for infants not for others. In some rural areas, breastfeeding brings out reasons for not being intimate. Women are concerned that if their husbands swallow their breast milk, they may be treated as siblings of their sons. This is a highly sensitive issue and it is difficult to invite the women to articulate about this.

Breastfeeding has a religious basis in Islam (Hawwas 1987). Religiously, it is recommended that the mother suckle her infant for 2 years. The infant's father has an obligation to support his wife through any circumstances that may affect breastfeeding. Even in the case of a divorce, fathers should provide shelter and financial support to the mother for as long as breastfeeding continues. According to Islam, Allah (God) recognises breast milk as the most wholesome food source for infants. In Islamic religion, fasting is recommended in the Koran (Kocturk 2002). All adult Muslims are expected to fast throughout the lunar month of Ramadan. Breastfeeding mothers, pregnant women, and women with menstruation bleeding are, however, legitimately not expected to fast during Ramadan. Pregnant, menstrual bleeding or lactating women are seen as weak, and hence are exempted from fasting. Ertem, Kaynak, Kaynak, and Ulukal (2001) reported that 50 percent of breastfeeding mothers were fasting during Ramadan, and 65 percent of them believe that breastfeeding mothers should not be fasting, and 12 percent of the mothers start supplementary foods during Ramadan (see also Gokdemirel, Gokcay, Bulut, & Atlan 2007).

According to the views of rural women, breastfeeding has an important value and should continue without interruption. In the rural region of Turkey, when a mother travels to a distant field for working, a neighbouring mother with an infant can breastfeed her baby. Sometimes, a sister or sister-in-law may get this duty of a 'wetnurse' (*sut anne* in Turkish). This creates a profound third-degree relationship. Breastfeeding creates a *'milk-right'* between the child and his/her wetnurse, who becomes his/her *'milk-mother'*, and incest prohibitions between the child, his/her wetnurse and all other children who had been breastfed by her (*milk-siblings*) applies. Sometimes fathers pay a little amount of money to the *milk-mother*, but many times this does not need payment. *'Milk siblings'* should be strong friends forever, and in some regions, milk-siblings cannot marry each other because they are seen as being a biological brother or sister. In urban areas, where neighbourhood or relative relationships are more diffuse, this kind of support mechanism is not apparent. This tradition has begun to wane in most Muslim communities including rural Turkey with the commercial introduction of bottle-feeding (see also Chapter 14 in this volume).

Despite recognition of the numerous benefits of breastfeeding and of exclusive breastfeeding (in which water, milk and other liquids or solid foods are not allowed), the rate of exclusive breastfeeding is low in Turkey (Yigit, & Tezcan 2003) and in the southern region. The reasons for this may be lack of support for breastfeeding by health care workers, emotional stress in mothers and perception of not having enough breast milk, and pressure from close relatives to introduce liquids or solid foods (Tuncel, Dundar, Canbaz, & Peksen 2006). Many mothers say that they do not produce enough milk and they believe that their infants need water or other non-milk liquids, so they have to supplement. Moreover, the number of mothers who are exclusively breastfeeding fell dramatically. In my research, nurses from primary health settings stated often that mothers-in-law have important effects on postpartum women. In the southeastern region of Turkey, most families are traditional extended families and couples live with husbands' parents, or they live in separate houses very close to parents-in-law. Mothers-in-law have important effects on infant growth, and most of the elderly women have beliefs that infants need water and that supplementary solid foods should be introduced earlier. This is similar to one of Islamic country, Nigeria, in Davies-Adetugba's study (1997). Young mothers in particular often find it impossible to ignore their elders or the pressures from their peers. Changing misinformation about nutrition is easier when mothers are younger, living in a nuclear family and far away from their mothers-in-law.

Mothers also are well aware of the contraceptive effect of breastfeeding, which has been recognised for thousands of years. Breastfeeding has been used for the prevention of pregnancy as a tradition in rural Turkey. Many mothers breastfeed their babies for a long period to prevent pregnancies. Mothers who do not have knowledge about the effect of contraceptive methods (like condom, IUD (Intra Uterine Device) or contraceptive pills), or who have no access to family planning services tend to use traditional methods. Some mothers do not want to use modern contraceptive methods for their concerns of adverse health effects. Those women would also use prolonged breastfeeding as a contraceptive method. However, many mothers do not know that the contraceptive effect of breastfeeding is limited for only 6 months. Conversely, sometimes mothers stop breastfeeding to become pregnant. In rural areas, people value procreation within marriage and fertility is highly praised. The southeastern region of Turkey is strongly patriarchal and the status of women is lower than those in other parts of Turkey. Having many children, especially boys, enhances the woman's status and is a source of prestige. It is believed that mothers who want to become pregnant should stop breastfeeding. They breastfeed for a short time in an attempt to increase birth rates. Furthermore, women consider pregnancy as a situation counteracting breastfeeding. It is believed that it is wrong for a pregnant woman to go on breastfeeding. Once a mother is pregnant, her milk belongs to the baby in her womb and pregnant women's milk, which is called 'spoiled milk', may be harmful to the suckling baby.

In the southeastern region, there is an important variable that influences breastfeeding practices. In this region, nearly 60 percent of the women are illiterate and most of the illiterate women do not know the official language of Turkish. Those women living in the rural southeastern region and do not know the official language, and hence have less chance to reach health education or breastfeeding medical advice. They also tend to adhere to their traditional ways. Practices that can negatively affect infant health, such as an early introduction of water or supplementary foods and discard of colostrum, are more likely to occur in these illiterate women.

18.3 Postpartum Affairs

The new mothers and their infants are vulnerable to infections, diseases and bad spirits. Certain beliefs, customs and taboos surround the postpartum period. Some foods are considered beneficial and some of them harmful. Foods accepted as harmful are restricted for mothers of newborn babies. In the rural areas, uncooked vegetables, fruits and cold water were considered to be dangerous by most women. During the postpartum period, mothers are forbidden to drink water for three or four days. Mothers or mothers-in-law insist on this tradition. It is believed that if a mother drinks water during this period, her abdomen would bulk, and she might be sick. It is also believed that uncooked vegetables and cold drinks could reduce the volume of breast milk and negatively alter the content of milk. On the contrary, nurses and midwives are insisting on drinking water for better milk production. Younger mothers may no longer follow the traditional practice.

Foods giving energy are encouraged during the perinatal period. After delivery, a traditional meal prepared of butter, eggs, and grape molasses is recommended for women. After giving birth, the movement of mothers is restricted for 40 days.

Mothers are assisted in her personal care and domestic affairs by her or husband's sisters.

In the region, the belief that the newborn baby and mothers are considered to be at risk caused by some supernatural powers is still prevalent. There are many traditional ways of protecting the newborn from the bad spirits. For instance, mothers with a newborn may keep a sharp metal device under their pillow to protect themselves and infant from these bad spirited 'gins'. During the first 40 days, it is believed that the 'grave of mother and newborn infant is open' (which means they are in risks of dying). Therefore, both mother and newborn should stay at home during this time, and stay away from other people's eyes in order to protect them from the bad effects of the evil eye. Many women hold a superstitious belief regarding *Albasması* (in English it means 'red catch'). *Albasması* refers to a woman who possesses malevolent powers, which can cause harm to postnatal women and newborn babies. *Albasması* is in fact a puerperal fever or childbed fever. According to Turkish traditions, women are confined at home for at least 40 days after childbirth. Both the woman and her baby should not be left alone at home in order to be protected from *Albasması*. To protect the mother and her baby from witches and evil forces, simple precautions are taken, and these include not leaving the new mother and her baby alone, putting the Koran, bread or garlic, for example, under their pillows, and not allowing other lactating women to enter their home (Şahin 1996; Santur 2005; Geckil, Sahin, & Ege 2009).

It is believed that newborns can easily become ill. Newborn babies and mothers should be kept warm. If women go outside during this period, they wear coats and head coverings often even the weather is warm. Mothers in my study stated that even winds raised by a bird's wing may cause newborn illness. Open windows is avoided to save newborn mothers from air flow. The implications of these statements are that newborns and mothers in the postpartum period need care and they have a significant risk of dying.

In the region, women think that contrasting colours can be used to counterbalance some diseases; often white and black are used. If a disease is believed to be caused by a 'white power', then it can be treated with 'black', and vice versa. For example, according to local beliefs, a baby's stomachache may be caused by the moon, which is called '*moon stroke*'. *Moon stroke* can be treated by painting an infant's face with black fume, in accordance with the belief, because the moon is white. Similar to this situation, the effect of black meconium can be treated by white sugary water. Because of this belief, most of the time sugary water is introduced to newborn baby by their mothers, before breast milk.

Nutritional rituals are the most popular practices for good health of mothers and infants. What mothers are fed has great importance for the breastfeeding of their infant. Most of the women eat a kind of dessert called *Bulamaç*, and drink a mixture of butter and grape molasses just after childbirth to enhance breast milk (Geckil et al. 2009). Family members, including husbands, are expecting mothers to breastfeed their infants and they tend to provide social support to breastfeeding mothers. See also Chapters 8 and 13 for postpartum practice in other parts of the world.

18.4 Prelacteal Feeding

According to the women, the newborn baby should be given sweet liquids, mostly with sugar in them. In most situations, the first food given to the newborn is water sweetened with sugar (sucrose) or grape molasses (*pekmez*). In different research projects conducted in Turkey, 6–20 percent of mothers introduce their infants to sugary water before breast milk (Vancelik, Sanci, Acemoglu, & Beyhun 2006; Akyuz et al. 2007). It is believed that such prelacteals cleanse the bowel of the newborn (see also Chapter 14 in this volume).

The organisation of health services has been recognised as a factor contributing towards the ability of a mother to breastfeed. Hospital practices may promote artificial feeding, for example, separation of the mother and infant after a Caesarean section, the routine use of artificial foods and attitudes of health professionals towards infant feeding methods. In the past decade, the proportion of delivery by a Caesarean section increased from 6 to 30 percent in Turkey (Koc 2003). A Caesarean section was reported as an important factor for late initiation of breastfeeding (Kutlu, & Marakoglu 2006; Akyuz et al. 2007). Often, the meeting time between the infant and mother takes place many hours after a Caesarean section. As a result of a Caesarean section and late contact with her baby, the flow of breast milk may be delayed (Smith 2007). When mothers failed to supply a reliable and adequate amount of breast milk, the cultural myth of 'insufficient milk supply' is rising, and they start to give artificial feedings. Unfortunately, several mothers whose breast milk flow is delayed are advised to give infant formulas for only few days by health professionals. However, this situation may play an important role on hindering breastfeeding.

18.5 Colostrum

Women have negative attitudes about giving colostrum to the newborn. In the southeastern region, in the local language mothers call colostrum '*mawu*' or '*fro*'. *Mawu* literally means 'new milk' and *fro* means 'dense milk' (Ergenekon, Elmaci, Ertem, & Saka 2006). *Mawu* or *fro* is always produced within the first 3 days of birth and that 'it should not be given to newborns'. Opinions on how long to wait before giving the breast varied: some suggested a waiting period of 3 to 6 *ezan* (Islamic prayer calls), or until the mother had taken a bath. Others suggested periods of up to 3 days.

Colostrum is often deemed unsuitable and harmful for babies (see also Liamputtong Rice 2000 and Chapter 1 in this volume). Mothers state that colostrum causes stomachache and infants dislike this milk (Ergenekon et al. 2006; Saka et al. 2005). Acik, Dinc, Benli, and Tokdemir (1999) reported that 27% of the mothers considered colostrum filthy and harmful for infants. In the region, most of the women state that 'colostrum looks like pus'. The view that it is necessary to remove this 'yellow, dirty milk' that had loitered inside the breasts throughout pregnancy is widespread. Mothers squeeze their breast to get rid of this first milk until white milk is produced and then they place a clean white piece of cloth on their breast. They make correlations between meconium and colostrum, indicating they are similar in their unwanted characteristics because both of them lasted around the same time. According to them, their practice is supported by religious leaders who advise them not to give breast milk for the first 3 days, and that yellowish milk may harm the newborn. Opinions such as the first milk 'can cause discomfort for the baby', 'make the baby ill or be harmful in some way', will make the baby 'swell up' or 'cause jaundice' are expressed. Meanwhile, the baby is fed with sugared cow's milk.

Although the view that colostrum should not be given to infants prevailed, some mothers, particularly those who are followed-up or educated by health workers, thought otherwise. During my research conducted in urban areas, some women stated that they knew the benefits of colostrums and considered it as the first vaccine for infants and believed that colostrum protects infants from many diseases. Besides their positive attitudes for colostrum, they also mentioned the difficulties of giving it. This is the reason that health professionals should give support to mothers of the newborn. Most of the young mothers claimed that in the early postpartum period milk did not flow easily and baby was hungry so the pressure from older women made difficult it to obey the rules advised by health professionals. See also Chapters 1, 14, 18 and 21 in this volume.

18.6 Weaning and Supplementary Food

The most common response in many interviews is that 'it is not necessary to give food if milk is enough; if milk is not enough we must feed'. The implication of this statement is that the longer and more you can breastfeed the child the better. Many mothers, by the second or third month, give small amounts of liquid meals (meals prepared with meat and vegetable) to develop the infants' taste capability. This is recommended by elder women such as mothers-in-law and is not considered as supplementary food by mothers. Exclusive breastfeeding for at least the first 6 months is rare in the region (less than 2 percent) (Yigit, & Tezcan 2003; Saka et al. 2005). The attitude towards supplementary food is positive. Some mothers are proud of themselves for having started supplementary food early. According to their opinions, supplementary foods should be introduced as early as possible (see also Chapter 14 in this volume).

Insufficient milk appears to be a major phenomenon. It prompts mothers to discontinue breastfeeding or introduce foods other than breast milk before 6 months. In the different reports, 30–50 percent of mothers showed this reason for stopping or early introducing supplementary foods (Irgil, Akis, Aydin, & Aytekin 2003; Tuncel et al. 2006). Insufficient milk is the result of biological, cultural and economic factors. Mothers stated that the longer one can exclusively breastfeed the child the better, but that sometimes breast milk is deemed to be insufficient for the infant. Mothers explained if a child still cries after breastfeeding, which is a sign that their breast milk is not enough for their babies. Unalan, Akgun, Ciftci, Boler, and Akman (2008) reported that in their study, 38 percent of the mothers who introduced supplementary foods earlier than 6 months gave the reason of '*crying baby although breastfed'* for early supplementary feeding. Frequently, they compared their infants with others (without much relevance to measures of their weight for height) and if they felt that their infant is smaller, which was also interpreted as another indication of not having enough breast milk. Some mothers thought that the ability to produce good milk was something women inherited from their mothers. They gave the reason for insufficient milk to their hereditary features. Working outside the home, being sad, stressed or exhausted, not eating enough are the other reasons cited for insufficient breast milk (see also Chapters 8, 9, 20 and 21 in this volume).

According to the Turkish women, mothers' nutrition is very important to increase the breast milk flow. Bostanci and colleagues (1996) state that there are several kind of traditional foods introduced to lactating mothers. Three of these are '*Kuymak*', '*Gömbe*', and '*Kaygana*'. '*Kuymak*' is prepared with cow milk, wheat flour, sugar and fresh butter. '*Gömbe'* is a flaky pastry prepared with sheep meat, hazelnut and fresh butter. '*Kaygana'* is a kind of omelette prepared with grape or mulberry molasses (*pekmez*), fresh butter and hen eggs. Most of these foods introduced to lactating mothers are heavy with calories. This is evident that in the region they give intensive value to nutrition of lactating mother both for her health and that of the infants.

Water is not perceived as a supplementary food by the mothers but a necessity for the maintenance of infant health. According to mothers' opinions, 'it is absolutely necessary to introduce water to the baby'. Internal organs need water to work properly, and infant's bowels may stick to each other if water is not given. In addition to water, different types of tea are also given. These include teas made with anise (*agastache foeniculum*) and 'meryemotu' (*avens,geum urbanum*), which are used to treat infant colic.

In the region, help is not available for those who cannot initiate successful breastfeeding. Several mothers are advised to give infant formulas for only few days after birth. By the time the flow of milk has been established, those mothers are expected to stop infant formulas. Attention needs to be paid to those who are advised infant formulas for a short period, because most of those who initiate infant formulas by medical advice may continue it.

Liquid prepared with rice flour, sugar and cow's milk or water is the most preferred supplementary food. Some women state that they are giving bisque with cow's milk as supplementary food. In low socio-economic regions, bread is preferred. Even in families with low socio-economic status, infant formulas are perceived as a higher societal class behaviour, and seen as a sign of prestige. In the southeastern region, women can easily reach 'illegal trade' infant formulas, which are imported from Iraq to markets. These formulas are called '*Iraq formulas'* and mothers prefer them because these formulas have no taxes so they are less expensive than other formulas.

Some women in my study explained that the reason they were giving infant formulas was advice they received from a physician. Although in Turkey one of the targets of Ministry of Health is to 'increase to 80 percent the percentage of infants exclusively breastfed up to 6 months by the year 2015', there is no sufficient laws to avoid advertisement of commercial formulas. Except for physicians working in Baby Friendly Hospitals, many physicians and other health professionals may promote formulas partially under the influence of such advertisements.

In the region, the sex of the child has a little effect on infant feeding pattern. In most of the studies, sex of the child was not a factor influencing initiation of breast milk (Cetin, Gunes, Karaoglu, & Ustun 2004; Eker, & Yurdakul 2006). However, according to women's opinions, mothers with son should be more careful in eating habits, because boys have more griping pain in their stomachs and boys need much nutritive materials than girls. Weaning with materials that have economic value is preferred by mothers for their son rather than girls. When they give formulas to their infants, they feel themselves that they are giving more importance to their infants. Mothers have preference for having male babies because mothers with male babies have greater prestige in family and they can obtain all kind of requirements easier. According to their opinion, if male babies have greater value, then they should be fed more expensive ways. Although we could not find difference between two genders by quantitative researches, during discussion meetings we faced the fact that mothers begin formulas earlier to male babies (cf Chapter 19 in this volume).

18.7 Cessation of Breastfeeding

In Turkey, pregnancy, infant's unwillingness, insufficient breast milk, illness of mother, illness of infant are the main factors shown by mothers for stopping breastfeeding (Aslan, Ozcebe, Bilir, Vaizoglu, & Subasi 2004). In the southeastern region of Turkey, fertility rate is very high. In my studies, I came across women who had never had a chance to menstruate, because they married at an early age, and were either pregnant or breastfeeding in the following years. In surveys regarding women's reproductive health, maximum pregnancy numbers were 12 or 13, in the region. More than half of the women decided to discontinue breastfeeding because they had become pregnant again. Pregnancy has a negative effect on breastfeeding, both biologically and culturally. Although it is not written in the Koran, women in the region consider pregnant women's breast milk as '*haram*'. In Islamic religion, food rules are contained within the concepts of *halal* and *haram*. *Halal* means lawful, permitted and recommended by the *sheria*. *Haram* is the opposite, meaning unlawful, prohibited. They consider pregnant women's breast milk as the right of the foetus. According to their beliefs, pregnant women's milk is forbidden religiously and this milk considered as 'spoiled milk'. Women make correlation between vomiting caused by pregnancy and sickness of an infant who might be exposed to milk from a pregnant mother.

An interesting but rare opinion against prolonged breastfeeding that emerged in my study is that if a child is breastfed for a long period, like more than 2 years, he/she will be imbecilc. This opinion conflicts with earlier results that they breast feed until they become pregnant again. According to the mothers' opinion, to be healthier, a child should eat solid foods, such as meals prepared with lamb. In contrast to these feelings, in practice, they breastfeed their infants for a long period to avoid a new pregnancy. When they consider breastfeeding as a contraceptive method, mothers continue to breastfeed more than 4 years.

Another reason to stop breastfeeding is when 'the child becomes too big', which is deemed he/she is old enough to stop. Illness of the mother is also a reason for ceasing breastfeeding. Ill mothers stop breastfeeding because they believe that sickness of mothers may harm the infant (cf Chapter 14 in this volume).

18.8 Conclusion

In Turkey, mothers give great value to breastfeeding, accepted as a natural and necessary way to nurture their infants. Nearly all mothers give breast milk to their infants. Breastfeeding is also highly valued by Islamic rules. Beside those positive beliefs and attitudes, there are some wrong practises. Particularly in rural Turkey, delayed initiation of breastfeeding, prelacteal feeding and failure to practice exclusive breastfeeding are widespread. Current beliefs and practices such as waiting three prayer call (*ezan*) to initiate breastfeeding or squeezing and discarding colostrum are strongly influenced by traditions. These are kept very much alive by elders such as mothers-in-law. Breastfeeding has also a religious basis in Turkey. In rural areas where fertility rates are higher, women stop breastfeeding to have new babies. However, pregnant women's breast milk is considered '*haram*' (not suitable in religious basis). The women are also well aware of the contraceptive effect of breastfeeding. The women and infants are believed to be vulnerable to spiritual powers. To avoid post delivery diseases and bad events, women and infants are kept from outside threats. Predominantly, foods with high energy are preferred to feed lactating mothers. Colostrum is deemed unsuitable and harmful for babies. Early introduction of supplementary foods is a frequently faced fact. Water or broths are not considered as supplementary foods. According to their beliefs, an initiation of supplementary foods is necessary for good development of the infants.

I contend that antenatal care visits stressing the importance of breastfeeding have an important influence on infant feeding practices. Day-by-day education programs in the region may affect or change mothers' behaviour and beliefs. Particularly in rural areas and in younger age mothers, exclusive breastfeeding, early initiation of colostrum and long duration of breastfeeding should be seen as a priority in an attempt to promote the health and well-being of newborn infants in Turkey.

References

Acik, Y., Dinc, E., Benli, S., & Tokdemir, M. (1999). The knowledge, attitudes of the women about breast milk and nutrition who has children aged 0 to 24 months in Elazig-Turkey. *Turkish Klinikleri Journal of Pediatrics, 8*, 53–62.

Akyuz, A., Kaya, T., & Senel, N. (2007). Determination of breastfeeding behaviors of mothers and influencing factors. *TAF Preventive Medicine Bulletin, 6*(5), 331–335.

Aslan, D., Ozcebe, H., Bilir, N., Vaizoglu, S., & Subasi, N. (2004). İnfant feeding practices and malnutrition in Van province. *Journal of Child Health, 4*(1), 16–23 (In Turkish).

Cetin, F., Gunes, G., Karaoglu, L., & Ustun, Y. (2004). Antenatal care receival initiating of breast-feeding and influential factors among mothers who gave birth at Turgut Ozal Medical Center. *Journal of Inonu University, 12*(4), 247–252.

Davies-Adetugba, A. A. (1997). Sociocultural factors and promotion of exclusive breastfeeding in rural Yoruba communities of Osun State Nigeria. *Social Science and Medicine, 45*(1), 113–125.

Eker, A., & Yurdakul, M. (2006). The knowledge and practices of mothers related to baby feeding and breastfeeding. *STED (Surekli Tip Egitimi Dergisi), 15*(9), 158–163.

Ergenekon, P. O., Elmaci, N., Ertem, M., & Saka, G. (2006). Breastfeeding beliefs and practices among migrant mothers in slums of Diyarbakir, in Turkey, 2001. *The European Journal of Public Health, 16*(2), 143–148.

Ertem, I. O., Kaynak, G., Kaynak, C., & Ulukal, B. (2001). Attitudes and practices of breastfeeding mothers regarding fasting in Ramadan. *Child Care Health and Development, 27*(6), 545–554.

Geckil, E., Sahin, T., & Ege, E. (2009). Traditional post partum practices of women and infant and the factors influencing such practices in South East Turkey. *Midwifery, 25*(1), 62–71.

Gokdemirel, S., Gokcay, G., Bulut, A., & Atlan, A. (2007). The effect of Ramadan fasting on breastfeeding. *Journal of Child Health, 7*(3), 177–181 (In Turkish).

Hawwas, A. W. (1987). Breastfeeding as seen by Islam. *Population Science, 7*, 55–58.

Irgil, E., Akis, N., Aydin, N., & Aytekin, N. (2003). Breastfeeding of infants in Gemlik. In *National Maternal and Child Health Congress Book* (p. 324). Ankara-Turkey: Ankara University Tip Fakultesi (In Turkish).

Koc, I. (2003). Increased cesarean section rates in Turkey. *European Journal of Contraception Reproduction Health Care, 8*(1), 1–10.

Kocturk, T. O. (2002). Food rules in the Koran. *Scandinavian Journal of Nutrition, 46*(3), 137–139.

Kramer, M. S., & Kakuma, R. (2002). *The optimal duration of exclusive breastfeeding: A systematic review*. WHO/NHD/01.08, WHO/FCH/CAH/01.23. Geneva: World Health Organization.

Kutlu, R., & Marakoglu, K. (2006). Evaluation of initiating, continuing, and weaning time of breastfeeding. *Marmara Medical Journal, 19*(3), 121–126.

Libbus, K., Bush, T. A., & Hockman, N. M. (1997). Breastfeeding beliefs of low income primigravidae. *International Journal of Nurse Study, 34*(2), 144–150.

Şahin, N. N. (1996). *The beliefs in İkiyamac village, Taşlıcay district of the City of Ağrı on pregnancy and birth and the impacts of these on mother and babies health*. Unpublished Master of Science Thesis, Hacettepe University Social Science Institute, Ankara, Turkey.

Saka, G., Ertem, M., Musayeva, A., Ceylan, A., & Kocturk, T. (2005). Breastfeeding patterns, beliefs and attitudes among Kurdish mothers in Diyarbakir, Turkey. *Acta Paediatrica, 94*(9), 1303–1309.

Samli, G., Kara, B., Unalan, P. C., Samli, B., Sarper, N., & Gokalp, A. S. (2006). Knowledge, beliefs and practices of mothers about breastfeeding and infant nutrition: A qualitative study. *Marmara Medical Journal, 19*(1), 13–20.

Santur, M. E. (2005). Birth traditions. Retrieved 20 December 2006, from http://www.folklor.org.tr/icerik/haber_detay.asp?id=34

Shaikh, U., & Ahmed, O. (2006). Islam and infant feeding. *Breastfeed Medicine, 1*(3), 164–167.

Smith, L. J. (2007). Impact of birthing practices on the breastfeeding dyad. *Journal of Midwifery Womens Health, 52*, 621–630.

Stewart-Knox, B., Gardiner, K., & Wright, M. (2003). What is the problem with breastfeeding? A qualitative analysis of infant feeding perception. *Journal of Human Nutrition and Diet, 16*(4), 217–218.

Tuncbilek, E., Kurtulus, E., & Hancioglu, A. (1999). *Nutrition of infants, children and mothers. Turkish National Health Survey 1998* (pp. 123–132). Ankara, Turkey: UNPF, Population Inst. Hacettepe University, Macro Int. Inc.

Tuncel, K. E., Dundar, C., Canbaz, S., & Peksen, Y. (2006). Research on breastfeeding status of children aged 0–24 months applied to a University Hospital. *Journal of CU Nursing Faculty, 10*(1), 1–6.

Unalan, P. C., Akgun, T., Ciftci, S., Boler, I., & Akman, M. (2008). Why do mothers attending a baby friendly mother and child health care unit start early solid food to their babies? *Turkish Archive of Pediatrics, 43*, 59–64.

Unsal, H., Atlıhan, F., Ozkan, H., Targon, S., & Hassoy, H. (2005). Breastfeeding attitudes and behavior in Turkish community and factors effecting breastfeeding practices. *Journal of Children Health Diseases, 48*(3), 226–233.

Vancelik, S., Sanci, N., Acemoglu, H., & Beyhun, E. (2006). Behaviors of mothers regarding breastfeeding. In *National Public Health Congress Book* (p. 7), Van-Turkey (In Turkish).

World Health Organization Secretariat (2002). Infant and young child nutrition: Global strategy on infant and young child feeding, Resolution WHA55/15. Geneva: World Health Organization. http://www.who.int/gb/EB_WHA/PDF/WHA55/ea5515.pdf (Accessed 25 Sept 2003).

Yigit, E. K., & Tezcan, S. (2003). *Infant feeding behavior and nutritional status of children: Turkish National Health Survey 2003* (pp. 141–55). Ankara, Turkey: Population Research Institute of Hacettepe University Press.

Chapter 19
Early Initiation of Breastfeeding and Its Beneficial Effects in Japan

Yuko Nakao and Sumihisa Honda

Contents

19.1 Introduction

In this chapter, we discuss early initiation of breastfeeding and its beneficial effects in Japan. According to the Association of Maternal Health in Japan (2007), the proportion of full breastfeeding has remained low since the 1970s. The proportion of full breastfeeding at 1 month was 71 percent in the 1960s; this figure decreased to 32 percent in the 1970s and has remained low ever since (42 percent in 2005) (Fig. 19.1).

On the other hand, according to a national birth-cohort study involving 53,000 babies in 2001 (Kaneko et al. 2006), the proportion of full breastfeeding, any breastfeeding and infant formula feeding at 6 months was 21, 93 and 6 percent, respectively. Using these reports as a background, Hashimoto (1998) comments on three changes: (1) from home delivery commonly supported by midwives to maternity clinic or hospital; (2) from breastfeeding to infant formula feeding and (3) from

Y. Nakao (✉)
School of Health Science, Nagasaki University, Sakamoto, Nagasaki 852-8520, Japan
e-mail: ynakao@nagasaki-u.ac.jp

P. Liamputtong (ed.), *Infant Feeding Practices*, DOI 10.1007/978-1-4419-6873-9_19,

© Springer Science+Business Media, LLC 2011

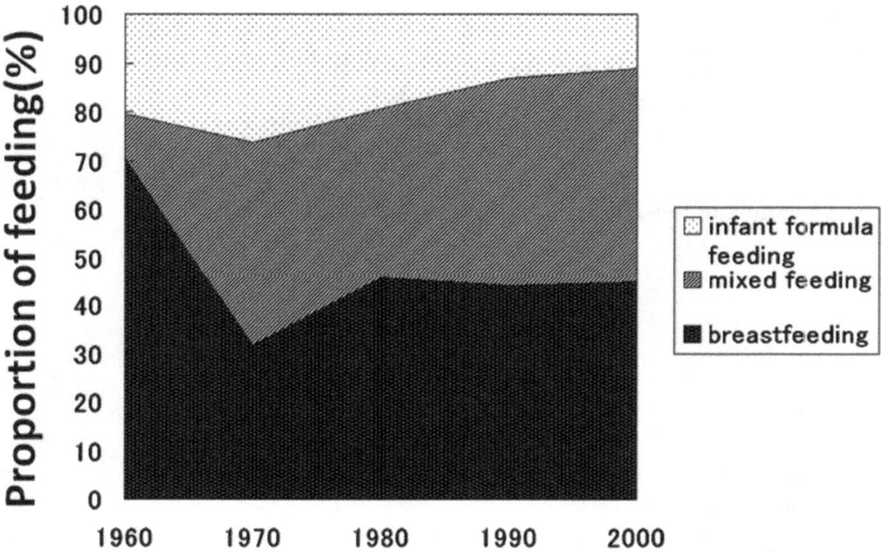

Fig. 19.1 Secular trend of feeding at 1 month in Japan, 1960–2005

the same room to a different room. This has resulted in the rapid reduction of breastfeeding to 32 percent in the 1970s. The World Health Organization (WHO) passed a resolution about infant nutrition and mother's milk childcare in 1974. In order to promote breastfeeding, the Ministry of Health, Labor and Welfare in Japan suggested the following: (1) newborn infants should be given only mother's milk for at least 1.5 months after birth: (2) mothers need to provide their infant only with mother's milk as much as possible; and (3) mothers should give their breast milk to their infants as much as possible, without changing to infant formula feeding, at 8 months or later. Although the proportion of mothers who breastfed exclusively recovered to 46 percent by 1980, with the promotion of breast treatment techniques by midwives, the same problems have continued.

Two meetings have become the pillar of breastfeeding promotion in Japan: the Japanese Society for Breastfeeding Research meeting in 1985 and the Japan Breastfeeding Association meeting in 1992. The Japan Breastfeeding Association has been entrusted with and performs the authorisation examination of the UNICEF Baby Friendly Hospital initiative.

Nakao, Moji, Honda, and Oishi (2008) describe that there were only 40 baby-friendly hospitals in Japan in 2005, which represents only 1.3 percent of the total number (2,933) of Japanese maternity hospitals. The Japan Breastfeeding Association (2009) recognised 56 baby-friendly hospitals in Japan in 2008. The proportion of mothers who breastfeed exclusively has, thus, remained low.

Early skin-to-skin contact promotes uterine contraction by stimulating maternal oxytocin production. It is well known that this helps control uterine bleeding. Furthermore, the maternal vagus nerve is stimulated by the baby's sucking, resulting in secretion of vasoactive intestinal peptide (VIP) and cholecystokinin (CCK).

These gastrointestinal hormones with anabolic actions change maternal digestive function for breastfeeding, as they result in efficient energy use. Moreover, VIP extends blood vessels, and it is considered to cause the breast to become red and warm. For both mother and child, extension of the breast blood vessels at the time of breastfeeding resulting in warmth is perceived as a comforting stimulus, and it is said that it becomes an important part of the mother–child interaction (Seo 2007). In addition, Mizui (2007) reports cases of pathological breast engorgement in mothers who did not start early breastfeeding.

In 1998, the World Health Organization summarised the findings of studies on the effects of early breastfeeding contact in Step 4 of *Evidence for the Ten Steps to Successful Breastfeeding,* which states that one should 'help mothers initiate breastfeeding within a half-hour of birth' (see also Chapters 10 and 14 in this volume). However, Moore, Anderson, and Bergman (2007) believe that there is controversy about the importance of first breastfeeding within 30 min after delivery. From observations in maternity hospitals, Widstrom et al. (1987) and Righard and Alade (1990) suggest that it is difficult for mothers to do this, as babies may not be ready to initiate suckling. Furthermore, Rowe-Murray and Fisher (2002) show that Caesarean section is a significant barrier to the implementation of Baby-Friendly Hospital Initiative Step 4. Therefore, it is important to discuss the timing of suckling after 30 min. In Baby-Friendly USA, Step 4 is interpreted and put in practice as less than 1 h. Nakao and colleagues (2008), using a self-administered questionnaire, reveal that commencement of early breastfeeding within 120 min after delivery was significantly associated with the continuation of full breastfeeding.

19.2 Issue of Supplemental Feeding

Exclusive breastfeeding is traditionally very rare in Japan. Warm water and/or sugar water are usually given in addition to breast milk (cf. Chapters 8, 9 and 12 in this volume). These liquids are given from a very early stage after birth and are frequently the first liquids given to a baby in the maternity hospital. Shimada and colleagues (2001) report that only breastfeeding was given in 15 percent, sugar water was added in 45 percent, infant formula was added in 29 percent, warm water was added in 5 percent, and an unknown supplement was given in 5 percent during the hospital or other medical facility stay in a total of 270 facilities and 6676 mothers. In our investigation, the first liquid was: breast milk, 133 (41.8 percent); infant formula, 50 (15.7 percent); sugar water, 66 (20.8 percent); and unknown supplement, 69 (21.7 percent). The contents of feeding during clinic or hospital stays were breast milk and sugar water, 86 (27 percent); breast milk, sugar water, and infant formula, 51 (16 percent); only breast milk, 44 (13.8 percent); breast milk and infant formula, 137 (43.1 percent). Ordinarily, lactation starts within 2 or 3 days after delivery. However, because some mothers have problems with their nipples, infant sucking, or stress, lactation is insufficient. Sugar water is then added as a water supplement (Horiuchi 1996).

Around 1930 in Japan, according to Oto (1982), many mothers and their families, while waiting for mother's milk for 1 or 2 days, gave *makuri* (a seaweed called *kainnsou*), the root of acoltsfoot, licorice juice or sugar water to rid the baby's body of eczema. The first breastfeeding was given not by the baby's natural mother but by a mother who had already started breastfeeding. In Japan, the custom was that a male baby was given mother's milk by a mother who had a female baby, and that a female baby was given mother's milk by a mother who had a male baby. This custom, called *chichiawase* (Mie Prefecture), *awasechichi* (Osaka Prefecture), *aichichi* (Okayama Prefecture) or *chikezichi* (Kochi Prefecture), was believed to allow male babies to grow up healthy and marry early. On the other hand, it was believed that the milk of a woman with an infant of the same sex would produce a rivalry between the children. In this way, those who were connected by the first breastfeeding were considered to have a relationship called *chizukeoya* or *chinomioya*, or temporarily becoming parent and child. The baby was associated with this *chizukeoya* throughout his or her life. It was thought that the mother's milk held a spiritual power for a child of the opposite gender (Oto 1982). The baby was believed to be given a strong spiritual power of hermaphrodite to grow up healthily.

After the 1930s, the importance of mother's milk for protecting the infant from diarrheal enteritis and as a secure nutrition source was recognised, because it was difficult to secure selected dairy products. Midwifery subsequently became involved in the promotion of lactation and preventing breast difficulties. In fact, midwives were more active than the mother and her family in promoting breastfeeding. Breast management or assistance with breastfeeding became part of the midwifery curriculum, and breast massage and early breastfeeding were carried out (Ito 1988; Tanigawa & Nishikawa 1981). However, the addition of supplements continues to the present.

19.3 Benefits and Issues of Kangaroo Mother Care

Kangaroo mother care was started in 1979 in Bogota, Colombia, by Dr. Edgar Rey and Dr. Heactor Martinez, in response to overcrowding (babies sharing incubators), insufficient resources (no monitoring equipment for oxygen and heart rate) and an extremely limited number of poorly paid nurses in the neonatal intensive care units, in which there was high morbidity and mortality among low-birthweight infants. The new home care, low-birthweight programme was based on the following principles: (a) discharge home without regard to weight once the baby's condition is stable and it has adapted to extrauterine life, thereby removing the baby from the disease-ridden hospital; (b) no artificial milk formula, only mother's milk supplemented with guava juice; (c) encouragement of early bonding by nursing the baby next to the mother's body between the breasts; and (d) maintenance of the baby in a head-up position. Using this approach, infants as immature as 32 weeks' gestation were successfully cared for at home (Whitelaw & Sleath 1985; Nathalie et al. 2005). Kangaroo mother care for low-birthweight infants was introduced in Japan in

Table 19.1 Beneficial effects of kangaroo care

Physiological effects
Body temperature maintenance
Stability of respiratory
Stability of circulatory
Relaxed state and increase in silent sleep
Promotion of mother' milk secretion
Psychological effects
Formation of attachment
Feeling of satisfaction
Realization as parent
Healing of delivery
Promotion of motherhood

1998. Kangaroo mother care has now expanded to include full-term infants in most Japanese maternity hospitals, since it has been shown to have both physiological and psychological benefits (Table 19.1) (Oishi et al. 2006).

Kangaroo mother care after delivery is also common in Japan. In our research, we also found that early skin-to-skin contact was performed with significantly early breastfeeding. In the practice of kangaroo care, which leads to early breastfeeding, Nakai and Hamasaki (2009) suggest that the temperature of the delivery room be adjusted to 24–26°C for comfort. If kangaroo care were performed in a cold room, the baby would have a low body temperature due to heat loss and blood sugar would be used up to produce heat, leading to hypoglycemia and adverse neurological effects. Takada (2007) suggests that when the mother perspires during delivery, she should be wiped using a dry towel to protect her baby from a low body temperature. It is important to prepare the delivery room environment to ensure that the mother and child are not cold during early skin-to-skin contact. Amniotic fluid also needs to be wiped off with a warm towel, and the newborn infant needs to be put gently on the mother's breasts, while waiting patiently for 1 h until the baby is likely to want to suckle.

In our study, breastfeeding within 2 h after delivery was related to maintenance of breastfeeding. Catecholamines are rapidly secreted within 120 min by the newborn infant; this period is called 'the newborn infant awakening term' in Japan (Hashimoto 2000). It is important to have a plan for kangaroo care within 2 h after birth.

19.4 The Study

A questionnaire was distributed by mail to all 391 mothers who were invited to participate in a physical examination of their 4-month-old infants between September and December 2003 in Nagasaki, southwestern Japan. The mothers were asked to answer the questionnaire voluntarily. Public health nurses collected the questionnaire on the day of the medical check-up. Three hundred and twenty-six mothers

(83 percent) responded to the questionnaire. Eight mothers who did not start breastfeeding during their stay in the clinic/hospital were excluded.

The questionnaire included time from birth to first breastfeeding, mothers' satisfaction with the first breastfeeding, method of feeding during their stay in the maternity hospital, method of feeding at 1 and 4 months after birth, characteristics of the mothers and babies, characteristics of delivery and characteristics of postpartum care. Early skin-to-skin contact was defined as the placing of the naked baby prone on the mother's bare chest within 2 h after delivery. The first breastfeeding was defined as the baby suckling at the breast directly for the first time after birth. The time from birth to first breastfeeding was classified into the following four groups: within 30 min, 31 to 120 min, 121 min to 24 h and more than 24 h. The proportions of fully breastfeeding mothers during their stay in the clinic/hospital, at 1 month, and at 4 months were compared among the four groups based on the time of the first breastfeeding.

In the present study, the following commonly used classification of feeding in Japan was used: (1) fully breastfeeding, which means that breast milk was given and infant formula was not given, regardless of whether other liquids and/or solid food were given; (2) any breastfeeding, which means including category 1 and that both breast milk and infant formula were given, regardless of whether other liquids and/or solid food were given; and (3) infant formula feeding, which means that formula was given and breast milk was not given, regardless of whether other liquids and/or solid food were given.

19.5 Effects of Breastfeeding

19.5.1 Early Breastfeeding

In all, 318 mothers participated; their mean age was 29.4 years (standard deviation 4.6 years); 93 percent of infants were term. Of the babies, 155 were males and 163 were females, and 17 percent of births were Caesarean sections. Bleeding at delivery of less than 500 ml was reported by 67 percent of mothers. Early skin-to-skin contact was reported by 20 percent. The proportion of mothers who breastfed within 30 min and within 31 to 120 min was 36 percent and 21 percent, respectively.

The proportions of mothers who initiated the first breastfeeding within 30 min and within 120 min were not significantly different by maternal age, baby's gender and parity. However, mothers who had babies with a gestational age of 36 weeks or less, had a Caesarean section or had bleeding of 500 ml or more during delivery initiated first breastfeeding significantly later than their respective controls. Early breastfeeding was disturbed by Caesarean section, premature delivery and severe bleeding during delivery. After excluding these 124 cases, early breastfeeding within 120 min was associated with breastfeeding in the first week ($p=0.006$) during the hospital or clinic stay, at 1 month ($p=0.006$) and at 4 months after birth ($p=0.004$) (Fig. 19.2). On the other hand, there was no significant difference in the proportion of mothers fully breastfeeding between the period within 30 min

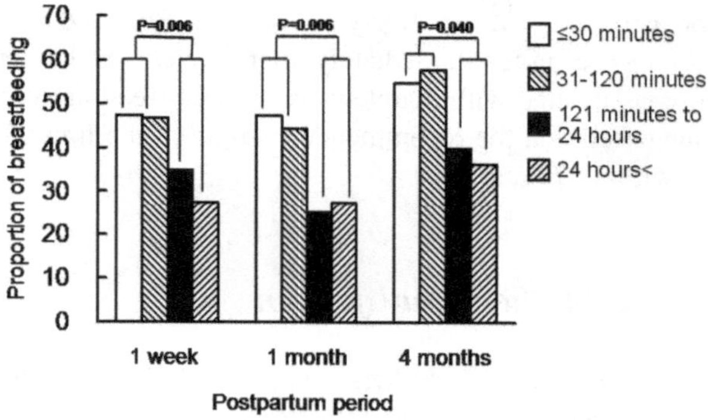

Fig. 19.2 Proportion of full breastfeeding by postpartum period

and that between 31 and 120 min at each time period. Moreover, the proportion of mothers with early breastfeeding was higher in those who had early skin-to-skin contact and in those who did not supplement feeding with sugar water or infant formula.

In order to determine the factors influencing the continuation of full breastfeeding, a multiple linear logistic model analysis was performed. The proportion of mothers who continued full breastfeeding at 4 months was 1.8-fold higher in those who breastfed within 30 min than in those who breastfed at more than 30 min, but the odds ratio was not significant. The proportion of mothers who continued full breastfeeding at 4 months was significantly higher in those who breastfed their baby within 120 min (OR 2.5) compared with those who breastfed at more than 120 min. The odds ratios for those who breastfed within 30 min (OR 1.8) and that for those who breastfed within 120 min (OR 2.5) were not significantly different.

Severe bleeding during delivery, premature delivery, and Caesarean section were obstacles for early breastfeeding. If it is possible to attempt early breastfeeding under these conditions, for example, by delaying routine neonatal procedures and keeping mother and baby in close proximity (Rowe-Murray, & Fisher 2002), we can further promote early breastfeeding. Mothers who initiated breastfeeding within 120 min maintained full breastfeeding during their stay in the clinic/hospital, as well as at 1 and 4 months after birth. The rate of decline in breastfeeding was significantly slower for infants who were first suckled early than for those who were first suckled later (Taylor, Maloni, & Brown 1986; Dyson, McCormick, & Renfrew 2005). The proportion of full breastfeeding mothers did not differ between first breastfeeding within 30 min and first breastfeeding within 31 to 120 min. Righard and Alade (1990) reports that infants require an average of 49 min in order to initiate breastfeeding through their own efforts and sucked for about 20 min. Widstrom et al. (1987) report that it takes 55 min for infants to start suckling after birth. On the other hand, Hashimoto (2000) describes the rapid secretion of catecholamines within 120 min by newborn infants, which is called the 'the newborn infant awakening term'. A previous study revealed that first breastfeeding within 120 min was significantly associated with skin-to-skin contact and extended the duration of subsequent breastfeeding (Mikiel-Kostyra, Mazur, & Boltruszko 2002). Breastfeeding does not need to be started immediately after delivery, as the first breastfeed within 120 min was associated with maintenance of breastfeeding for up to 4 months. It might be suggested that the recommended timing of the first breastfeed should be extended to within 120 min.

19.5.2 Mothers' Satisfaction

The proportion of mothers who were satisfied with the first breastfeeding was higher among those who breastfed within 120 min than among those who breastfed more than 120 min after birth. The proportion of satisfied (including slightly satisfied) mothers among those who first breastfed their baby within 120 min was 88.8 percent, and among those who breastfed more than 120 min it was 73.6 percent (Fig. 19.3). Some mothers responded to our questionnaire and described their feelings about breastfeeding as 'I felt motherly love', 'I had greater pleasure with childbirth' and 'I felt calm'. Early breastfeeding helped to calm the mothers and make them feel relaxed. There was no significant difference in the proportion of mothers' satisfaction in the first breastfeeding between within 30 min and 31 to 120 min. The mother who has early contact with her baby and initiates breastfeeding after delivery might have enhanced maternal behavior compared with the mother who does not (Widstrom et al. 1990). Contact with the baby immediately after birth promotes a closer relationship between mother and baby. Moreover, Nakamura and Yamanouchi (2000) suggest that early initiation of breastfeeding gives the mother

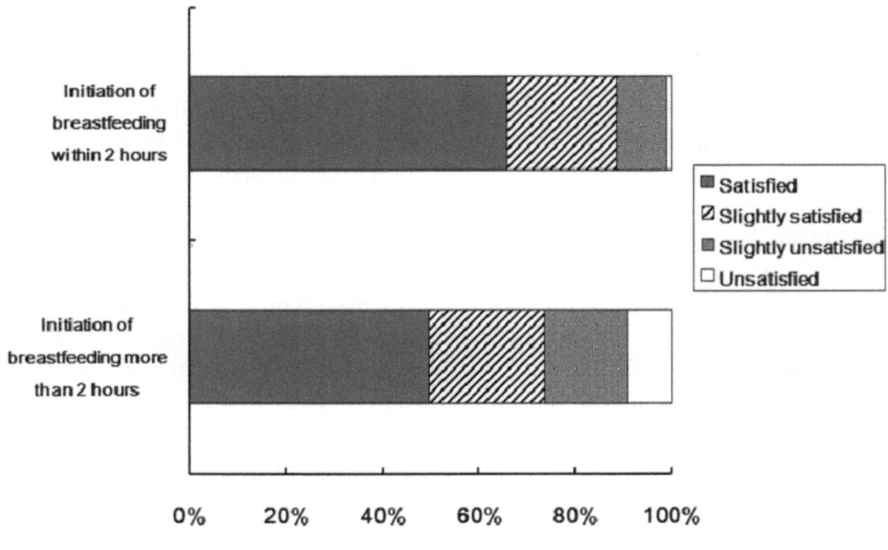

Fig. 19.3 Proportion of satisfied mothers among those who first breastfed their baby within 2 h and those who breastfed after more than 2 h

a strong sense of satisfaction. In our study, maternal satisfaction with first breastfeeding was also associated with early initiation of breastfeeding within 120 min. According to Horiuchi (2007), one mother told of her experience when her baby suckled her nipple: 'The feeling of my baby suckling was like the sound of a beating heart', a description of the child's vitality.

Horiuchi (2007) also describes the mothers' narratives about the experience of kangaroo mother care at 30, 60 and 120 min after delivery. Mothers who held their babies for 30 min described having severe pains, but when they held their babies, they were able to realize and express their love. Mothers who held babies for 60 min vividly described the feeling of cooperation between mother and child and the baby's sucking power. Mothers who held their babies for 120 min described their confidence as parents. Early breastfeeding not only increased the proportion of mothers maintaining full breastfeeding but also produced positive mental effects in the mothers.

19.6 Infant Gender and Maintenance of Breastfeeding

In the present study, it was interesting to find that the proportion of mothers who continued full breastfeeding at 4 months was significantly higher (by about twofold) for female infants than for male infants. This is in contrast to previous studies. A previous study in Latin American countries (Brazil, Honduras, and Mexico) reported that male infants were significantly more likely to have early cessation of exclusive breastfeeding (Perez-Escamilla et al. 1995). Another study in Greece analysed factors affecting intention to breastfeed and found that male gender was associated with negative attitudes to breastfeeding (Ladomenou, Kafatos, & Galanakis 2007). It is possible that mothers may think that male infants need more nutrition than female infants, and they may add infant formula earlier. On the other hand, a study in China (Graham, Larsen, & Xu 1998) reported that girls were breastfed for a significantly shorter period than boys because of a cultural preference for sons. Messner, Lalakea, Aby, Macmahon, and Bair (2000) suggest that mothers with ankyloglossia had more difficulties with breastfeeding. Ankyloglossia is defined as nipple pain lasting longer than 6 weeks and/or difficulty of the baby latching onto the breast, which is more common in males than in females. The higher frequency of medical problems in male infants might have been related to the lower proportion of full breastfeeding among males at 4 months.

19.7 Conclusion

In Japan, home delivery was popular in the 1960s, supported primarily by *josanpu* (midwives). After delivery, the baby was given a bath in the traditional tub (*tarai*) and taken to the mother's side. When the infant wanted breastfeeding, it was immediately placed at the mother's nipple. Mother and child always slept in the same bed (Japanese-style futon) until the mother recovered.

However, in the 1970s, the place of delivery changed from the home to the maternity clinic or hospital. The baby is given a bath using a tub after delivery, the routine neonatal procedures, such as height, weight, head and chest measurements, are performed, and then the baby meets the mother for a short time. The baby is then separated from the mother and observed in the nursery. There is enough time to enhance bonding between the mother and child, but medical personnel separate them to protect against infections.

Even now, the Japanese tradition of bathing a baby immediately after birth continues to a certain extent, after which routine neonatal procedures are performed. To try kangaroo care immediately after birth, it is very important to allow the baby a chance to suckle. The delivery room environment must be appropriate, with the proper room temperature, and the mother and infant should not be separated after birth unless there is an unavoidable medical reason. We suggest that the baby should be with the mother continuously from birth and be allowed to suckle spontaneously at the breast whenever the baby shows signs of readiness to do so. This should be continued for at least 2 h. Thus, breastfeeding should provide the baby's first liquid.

As mentioned above, since early initiation of breastfeeding has many beneficial effects, it is important to provide sufficient support for early breastfeeding and not separate mother and child.

References

Baby-Friendly USA. The ten steps to successful breastfeeding. MCHB 03-0232P. Retrieved July 15, 2009, from http://www.babyfriendlyusa.org/eng/docs/BFUSAreport.pdf

Dyson, L., McCormick, F., & Renfrew, M. (2005). Interventions for promoting the initiation of breastfeeding (Cochrane Review). *Cochrane Database Systematic Review, 18*(2), CD001688.

Graham, M. J., Larsen, U., & Xu, X. (1998). Sons preference in Anhui Province, China. *International Family Planning Perspectives, 24*(2), 72–77.

Hashimoto, T. (1998). *The promotion policy study of maternal feeding*. Ministry of Health and Welfare mental-and-physical-disorder research report, pp. 112–115 (in Japanese).

Hashimoto, T. (2000). Breastfeeding. *The Japanese Journal of Neonatal Care, 13*(12), 10–17 (in Japanese).

Horiuchi, T. (1996). The problem of the mother and child stayed in the same hospital room and added sugared water. *Journal of Japan Society for Premature and Newborn Medicine, 8*(3), 81 (in Japanese).

Horiuchi, T. (2007). Breast-feeding – It's a world of narrative. *Journal of Japan Breast Feeding Association, 1*(2), 59–70 (in Japanese).

Ito, T. (1988). Service for a resident of professional organization. In T. Ito (Ed.), *Steps of 60-years* (pp. 68–72).Tokyo: Japanese Midwives' Association (in Japanese).

Japan Breastfeeding Association. About Baby Friendly Hospital (BFH) in Japan. Retrieved June 5, 2009, from http://www.bonyuweb.com/shoukai/about_bfh.htm (in Japanese).

Kaneko, A., Kaneita, Y., Yokoyama, E., Miyake, T., Harano, S., Suzuki, K. et al. (2006). Factor associated with exclusive breast-feeding in Japan: For activities to support child-rearing with breast-feeding. *Journal of Epidemiology, 16*(2), 57–63.

Ladomenou, F., Kafatos, A., & Galanakis, E. (2007). Risk factors related to intention to breastfeed, early weaning and suboptimal duration of breastfeeding. *Acta Paediatrica, 96*(10), 1441–1444.

Messner, A. H., Lalakea, M. L., Aby, J., Macmahon, J., & Bair, E. (2000) Ankyloglossia: Incidence and associated feeding difficulties. *Archives of Otolaryngology—Head & Neck Surgery, 126*(1), 36–39.

Mikiel-Kostyra, K., Mazur, J., & Boltruszko, I. (2002). Effect of early skin-to skin contact after delivery on duration of breastfeeding: A prospective cohort study. *Acta Paediatrica, 91*(12), 1301–1306.

Mizui, M. (2007). Change of mamma and breastfeeding within 1 week after birth and support. In Y. Kanahara (Ed.), *Standard of breastfeeding support* (pp. 157–165). Tokyo, Japan: Igaku-syoin Publications (in Japanese).

Moore, R. E., Anderson, G. C., & Bergman, N. (2007). Early skin-to-skin contact for mothers and their healthy newborn infants (Cochrane Review). *Cochrane Database System Review, 3*, CD003519.

Nakai, H., & Hamasaki, M. (2009). The risk-free interpretation of "Ten Steps to Successful Breastfeeding". *Journal of the National Institute of Public Health, 58*(1), 51–55.

Nakamura, K., & Yamanouchi, T. (2000) Early breastfeeding and the meaning. *The Japanese Journal of Neonatal Care, 13*(12), 156–61 (in Japanese).

Nakao, Y., Moji, K., Honda, S., & Oishi, K. (2008). Initiation of breastfeeding within 120 minutes after birth is associated with breastfeeding at four months among Japanese women: A self-administered questionnaire survey. *International Breastfeeding Journal, 3*(1). Retrieved January 20, 2009, from URL:http://www.internationalbreastfeedingjournal.com/content/3/1/1

Nathalie, C., Juan, G. R., Jelka, Z., Adriano, C., Zita, F., Rejean, T., et al. (2005). Kangroo mother care: 25 years after. *Acta Pediatrica, 94*, 514–522.

Oishi, M., Asada,S., Kuroki, E., Date, K., Miyama, C., & Nakao, Y. (2006). The method and results of kangaroo care in Japan: Search of literature. *Health Science Research, 19*(1), 21–26 (in Japanese).

Oto, Y. (1982). *The folklore of child*. Tokyo, Japan: Soudobunka (in Japanese).

Perez-Escamilla, R., Lutter, C., Segall, AM., Rivera, A., Trevino-Siller, S., & Sanghvi, T. (1995). Exclusive breast-feeding duration is associated with attitudinal, socio-economic and biocultural determinants in three Latin American countries. *American Institute Journal of Nutrition, 125*(12), 2972–2984.

Righard, L., & Alade, M. O. (1990). Effect of delivery room routines on success of first breast-feed. *The Lancet, 336*, 1105–1107.

Rowe-Murray, H. J., & Fisher, J. R. W. (2002). Baby friendly hospital practices: Cesarean section is a persistent barrier to early initiation of breastfeeding. *Birth, 29*(2), 124–131.

Seo, T. (2007). Meaning of early attachment. In Y. Kanahara (Ed.), *Standard of breastfeeding support* (pp. 148–151). Tokyo, Japan: Igaku-syoin (in Japanese).

Shimada, M., Watanabe, H., Toda, R., Nakane, N., Kamiya, S., Agata, T. et al (2001). A Relationship between Breast-feeding Care in Hospital and breast-feeding at 1-month Postpartum: a National Survey on Breast-feeding. *The Journal of Child Health, 68*(1), 749–756 (in Japanese).

Takada, E. (2007). Support of early skin to skin contact. In Y. Kanahara (Ed.), *Standard of breastfeeding support* (pp. 152–156). Tokyo, Japan: Igaku-syoin (in Japanese).

Tanigawa, I., & Nishikawa, Y. (1981) *Folklore of traditional delivery house in Japan*. Tokyo, Japan: Kokusho (in Japanese).

Taylor, P. M., Maloni, J. A., & Brown, D. R. (1986). Early sucking and prolonged breast-feeding. *American Journal of Disease of Children, 140*(2), 151–154.

Whitelaw, A., & Sleath, K. (1985). Myth of the marsupial mother: Home care of very low birth weight babies in Bogota, Colombia. *The Lancet, 1*(8439), 1206–1208.

Widstrom, A. M., Ransjo-Arvidson, A. B., Christensson, K., Matthiesen, A. S., Winberg, J., & Uvnas-Moberg, K. (1987). Gastric suction in healthy newborn infants: Effects on circulation and developing feeding behaviour. *Acta Paediatrica Scandinavica, 76*, 566–572.

Widstrom, A. M., Wahlberg, V., Matthiesen, A., Eneroth, A. P., Uvnas-Moberg, K., Werner, S., et al. (1990). Short-term effects of early suckling and touch of the nipple on maternal behaviour. *Early Human Development, 21*, 153–163.

Chapter 20
Socio-cultural Factors Influencing Infant Feeding Patterns Within 6 Months Postpartum in Rural Vietnam

Dat Van Duong

Contents

20.1 Introduction

According to the World Health Organization, malnutrition contributes directly or indirectly 60 percent to the 10.9 million deaths annually amongst children under five (WHO 2003). In Vietnam, despite the recent improvement in national health indicators, malnutrition in children under 5 years old remains a major public health concern. With 30 percent of children under 5 years of age malnourished in terms of weight-for-age, and 33 percent undernourished in terms of height-for-age, Vietnam has one of the highest child malnutrition rates in Southeast Asia (National Institute of Nutrition & UNICEF 2003).

Inappropriate infant feeding practice is an important factor contributing to the malnutrition of children (Ighogboja 1992; Madzingira 1995). In Vietnam, although the WHO has recommended that infants should be exclusively breastfed for the first 6 months with the introduction of appropriate complementary foods and continued

D. Van Duong (✉)
United Nations Population Fund in Vietnam, UN Apartment Building, 2E Van Phuc Compound, Kim Ma Street, Ba Dinh District, Hanoi, Vietnam
e-mail: dat@unfpa.org.vn

P. Liamputtong (ed.), *Infant Feeding Practices*, DOI 10.1007/978-1-4419-6873-9_20,

© Springer Science+Business Media, LLC 2011

breastfeeding thereafter (WHO 2001), recent studies showed that only 31 percent of infants aged less than 2 months were exclusively breastfed; and after the fifth month, no infant was being exclusively breastfed. There has been a decreasing trend of exclusive breastfeeding in favour of an early introduction of complementary food. Typically, the proportion of infants under 4 months old who are exclusively breastfed has reduced from 27 percent in 1997 to 20 percent in 2002 (Committee for Population Family and Children 2003).

Factors influencing breastfeeding have been investigated in the international literature. Mother-related factors such as employment and perceived insufficient breast milk, and infant-related factors were reported (Bulk-Bunschoten, van Bodegom, Reerink, Pasker-de Jong, & de Groot 2001; McCarter-Spaulding & Kearney 2001; Moffat 2002). Breastfeeding could be influenced by health providers (DiGirolamo, Grummer-Strawn, & Fein 2003) and marketing of the formula industry (Adair, Popkin, & Guilkey 1993). In addition, cultural environment was found to affect breastfeeding practice (Kendall-Tackett & Sugarman 1995; see also Chapters 6, 7, 8, 9, 13, 14, 17, 18 and 19 in this volume).

It is known the factors affecting breastfeeding may operate differently across countries (WHO 1998). Despite the alarming decline in exclusive breastfeeding rate in Vietnam, there have been few studies specifically focused on determinants of breastfeeding (Morrow 1996; Doyle 2001; Ministry of Health of Vietnam 2001; Dearden et al. 2002). Moreover, their applications are rather restrictive due to either small sample size (Morrow 1996; Dearden et al. 2002) or limitations in data analysis (Doyle 2001; Ministry of Health of Vietnam 2001). In this study, I explore factors influencing breastfeeding practices within the first 6 months postpartum amongst women residing in the rural Northern Central region of Vietnam using a combination of qualitative and quantitative methods. Exclusive breastfeeding is defined as feeding infants by only breast milk from the mother or a wetnurse, or expressed breast milk, but no other liquids or solids with the exception of drops or syrups consisting vitamins, mineral supplements, or medicine (WHO 1996).

20.2 The Study

This study was conducted in Quang Xuong District, Thanh Hoa Province, located 150 km south of Hanoi. Quang Xuong District is divided into 41 communes, of which nine are coastal and 32 lowland, with a total population of 240,000. The population growth rate for Quang Xuong was 1.6 percent in the national census of 1999. The district is representative of the Northern Central Vietnam according to demographic and health indicators (Quang Xuong District Health Service 2000).

The study consisted of two phases. A longitudinal study was first conducted during August 2002–May 2003. A sample of 463 rural women who gave birth during August–October 2002 was enrolled in the study. For the initial survey, participants were interviewed within the first week after delivery. Research assistants were given information about deliveries by district and commune health authorities. For those who delivered in the District Hospital (DH), research assistants interviewed them during their post partum period in the hospital. For those who delivered either at a commune health centre (CHC) or at home attended by a Traditional Birth Attendant (TBA), interviews were conducted at CHCs or at the home of participants. Participants were consecutively selected until the required sample size for sufficient statistical power (80 percent) was attained. They were then followed up at home during weeks 16 and 24. In the surveys, participants were asked information relating to infant feeding practice within the past 24 hours. In the initial survey, the weight of infants at birth was based on the recall of the mothers while in the follow-up surveys, their weight was scaled by the research assistants immediately after the interview.

In the second phase, 16 focus group discussions were undertaken during May–June 2004. The objective was to obtain complementary information not available from the quantitative surveys. These included women within the first 6 months post-partum (six groups), men whose partners were within the first 6 months postpartum (six groups), and commune health workers (four groups). The size of the groups ranged between 6 and 8 people. The focus group discussions were conducted in Vietnamese by myself and a research assistant.

For the quantitative surveys, the structured questionnaires used were adapted from those of Scott et al. (Scott 1997; Scott, Landers, Hughes, & Binns 2001). Both quantitative and qualitative instruments were pre-tested for cultural sensitivity prior to actual data collection.

Participants were informed about the purpose of the study and asked to give their formal consent to participation. The protocol followed the ethical principles of the Helsinki Declaration (World Medical Assembly (WMA) 1996) and the National Health and Medical Research Council of Australia (NHMRC 1999), and was approved by the local health authorities and the Human Research Ethics Committee of Curtin University.

20.3 Results

20.3.1 Demographic Characteristics

The initial survey included 463 women, with high participation rates at the follow-up surveys; only 3 participants at week 16 and 4 participants at week 24 missed the interviews. The average age of the cohort was 26.40 years at baseline survey (SD=4.97). About 47 percent of them had monthly family income between VND 500,000 and 1,000,000, and about 40 percent between VND 200,000 and 500,000 (US$1 ≈ VND 15,500). More than half of them passed lower secondary school, 8.2 percent passed high school and 6.3 percent had diploma or university degree while 18 percent did not complete primary school or never attended

Table 20.1 Demographic characteristics of respondents

Characteristics	
n	463
Age	
Mean (SD)	26.40(4.97)
Household income (log-transformed)	
Mean (SD)	13.05(0.66)
Occupation	
Farmer	62.9
Non-farmer	37.1
Education	
Tertiary/university	6.3
High school	8.2
Secondary school	56.8
Primary school	11.1
Not complete primary school	10.2
Never attend school	7.4

school. About 63 percent of the participants identified themselves as farmers (see Table 20.1).

20.3.2 *Infant Feeding Patterns*

Within a week after delivery, 98.3 percent of the respondents had initiated breastfeeding, with 73.6 percent of the mothers initiating within the first hour. Colostrum or breast milk was fed to 85.6 percent of babies as the first meal while the remaining 14.4 percent were given a fluid other than breast milk. Most babies were fed according to their needs (96.7 percent), with an average of 10 times within 24 hours during the first week after birth.

At week 1, exclusive breastfeeding was practised by 83.6 percent of the mothers while the rest fed breast milk together with some complementary foods or exclusively bottle-fed their babies. The complementary foods used included sugar solutions, fruit juice, porridge, and even steamed rice. In most cases where solid food was prematurely introduced to babies, the deliveries took place at home with assistance of a traditional birth attendant. About 7 percent of the mothers introduced formula to their babies, including 1.7 percent (8 cases) who exclusively bottle-fed. 'Suggested by relatives or friends', 'bottle-feeding is easier', 'did not like breastfeeding' and 'had to work after delivery' were the common reasons given for choosing formula and/or other complementary foods.

Table 20.2 shows the feeding patterns when infants were 1, 16 and 24 weeks old. The complementary feeding rate increased from 16.4 percent at week 1 to 56.5 percent at week 16 and nearly 100 percent at week 24. The rate of breastfeeding together with drinkable and solid food such as porridge or steamed rice increased considerably at weeks 16 (23.5 percent) and 24 (61 percent). For breastfeeding

Table 20.2 Feeding patterns for infants at weeks 1, 16 and 24

	Week 1		Week 16		Week 24	
	n	(percent)	*n*	(percent)	*n*	(percent)
Exclusive breastfeeding	387	(83.6)	200	(43.5)	2	(0.4)
Breastfeeding together with bottle-feeding	22	(4.7)	46	(10.0)	1	(0.2)
Breastfeeding together with drinkable food	21	(4.5)	23	(5.0)	112	(24.4)
Breastfeeding together with solid and drinkable food	22	(4.8)	108	(23.5)	280	(61.0)
Bottle-feeding only	8	(1.7)	1	(0.2)	1	(0.2)
Bottle-feeding together with solid and/or drinkable food	0	(0)	80	(17.4)	61	(13.4)
Other types	3	(0.7)	2	(0.4)	2	(0.4)
N	463		460		459	

together with home cooked rice solution (*nuoc chao*[1]) and other drinkable food, the proportion was similar between weeks 1 and 16 (about 5 percent), but rose sharply to 24.4 percent at week 24. The rate of formula and cow milk together with solid and other drinkable food increased at week 16 (17.4 percent), but slightly declined at week 24 (13.3 percent). Exclusive bottle-feeding with formula or cow milk accounted for a very small proportion of the participants at the initial and follow-up surveys.

20.3.2.1 Formula and Milk Feedings

The use of formula for infants increased from 4.4 percent at week 1 to 16.2 percent at week 16, but decreased to 6.3 percent at week 24. Local formulas *Dielac* and *Ridielac* were the most widely consumed (76 percent) whereas imported brands were not popular. Cow milk and other milks used at week 1, week 16 and week 24 were 2.5 percent, 12.2 percent and 7.4 percent, respectively. 'Influence of formula advertisement' and 'follow other people who used formula in health setting' were the most common reasons for choosing these two formulas, which accounted for 53 percent and 27 percent of the total responses, respectively. Most of the participants (98 percent) were exposed to commercial advertisement of formula through the mass media, especially television.

20.3.2.2 Drinkable Food

Water, fruit juice and rice solution (*nuoc chao*) were the most common drinks for infants at weeks 16 and 24: water was used by 57.1 percent and 90.4 percent of

[1] *Nuoc chao* is often made by boiling a small cup of rice with two or three bowls of water for about one hour. It is then filtered through a piece of thin fabric. Other ingredients such as salt or sugar are sometimes cooked together with rice.

subjects, fruit juice by 14.7 percent and 19.4 percent, rice solution by 5.0 percent and 24.4 percent, respectively.

20.3.2.3 Solid Food

Solid food was introduced very early to infants by 4.8 percent of the cohort at week 1. The use of formula and cow milk decreased, while the use of solid food increased significantly from 40.9 percent at week 16 to 74.3 percent at week 24 (p<0.01). In all cases, home-cooked meals were used to feed infants.

20.3.2.4 Ingredients of Home-Cooked Food

Three popular types of home-cooked solid food were rice porridge (*chao dac*)[2], rice-floured porridge (*bot*)[3] and steam rice. The main ingredients used to prepare these were rice, meat and egg. Over 40 percent of cases used monosodium glutamate to cook food for their infants.

20.3.2.5 Feeding Frequency

In all three surveys, over 95 percent of infants were fed on demand. The mean number of feeds within 24 hours reduced slightly over time: 10.2 times (SD=3.2) at week 1, 9.7 (SD=3.4) at week 16, and 9.2 (SD=2.5) at week 24. For those infants whom solid food was introduced to, they were fed more than twice per day.

20.3.3 Factors Influencing Infant Feeding Practices

20.3.3.1 Mother-Related Factors

Education Level

Results from logistic regression analysis show that mother's education level is an important factor that can influence her infant feeding practice. Education is a statistically significant determinant of mother feeding practice at week 16 and 24, but not at week 1. Table 20.3 showed that mothers who completed secondary school or higher were more likely to practice exclusive breastfeeding than those completed primary school or had a lower education (OR=6.45). Similarly, for woman who had achieved a high education level, there was less chance of feeding her infant with solid food (OR 0.35 at week 16 and 0.28 at week 24).

---

[2]*Chao dac* is often made by boiling two small cups of rice with two or three bowls of water for about one hour. Other ingredients such as minced meat, fish sauce, salt or sugar are sometimes cooked together with rice.

[3]*Bot* is made by mixing three spoons of rice flour in a bowl of water. It is then cooked for about 15 minutes. To enrich nutrition of *bot*, it is generally advised to boil bones or meats for one or two hours and use this broth to mix with rice flour. Egg is recommended to stir into *bot* for five minutes before the cooking finished.

Table 20.3 Factors that influence infant feeding practice at weeks 1, 16 and 24 postpartum

	Exclusive breastfeeding at week 1		Exclusive breastfeeding at week 16		Introduction of solid food at week 16		Introduction of solid food at week 24	
Variables	Odd ratio	95 percent CI	Odd ratio	95 percent CI	Odd ratio	95 percent CI	Odd ratio	95 percent CI
Mother-related factors								
Education								
Primary school or lower			1		1		1	
Secondary school or higher			6.45**	2.75–15.09	0.35**	0.19–0.64	0.28**	0.10–0.54
Occupation								
Non-farmer							1	
Farmer							0.52*	0.18–0.95
Feeding preference								
Other methods	1							
Breastfeeding	3.52*	1.21–10.28						
Mother make own decision on breastfeeding								
No			1					
Yes			2.14*	1.09–4.13				
Feeding problems of mother								
At least one problem	1							
No problem	4.54**	1.61–12.85						
Feeling uncomfortable to breastfeed in pubic places								
No			1					
Yes			0.45**	0.25–0.80				

Table 20.3 (continued)

Variables	Exclusive breastfeeding at week 1		Exclusive breastfeeding at week 16		Introduction of solid food at week 16		Introduction of solid food at week 24	
	Odd ratio	95 percent CI	Odd ratio	95 percent CI	Odd ratio	95 percent CI	Odd ratio	95 percent CI
Infant-related factors								
What baby was first fed								
Other foods	1							
Colostrum/breast milk	2.71*	1.28–7.46						
Health problems of infants								
No					1			
Yes					1.91**	1.18–3.10		
Father-related factors								
Occupation								
Non-farmer			1		1			
Farmer			2.11*	1.17–3.81	0.47**	0.28–0.80		
Feeding preference								
Other methods	1		1		1			
Breastfeeding	5.37**	1.64–17.60	4.92*	2.43–9.98	0.38**	0.20–0.75		
Satisfaction with baby's sex								
Not satisfied/neutral opinion							1	
Satisfied							0.30**	0.17–0.53
Close relatives- and friend-related factors								
Feeding practices of friends								
Other methods	1						1	
Breastfeeding	3.65**	1.34–9.97					0.41*	0.16–1.10
Feeding preference of mother-in-law								

Table 20.3 (continued)

Variables	Exclusive breastfeeding at week 1		Exclusive breastfeeding at week 16		Introduction of solid food at week 16		Introduction of solid food at week 24	
	Odd ratio	95 percent CI	Odd ratio	95 percent CI	Odd ratio	95 percent CI	Odd ratio	95 percent CI
Other methods							1	
Exclusive breastfeeding							0.18*	0.04–0.75
Socio-economic factors								
Living status								
Living in extended family					1		1	
Living independently					1.71*	1.05–2.79	1.76	1.01–3.06
Family income							1.47**	1.29–1.67
Having sufficient food during the year								
No			1					
Yes			4.16*	1.02–9.83				
Medical-related factors								
Delivery methods								
Caesarean section	1				1			
Normal delivery	18.52**	5.47–62.71			3.29*	1.02–10.60		
Delivery settings								
At home	1							
At district hospital	6.80**	2.73–16.92						
At commune health centre	2.31	0.84–6.35						

$^{*}p < 0.05$, $^{**}p < 0.01$

Knowledge of Lactation Mechanism and Nutrition

Women generally did not have sufficient knowledge of the milk production mechanism. By week 24, about 65 percent of surveyed women believed that feeding formula to 1-month-old baby would not reduce the amount of milk produced by the mother. Qualitative data from focus groups revealed their perception that breast milk would have good quality only if mothers consumed sufficiently high-protein foods. Diet for mothers seemed poor, partly due to lack of understanding of postnatal nutrition. Some women said they had good nutrition within few weeks after delivery. After that they often had the same meal as other family members. We also found that some women did not eat fish, fresh vegetable and fruit as they were afraid that this food could deteriorate quality of breast milk and cause diarrhoea for infants. The lack of understanding of postnatal nutrition and lactation mechanism resulted in early introduction of complementary foods to infants, as evident from the following example:

> I have a lot of milk but it is very thin, because I cannot afford meat everyday. My baby is so small, so I gave him some rice solution and it seems good. (A woman, aged 26)

One woman shared with the researcher her breastfeeding experience:

> Three weeks after delivery, I started losing my milk. The milk was reduced day by day. I did not know what I had to do to get the milk returned. My mum said my body is not suitable for making breast milk and advised me to give up. By the second month, I totally lost the milk and raised the child with *nuoc chao* and sweetened milk. (A woman, aged 23)

In addition, the concern of having insufficient breast milk was common amongst non-exclusive breastfeeding women. At week 24, 97 percent of the surveyed women believed that formula is necessary whenever they cannot produce enough milk. They appeared to lack adequate knowledge and skills to stimulate lactation. Eating more pork feet cooked with green papaya was often advised as a workable remedy, while some cases ended up with complementary feeding of infants.

> I wanted to fully breastfeed my baby but I could not, even I tried to eat as much as I could. Breast milk was not enough for the baby and she cried for a whole day. I gave up after five days and started giving her some rice porridge. (A woman, aged 19)

Qualitative data suggested that some mothers were confused about 'exclusive breastfeeding'. They perceived exclusive breastfeeding as not giving solid and semi-solid foods to infants, but water, fruit juice, sugar solution and even formula milk were permissible.

> In the clinic, they told me how to exclusively breast my baby for at least 4 months. But I did not know that I should not give him water or cow milk. I though doctor meant I should not give him steamed rice. (A woman, aged 24)

Employment

At week 24, logistic regression analysis indicated that there was less likelihood for the infant to be fed with solid food if the mother was a farmer (OR=0.52).

Qualitative discussions found that women returned to work very early after delivery. At week 16, most of the women (95 percent) already returned to their usual work. Their workload was unlikely to reduce during postnatal period, especially at planting and harvesting seasons. If their house is close to the field, they could go home at lunchtime to feed their babies.

> It is normal here for women to return to work just one or two months after delivery... For my case, I can fully breastfeed my son at night. But at daytime, I could only feed him two times. My mother-in-law gives him some rice solution while waiting for me to come back. (A woman, aged 28)

Discomfort of Breastfeeding in Public Places

Logistic regression analysis indicated that if women did not feel comfortable to breastfeed their child in public places, they were unlikely to maintain exclusive breastfeeding practice (OR=0.45). In group discussions, women also addressed their embarrassment of showing their breast during breastfeeding.

> I have to give breast milk to my baby in the fish market. It is the only option as I have to work. It is really embarrassed that nearly everybody watched me. I often used a *non* [a hat] to hide the head of the baby and put my eyes to other directions, but I still felt some men were watching us. (A woman, aged 26)

Health-Related Conditions

During the first week, 15.6 percent of mothers reported at least one health problem related to breastfeeding, such as inverted nipples, cracked or sore nipples, or not having enough milk or colostrum for their baby. At week 16, 8 percent of women experienced at least one breastfeeding-related problem compared to 12 percent of women at week 24. The main problems were 'inverted nipples', 'cracked or sore nipples', 'not enough milk for babies' and 'pain when breastfeeding'. Logistic regression analysis found that the health condition of mothers significantly affected breastfeeding patterns at week 1, but not at weeks 16 and 24. Data suggested that at week 1, mothers who faced difficulties in breastfeeding were less likely to practice exclusive breastfeeding (OR=4.54). In addition, qualitative data suggested that when women were ill, they were very concerned of the low quality and quantity of breast milk, especially if they took medicine such as antibiotics.

> ...My wife got cough and fever and I bought for her antibiotics. She was very sick and I could smell antibiotics in her sweat. We decided not to give our son breast milk as it is contaminated with antibiotics and could harm his health. (A man, aged 38)

Other Factors

Logistic regression results suggested that feeding preferences of the mother could also influence her decision on exclusive breastfeeding at week 1 (OR=3.52). Moreover, when mothers made their own decision on breastfeeding, their babies were likely to be exclusively breastfed at week 16 (OR=2.14). Qualitative data further indicated that due to financial constraints,, exclusive breastfeeding seemed a practical and economical choice for many mothers. However, to maintain exclusive breastfeeding they needed ongoing motivation from close relatives and health workers.

> I experienced loosing milk for four days. I was so worried and wanted to give my baby some *nuoc chao* [rice solution]. But my mother-in-law and husband always comforted me and told me to be patient. They took care of my baby so I could sleep... A commune nurse visited me at home. She gave me a vacuum and instructed me how to use it. Thank God, after some days, milk came back. (A woman, aged 30)

Although some women were fully aware of the significance of breast milk for the development of the child, after struggling with insufficient milk and hardship, they started giving infants complementary food. The story of the following woman is a typical example:

> I believed that breastfeeding is good. I used to exclusively breastfeed my first son for six months. But for this time, I am not able to do it because I have to work far from home. It takes at least one hour walking from home to our [rice] field so I am not able to breastfeed my baby during working hours. A village activist from village Women Union suggested me to take the milk out and keep it in a cool place so that my mother could feed him during my absence. However, I do not have a fridge at home. I am afraid that my child could have diarrhoea. (A mother, aged 31)

20.3.3.2 Infant-Related Factors

Sex of Infant

Of the 463 babies born during the study period, 54.3 percent were male and 43.7 percent female. While there was no evidence suggesting that sex of infant could significantly influence exclusive breastfeeding practice of mothers during the first 6 month postpartum, logistic regression analysis still indicated that if a father was satisfied with infant's sex, less possibility for the infant to be fed with solid foods by week 24 (OR=0.30).

Physical Development of Infants

The average weight of babies at birth was 3,098 grams (SD=357). Infants who were exclusively breastfed tended to be heavier than those fed with complementary foods. At week 16, the average weights were 6,890 grams (SD=0.765) for those exclusively breastfed, 6,730 grams (SD=0.847) for those complementarily fed with drinkable food and 6,710 grams (SD=0.841) for those complementarily fed with solid and semi-solid food. Similar results were also found at week 24. However, significant differences were observed at week 24 (p<0.01), but not at week 16. Logistic regression analysis also indicated that at week 24 the satisfaction of mother with the weight of the infant could lead to continue breastfeeding (OR=4.27).

Infant Health Problems

At week 1, 6 percent of the infants were reported to have health problems, especially respiratory tract related conditions. At week 16, 38 percent of the infants were reported having at least one health problem, mainly respiratory tract-related conditions (90 percent), fever (43 percent), and diarrhoea (13 percent). At week 24, 42 percent of infants were reported to have at least one health problem, mainly respiratory tract-related conditions (92 percent), fever (65 percent), and diarrhoea (26 percent). At week 16, infants who were exclusively breastfed reported significantly less health problems than non-exclusive breastfed infants ($p<0.01$). However, logistic regression analysis found that the health condition of infants did not significantly affect breastfeeding patterns.

Nevertheless, qualitative data suggested that infant's temperament could influence the breastfeeding decision of mothers. The cry of infants or their demand for milk at night could exhaust the mothers who need to work in the field from the early morning. Some mothers then decided to give babies complementary food so that the child could sleep well.

> My son cried for milk several times at night that made me so tired because I had to work at six o'clock in the morning. He was hungry and could not sleep. As recommended by our neighbour, I gave him porridge twice per day that really make him full and quiet at night. I think it is not too bad idea. (A mother, aged 24)

20.3.3.3 Father-Related Factors

At week 16, it appears that for those fathers who were farmers their infants were more likely to be exclusively breastfed and less likely to be fed with solid foods (ORs are 2.11 and 0.47, respectively). Similarly, if the father preferred breastfeeding, there was higher chance for the infant to be exclusively breastfed at weeks 1 and 16 and less fed with solid foods at week 16. Logistic regression analysis found ORs 5.37, 9.42 and 0.38 respectively. During group discussions, some men expressed their interests in breastfeeding. Although they were aware of the advantages of breastfeeding to the healthy development of infants, their actual assistance to infant feeding was limited. It is a traditional norm that men should not involve with infant feeding because it is a 'women's job'. Men could share with the workload of women in the field but not housework. In addition, after replanting and harvesting periods, men in Quang Xuong district often worked outside the village for additional incomes for the family. Most works are relatively mobile and they often do not bring their wife with them. Women stay at home to take care of children, parents-in-law as well as farming works.

> I think breastfeeding is good because it is simple and natural. But I let my wife decide how to feed the baby. She should know how to take care of children. I know nothing about it. . .. My job is to earn living for the whole family. I return home during weekend every two weeks and could not help much for my wife. I just give her money and she manages the whole thing. (A man, aged 31)

20.3.3.4 Close Relative- and Friend-Related Factors

Data showed feeding practices of friends could influence their decision on exclusive breastfeeding and introduction of solid foods. Logistic regression analysis suggested that if mother's friends practiced exclusive breastfeeding, it is likely that she would exclusively breastfeed her baby at week 1 and unlikely introduce solid foods for the child at week 24 (ORs 3.65 and 0.41, respectively).

Similarly, feeding preference of close relatives could influence on infant feeding practice of the woman. Statistics showed that if a mother-in-law preferred exclusive breastfeeding, it is unlikely her daughter in-law would introduce solid foods to the infant at week 24 (OR=0.18).

Traditionally, grandmothers often serve as a carer for both mother and infant in the first few months after delivery. The grandmother would help cooking and washing dirty clothes of the mother and baby. She also helps her for some other house works such as shopping and taking care of other children. The traditional meals she cooks could be of high rich protein (for instance, *chao* cooked with chicken or pork) that may support the lactation process. However, she may give her very poor nutrition meals (such as steam rice with dried salt) for a couple of weeks with a traditional belief that these foods can bring better physical and spiritual power for both the mother and the baby. The woman would find difficult to oppose the cooking decision of her mother-in-law, especially when she was newly married and financially dependent to her husband's family. A man could feel comfortable to work away from home for a long time as he traditionally believes that he wife and baby are well taken care by his mother. Even when his wife complains to him about the tasteless meals, he may find difficult to ask his mother to change the recipe: caring a postnatal woman and a baby is a simple task of a grandmother why a good man has to be bothered with?

It is cultural expectation that mothers should learn from the experience of grandmothers. However, grandmothers may not necessarily have an adequate knowledge of infant feeding, leading to potentially conflicting situations. The following case is an illustration:

> I am not comfortable with the way my mother-in-law gave porridge to my daughter. But it is very hard to talk with her about it, as she would be very disappointed. Old people often turn a small issue into a complicated matter. My husband will not be satisfied about it. (A woman, aged 27)

Traditional factors also had strong influence on infant feeding practice of mother. For instance, the infant was likely to be fed with solid food when the parents lived independently compared to those who lived with their extended family (ORs at weeks 16 and 24 were 1.71 and 1.76 respectively). While a mother-in-law and other relatives in the extended family would provide useful support to the mother during the postnatal period, they may impose their own traditional feeding practices and health beliefs (that could be backwards and harmful) and the mother may be in a vulnerable position to decline their support. On the other hand, living separately from parents-in-laws gives opportunities for the mother to practice infant's feeding in her own way or at least she would eat whatever she likes without a controller.

> I stayed with my mother-in-laws for two weeks after delivery and it was really a disaster when she requested me to follow a special diet scheme that I could eat only steam rice with dried salt and very salted fishes. I was advised not to take bath for at least two months. I

really wanted to eat raw vegetables but she did now allow it. I was not allowed to have a bath for at least a month although it was a very hot summer. I understand that my mother-in-law loved me and really wanted to take care of myself. I tried to eat whatever she gave me because I did not want to upset her...... I am so happy that she stayed only for two weeks with us. Then I could cook and eat whatever I want. (A woman, aged 24)

20.3.3.5 Health Setting-Related Factors

Statistical data recommended that at week 1 postpartum, women who had a vaginal delivery tended to have a much higher rate of exclusive breastfeeding than those who underwent caesarean section (OR=18.52). However, data also indicated that women who experienced a normal delivery was more likely to introduce solid foods for their infant at week 24 than those who underwent caesarean section (OR=3.29).

In addition, mothers who delivered at district hospital and commune health centre were more likely to practice exclusive breastfeeding, compared to those delivered at home and being attended by a traditional birth attendant. The odds ratios were 6.8 and 2.3, respectively. In the initial survey, for women who delivered at a health setting, 79.6 percent reported being encouraged by health workers to breastfeed their infants immediately after birth, and 76.1 percent feeding on demand during their stay in the hospital or commune health centres. However, only 22 percent of the respondents reported receiving information, education and communication materials on breastfeeding, 37.6 percent receiving demonstrations on breastfeeding and 7.5 percent having individual consultation or discussion with health workers about breastfeeding.

In group discussions with health workers, we learned that a national breastfeeding programme had been implemented in Quang Xuong District in recent years. However, very little training on breastfeeding counselling was given to health workers. Moreover, supportive supervision from the district hospital to commune health workers on this issue was limited. Therefore, despite the dissemination of the national guidelines on breastfeeding, many health workers either lacked the basic knowledge and skills of breastfeeding counselling or were not confident of providing coaching in the daily practice.

Some health workers seemed not convinced of the values of breastfeeding. In a commune health centre, we saw a woman bottle-feeding her baby just two days after delivery. All health workers knew it, but did not do anything to convince the woman to exclusively breastfeed the infant.

The practice of Traditional Birth Attendants (TBAs) was observed in the communes in this study. In each commune there were three to six TBAs. TBAs have good credibility in the community. They typically have practised for many years and attended generations of deliveries in the commune. Some women expressed that TBA did not work just for money as they had a 'good heart' and the 'kindness of a mother'. They would attend the delivery upon being called, and received whatever the family gave them in return: a dozen eggs, a small amount of money, or simply assisting the TBA's family during the harvesting season. In case the delivery was attended by a TBA, very few women received information on infant feeding from this provider (26 percent). However, information provided by TBAs was often insufficient or inadequate.

> She [a TBA] told me to give rice solution or porridge for my baby after three months so that the child would have strong bones. (A woman, aged 34)

In Quang Xuong district, Women Union – a community-based organisation which supports to enhance the role of women in the society – was very active and had its network in each village. Women Union activists worked closely with CHCs to outreach mothers for health education including breastfeeding. Unfortunately, they did not possess sufficient knowledge and skills on breastfeeding counselling.

> Women Union was very active in health education to the community. However, they do not know how to do it properly. At our monthly meeting, we sometimes teach them how to talk to women about breastfeeding. But they still insist doing it in their own way [traditional practices] rather than following our advice. (A commune doctor, aged 38)

20.3.3.6 Socio-economic Factors

Poverty is another significant determinant of breastfeeding. Logistic regression analysis indicated possible association between the family income and feeding solid food (OR=1.47). It was also found that when a family had sufficient food during the year, it is likely for the baby to be exclusively breast-fed (OR=4.16). Nevertheless, in the qualitative component, some women expressed their wish to have formula but were unable to purchase such products due to financial constraints, as a package of formula could cost 10 percent of the family's monthly income.

> Since the baby was born, we bought only three packages of 'Dielac' [a locally produced formula]. We could not afford more, as the milk was so expensive. (A mother, aged 28)

For low breastfeeding rate, it is often generally blamed milk's industry to put pressure on women to use formula through commercial campaigns. However, even long time before milk products are wildly introduced in a rural area such Quang Xuong district, solid and semi-solid foods (mainly made from rice) had been already given to infants in a very early period of their life. Local people have strong beliefs on nutritious value of rice. Rice helped to grow generations of Vietnamese for thousands years and it could help to grow infants in both physical and spiritual aspects. In other words, premature introduction of complementary foods to infants had been culturally rooted phenomenon.

20.3.3.7 Influence of Commercial Advertisement

The use of formula and/or cow milk for infants increased from 6.4 percent at week 1 to 13.7 percent at week 24. Most of the women in the study were exposed to commercial advertisement of formula through the mass media (98 percent). Commercial advertisement of formula often portrayed an urban wealthy couple with a healthy and clever baby, and that formula could provide the super nutrients for proper infant development that really influenced women's perception and practice of breastfeeding.

By February 2006, Ministry of Health issued Decree 25 that does not allow advertising formula for children under 12 months old. Nevertheless, this decree is not efficiently reinforced in practice and the milk's companies always find a way to deliver biased messages of over-positive outcomes of formula to clients. For instance, by regulation, representatives of milk's companies are not allowed to meet health workers or mothers at health care settings, they still regularly contact them. Existence of formula's advertisement and logos in obstetric and pediatric care facilities are a clear example of this practice. Logo of formulas is also labeled in the furniture, toys and other equipment in kindergartens and facilities for children. In addition, although selling formula in health care settings is not allowed by Ministry of Health, different types of formula are still available in canteens of pediatric and obstetric facilities. Even biased advertisement on positive outcomes of formula is also seen in the cover of medical handbooks for mothers and infants issued by hospitals.

A common marketing approach of milk's companies is inviting mothers to attend seminars that advertise formula. Well-known health professionals are invited to convince mothers to use formula for their children. Free samples of substitutes are often provided for mothers to encourage their future use for their babies. Marketing efforts of formula's industries actually have a profound impact to mothers on their feeding practice to their infants.

20.4 Conclusion

Although the rates of breastfeeding initiation and exclusive breastfeeding were high at week 1, the rate of exclusive breastfeeding sharply decreased at week 16 and week 24. On the other hand, complementary food was commonly used to feed infants at a very early stage. This trend is consistent with findings of other research in Vietnam and elsewhere (Bronner et al. 1999; Sellen 2001; Committee for Population Family and Children 2003). However, the exclusive breastfeeding rates estimated in my study were higher than those of other studies in the same year. The 2002 Demographic and Health Survey found that only 31 percent of infants less than 2 months of age were exclusively breastfed. The rate declined rapidly to 12.1 percent when infants were 2–3 months of age, and 7.7 percent when they became 4–5 months of age. Another national nutrition survey in 2002 based on a sample of 1,500 children from 30 communes reported the proportion of infants less than 4 months of age exclusively breastfed accounted for 29.2 percent (National Institute of Nutrition & UNICEF 2003). It is noted that while the disparities in health indicators among geo-ecological regions of Vietnam were relatively large, the 2002 Demographic and Health Survey used a very small sample when calculating the national exclusive breastfeeding rate. This longitudinal study, on the other hand, utilised a cohort sample representative of the rural North Central region of Vietnam to estimate the rates. The interviews conducted at regular intervals had allowed us to measure changes in infant feeding with reasonable accuracy.

This study found women's education could positively influence breastfeeding patterns, unlike previous studies (Nath & Goswami 1997; Abada, Trovato, & Lalu 2001). It may be argued that the decline of the initiation and duration of breastfeeding is an inevitable consequence of modernisation (see also Chapters 9, 15, 16 and 21 in this volume). Higher education is associated with the adoption of modern ideas often leading to the abandonment of traditional practice including breastfeeding (Abada et al. 2001).

In rural Vietnam, women contribute a major part of the family labour force. In Quang Xuong district, by week 16, nearly all mothers had already returned to normal work while still taking care of their infants. Pressure of workload at the early postpartum stage is likely to prevent mothers from practising exclusive breastfeeding. Feeding infants with complementary food, especially with solid food, gave mothers more time to earn living for the family. Studies in developing countries also showed an inverse relationship between employment and breastfeeding (Bamisaiye & Oyediran 1983; Launer 1993; Lakati, Binns, & Stevenson 2002; see Chapters 7 and 8 in this volume).

Poverty is an important factor to encourage breastfeeding amongst rural women (Morrow 1996). Although financial constraints may prevent women from buying formula, infants are likely to be fed with home cooked food at the early stage. Despite the economic reforms that have taken place in recent years, most women in rural Vietnam are not covered by any social insurance schemes and do not have maternal leave. The pressure to earn a living to support the family makes exclusive breastfeeding difficult in practice (cf Chapter 8 in this volume).

Evidence also suggested that whenever a woman did not live in an extended family where workload was often shared with other family members, it was likely for her infants to be fed with solid food. Within a historically Confucian culture, the breastfeeding practice of rural Vietnamese women is expected to be influenced by husband and senior members of the family. Although 80 percent of participants reported they could make the decision themselves on breastfeeding practice, we still found that husband and maternal mother could substantially influence their decision on this issue, as the breastfeeding practices of friends. This finding is consistent with the literature that attitudes of spouse (Scott et al. 2001), parents (Sharps, El-Mohandes, Nabil El-Khorazaty, Kiely, & Walker 2003) and relatives (Kendall-Tackett & Sugarman 1995) play an important role in determining the initiation and duration of breastfeeding (see Chapter 3 in this volume).

Media is pervasive and powerful and has the potential to affect social norms about breastfeeding and decision-making (Bentley, Dee, & Jensen 2003: see also Chapter 3 in this volume). This study found that 98 percent of the respondents were exposed to formula commercials via the mass media. Of the mothers who used formula for their babies, about 53 percent decided to buy a particular brand after seeing the commercial advertisement, and 27 percent followed the bottle-feeding experiences of others, despite considerable efforts have been spent in providing a supporting environment for breastfeeding at health settings. The Ministry of Health of Vietnam issued a national regulation on the marketing of breast milk substitutes in 1994 in which advertisements of formula directly targeting infants under 6 months of age are not allowed in any of the mass media. However, the marketing advertisement most often seen in Vietnamese television portrays a small baby together with a 'miracle' formula and the nature of the message indirectly encourages mothers to use formula for young infants.

Health providers had a considerable impact on breastfeeding practices. Women who delivered at home with a traditional birth attendant were less likely to receive appropriate instruction on breastfeeding. Although breastfeeding is recommended to commence immediately after birth (American Academy of Pediatrics 1997; Kramer & Kakuma 2002), the initiation rate of breastfeeding within the first hour by this group was only 24.6 percent, compared to 73.6 percent and 85 percent, respectively, for babies delivered at district hospital and commune health centre.

To maintain exclusive breastfeeding practice, women seemed to need further motivation from health providers. However, health providers generally lacked the necessary knowledge and skills for practical counselling. Similar results were reported in other countries (Adair et al. 1993; Lazzaro, Anderson, & Auld 1995; Dillaway & Douma 2004). Studies indicated that lack of administrative support and supervision of health worker's performance could cause the failure of a breastfeeding programme (Stokamer 1990).

In conclusion, this study examined factors influencing breastfeeding patterns in rural Vietnam. To improve the breastfeeding situation, the implementation of national guidelines on breastfeeding should be further reinforced by providing appropriate training and supportive supervision to health workers. There is also a need for effective programmes to support the working mothers to exclusively breastfeed their infants through the community mobilisation. Health education on breastfeeding should target at both mother and father taking into account local socio-cultural features.

References

Abada, T. S., Trovato, F., & Lalu, N. (2001). Determinants of breastfeeding in the Philippines: A survival analysis. *Social Science and Medicine, 52*(1), 71–81.

Adair, L. S., Popkin, B. M., & Guilkey, D. K. (1993). The duration of breast-feeding: How is it affected by biological, sociodemographic, health sector, and food industry factors? *Demography, 30*(1), 63–80.

American Academy of Pediatrics (1997). *Breastfeeding and the use of human milk. American Academy of Pediatrics*. Work Group on Breastfeeding. *Pediatrics, 100*(6), 1035–1039.

Bamisaiye, A., & Oyediran, M. (1983). Breastfeeding among female employees at a major health institution in Lagos, Nigeria. *Social Science and Medicine, 17*(23), 1867–1871.

Bentley, M. E., Dee, D. L., & Jensen, J. L. (2003). Breastfeeding among low income, African-American women: Power, beliefs and decision making. *Journal of Nutriton, 133*(1), 305S–309S.

Bronner, Y. L., Gross, S. M., Caulfield, L., Bentley, M. E., Kessler, Jensen, J., et al. (1999). Early introduction of solid foods among urban African-American participants in WIC. *Journal of the American Dietetic Association, 99*(4), 457–461.

Bulk-Bunschoten, A. M., van Bodegom, S., Reerink, J. D., Pasker-de Jong, P. C., & de Groot, C. J. (2001). Reluctance to continue breastfeeding in The Netherlands. *Acta Paediatrica, 90*(9), 1047–1053.

Committee for Population Family and Children (2003). *Demographic and health survey 2002.* Hanoi: Committee for Population Family and Children.

Dearden, K. A., Quan Le, N., Do, M., Marsh, D. R., Pachon, H., Schroeder, D. G., et al. (2002). Work outside the home is the primary barrier to exclusive breastfeeding in rural Viet Nam: Insights from mothers who exclusively breastfed and worked. *Food and Nutrition Bulletin, 23*(4), 101–108.

DiGirolamo, A. M., Grummer-Strawn, L. M., & Fein, S. B. (2003). Do perceived attitudes of physicians and hospital staff affect breastfeeding decisions? *Birth, 30*(2), 94–100.

Dillaway, H. E., & Douma, M. (2004). Are pediatric offices ′supportive′ of breastfeeding? Discrepancies between mothers′ and health care professionals′ reports. *Clinical Pediatrics, 43*(5), 417–430.

Doyle, N. (2001). Key family practices: Building better child-care-interventions. Hanoi: Ministry of Health.

Ighogboja, S. I. (1992). Some factors contributing to protein-energy malnutrition in the middle belt of Nigeria. *East African Medical Journal, 69*(10), 566–571.

Kendall-Tackett, K. A., & Sugarman, M. (1995). The social consequences of long-term breastfeeding. *Journal of Human Lactation, 11*(3), 179–183.

Kramer, M., & Kakuma, R. (2002). The optimal duration of exclusive breastfeeding – A systematic review. Geneva: World Health Organization.

Lakati, A., Binns, C., & Stevenson, M. (2002). The effect of work status on exclusive breastfeeding in Nairobi. *Asia Pacific Journal of Public Health, 14*(2), 85–90.

Launer, L. J. (1993). The work patterns of lactating women in Madura. *Social Science and Medicine, 37*(4), 555–563.

Lazzaro, E., Anderson, J., & Auld, G. (1995). Medical professionals′ attitudes toward breastfeeding. *Journal of Human Lactation, 11*(2), 97–101.

Madzingira, N. (1995). Malnutrition in children under five in Zimbabwe: Effect of socioeconomic factors and disease. *Social Biology, 42*(3–4), 239–246.

McCarter-Spaulding, D. E., & Kearney, M. H. (2001). Parenting self-efficacy and perception of insufficient breast milk. *Journal of Obstetrics, Gynecologic, and Neonatal Nursing, 30*(5), 515–522.

Ministry of Health of Vietnam (2001). *Key family practices of mothers of children under 5 years old in nine target districts*. Hanoi: Ministry of Health of Vietnam.

Moffat, T. (2002). Breastfeeding, wage labor, and insufficient milk in peri-urban Kathmandu, Nepal. *Medical Anthropology, 21*(2), 207–230.

Morrow, M. (1996). Breastfeeding in Vietnam: Poverty, tradition, and economic transition. *Journal of Human Lactation, 12*(2), 97–103.

Nath, D. C., & Goswami, G. (1997). Determinants of breast-feeding patterns in an urban society of India. *Human Biology, 69*(4), 557–573.

National Institute of Nutrition & UNICEF (2003). *Vietnam 2000–2002: A review of the nutrition situation*. Hanoi: National Institute of Nutrition & UNICEF.

NHMRC (1999). *National statement on ethical conduct in research involving humans*. Canberra: NHMRC.

Quang Xuong District Health Service (2000). *Quang Xuong District health report, March 2000.* Thanh Hoa, Vietnam.

Scott, J. A. (1997). *Determinants of the initiation and duration of breastfeeding*. Perth: Curtin Univeristy of Technology.

Scott, J. A., Landers, M. C., Hughes, R. M., & Binns, C. W. (2001). Factors associated with breastfeeding at discharge and duration of breastfeeding. *Journal of Paediatrics and Child Health, 37*(3), 254–261.

Sellen, D. W. (2001). Comparison of infant feeding patterns reported for nonindustrial populations with current recommendations. *Journal of Nutriton, 131*(10), 2707–2715.

Sharps, P. W., El-Mohandes, A. A., Nabil El-Khorazaty, M., Kiely, M., & Walker, T. (2003). Health beliefs and parenting attitudes influence breastfeeding patterns among low-income African-American women. *Journal of Perinatology, 23*(5), 414–419.

Stokamer, C. L. (1990). Breastfeeding promotion efforts: Why some do not work. *Internatinal Journal of Gynaecology and Obstetrics, 31*(Suppl 1), 61–65; discussion 67–68.

World Health Organization (1996). *WHO global data bank on breastfeeding*. Geneva: World Health Organization.

World Health Organization (1998). *Evidence for the ten steps to successful breastfeeding*. Geneva: World Health Organization.

World Health Organization (2001). *The optimal duration of exclusive breastfeeding*. Report of an expert consultation. Geneva: World Health Organization.

World Health Organization (2003). *Global strategy for infant and young child feeding*. Geneva: World Health Organization.

World Medical Assembly (WMA) (1996). *Declaration of Helsinki*, Adopted by the 18th World Medical Assembly, Helsinki, Finland, June 1964, and amended by the 29th World Medical Assembly, Tokyo, Japan, October 1975, the 35th World Medical Assembly, Venice, Italy, October 1983, the 41st World Medical Assembly, Hong Kong, September 1989 and the 48th General Assembly, Somerset West, Republic of South Africa, October 1996.

Chapter 21
Infant Feeding Following Migration: Attitudes and Practices of Women Born in Turkey and Vietnam After Migration to Australia

Helen L. McLachlan and Della A. Forster

Contents

21.1 Introduction

Migration is increasing throughout the world and large numbers of women give birth in a country in which they were not born. In Victoria, Australia, approximately 17 percent of all women giving birth, are born in non-English-speaking countries, and an unknown proportion of Australian-born women, possibly an equivalent number, are of non-English-speaking background (Consultative Council on Obstetric and Paediatric Mortality and Morbidity 2008). Women born in Asia and the Middle East contributed to 10.5 percent and 2.2 percent, respectively, of all births in Victoria in

H.L. McLachlan (✉)
Division of Nursing and Midwifery and Mother and Child Health Research, La Trobe University, Bundoora, Victoria, Australia 3086
e-mail: h.mclachlan@latrobe.edu.au

P. Liamputtong (ed.), *Infant Feeding Practices*, DOI 10.1007/978-1-4419-6873-9_21,

© Springer Science+Business Media, LLC 2011

2006, with women born in Vietnam comprising the highest proportion (Consultative Council on Obstetric and Paediatric Mortality and Morbidity 2008).

The World Health Organization (2001) recommends that all infants should be exclusively breastfed from birth to 6 months of age followed by continued breastfeeding and the gradual introduction of solids. Despite this recommendation, there is marked variation in breastfeeding rates in different countries (UNICEF 2009), and in Australia, many women do not breastfeed for the recommended period of time (Amir & Donath 2008). For some cultural groups, migration to a new country is associated with a reduction in both initiation and duration of breastfeeding (Manderson & Mathews 1981; Henderson & Brown 1987; Nguyen et al. 2004; Rossiter 1992a; Yelland, Small, Lumley, Liamputtong Rice, Contronei, et al. 1998; Golin, Marzarib, & Zanardo 2003; Yelland, Small, Krastev, et al. 2003; Gibson-Davis & Brooks-Gunn 2006).

In this chapter, we will briefly discuss breastfeeding practices in Australia, Turkey and Vietnam, and then report on a study which explored the initial infant feeding attitudes and practices of the three groups of women from these countries who gave birth in Victoria, Australia: a group of women born in Vietnam, a group born in Turkey and a third group born in Australia.

In Australia, most women commence breastfeeding, with initiation rates of around 88 percent, although by 6 months less than 50 percent of infants are receiving any breast milk, with women from lower socio-economic groups less likely to breastfeed than those from higher socioeconomic groups (Amir & Donath 2008). This is similar to other countries; a 2005 systematic review of interventions to increase breastfeeding found that 'in all countries breastfeeding initiation rates are closely related to social class, income and education levels' (Dyson, McCormick, & Renfrew 2005). The Australian breastfeeding figures have not changed in the past 20 years despite many strategies to increase breastfeeding, and the pattern prior to this was similar to many developed countries – that the proportion of women breastfeeding declined steadily from the early 1940s (Wiles 1984; Jones, West, & Newcombe 1986) with that trend not reversing until the 1970s, and possibly later in the United States (Piper & Parks 1996).

Traditionally, in Turkey almost all women breastfeed (Neyzi et al. 1991; Alikasifoglu et al. 2001; Hizel, Ceyhun, Tanzer, & Sanli 2006; Camurdan et al. 2008; Karacam 2008; Yesildal et al. 2008) and in traditional Turkish society, breast milk is considered 'holy' (Hizel et al. 2006). According to the WHO Global Bank on Breastfeeding and Complementary feeding, 96 percent of women in Turkey commence breastfeeding (World Health Organization 2009) and the Quran encourages women to breastfeed their children for 2 years (Gatrad 1994; Ali 1975). Turkey continues to have strong traditional beliefs in relation to breastfeeding practices – in terms of both the benefits and the harms of breast milk (Hizel et al. 2006). A large cross-sectional study exploring traditional breastfeeding beliefs in Turkey reported that one third of participants believed the evil eye could harm the mother's breast milk, and thirty one percent of women reported that some mothers' milk can be harmful to babies (Hizel et al. 2006). See also Chapter 18 in this volume.

Despite the widespread support for breastfeeding and the high rates of breastfeeding initiation in Turkey, rates of exclusive breastfeeding are low and early introduction of solids is common (Hizel et al. 2006; Camurdan et al. 2008; Karacam 2008; Yesildal et al. 2008). Reported reasons for this include maternal employment (Yilmaz, Gurakan, Akgun, & Ozbek 2002; Camurdan et al. 2008); women's perception that they do not have enough milk (Camurdan et al. 2008; Yesildal et al. 2008) and formula supplementation in hospital (Alikasifoglu et al. 2001). Differences in duration of breastfeeding by gender have been reported with male infants fed longer than female infants (Yesildal et al. 2008).

Little is known about breastfeeding initiation and attitudes of Turkish women to infant feeding following migration to a new country. One Australian study reported high initiation rates (97 percent), but that two thirds of these women had stopped breastfeeding by 2 months (Yelland, Small, Lumley, & Liamputtong Rice 1997). A study conducted in Sweden found that Turkish women were less likely to breastfeed following migration with early weaning common and a change in traditional attitudes to breastfeeding (Kocturck & Zetterstrom 1986).

In Vietnam, most women breastfeed. The 2002 Vietnam Demographic Health Survey reported that 98 percent of women breastfed their baby (Committee for Population Family and Children 2003). Exclusive breastfeeding is less common, however, with rates around 21 percent at 4–6 months (UNICEF). Many infants are fed sugar water or sweetened condensed milk during the first days of life (Morrow 1996; Almroth, Arts, Quang, Hoa, & Williams 2008; see Chapter 20). Reasons for low rates of exclusive breastfeeding in Vietnam include poor knowledge of the benefits of exclusive breastfeeding by health professionals (Almroth et al. 2008); the influence of family members and friends, i.e. suggesting that breast milk alone is insufficient and that substitutes added value (Almroth et al. 2008; Duong, Binns, & Lee 2004; Duong, Lee, & Binns 2005); lower levels of education (Liubai, Doan Thi Phuong, Nguyen-Thi, & Hiroshi 2002; Duong et al. 2005); maternal employment (Duong et al. 2005) and the introduction of formula in hospital (Liubai et al. 2002). See also Chapter 20 in this volume.

Despite the high rates of breastfeeding initiation in Vietnam, a number of studies have reported that women born in Vietnam who have migrated to a new country have lower breastfeeding rates following migration (Mathews & Manderson 1980; Henderson & Brown 1987; Fishman, Evans, & Jenks 1988; Rossiter 1992a, b; Rossiter, Ledwidge, & Coulon 1993; Tuttle & Dewey 1994; Yelland et al. 1998; Rossiter & Yam 2000; Yelland et al. 2003).

Attitudes and practices towards feeding colostrum (the early breast milk produced in the first few days after the birth) to newborn babies differ by cultural group. Despite the unequivocal benefits of colostrum, the practice of withholding it from the newborn is widespread and variation exists between countries regarding length of time and reasons for withholding it (Morse, Jehle, & Gamble 1990; Liamputtong Rice 2000; Liamputtong 2007). We could not identify any studies that reported Australian *not* feeding colostrum to their babies. However, in Turkey approximately one third of women report that colostrum should not be fed to their babies (Hizel et al. 2006), and in Vietnam, colostrum is often discarded (Mathews & Manderson 1980; Rossiter 1992a).

Given the importance of exclusive breastfeeding from birth, and the fact that women who migrate might have altered infant feeding practices, we wanted to explore infant feeding among two of the most prevalent migrant groups giving birth in our community. We, therefore, conducted a study describing and comparing the early breastfeeding practices of Australian, Turkish and Vietnamese women giving birth in Australia, and exploring cultural differences in the groups' attitudes to breastfeeding. These three groups of women were selected for the study because of differences in cultural background and because women from Turkey and Vietnam are large minorities in the population of women giving birth at The Royal Women's Hospital (RWH) in Melbourne, where the study was conducted. The hospital is a tertiary hospital with approximately 6500 births per year.

21.2 The Study

Three hundred women who had given birth at the RWH were included in the study: 100 Turkish-born, 100 Vietnamese-born and 100 Australian-born. To be eligible, Australian women had to have an English-speaking background, defined as at least one parent born in Australia. Only women who had a normal vaginal birth without any major medical problems (such as severe pre-eclampsia/eclampsia, severe postpartum haemhorrhage, severe psychiatric disturbance, pulmonary embolus), who had given birth to a healthy baby (not admitted to neonatal nursery) and were booked as public patients, were eligible for inclusion into the study.

All Turkish, Vietnamese and Australian women who gave birth at the RWH during the recruitment period were identified by a confidential, computer-generated report which identified country of birth. Women were then approached while they were in hospital after the birth, the study explained, and then if they agreed to participate they signed a consent form and an interview time was arranged. If the woman did not speak English, hospital interpreters or sometimes relatives explained the study, gained consent and arranged an interview time. We aimed to approach all eligible Turkish-born and Vietnamese-born women. In order to be sure that Australian women were recruited at a similar rate and over the same time period as the other women in the study, for each Turkish woman recruited to the study, the following Australian woman who gave birth and who met the eligibility criteria were approached and offered participation.

Women were interviewed in hospital, between 24 hours after the birth and discharge from hospital which was on average three days for primiparas and two days for multiparas. The interviews were conducted in a quiet place on the postnatal ward of the hospital. Vietnamese- and Turkish-speaking women were interviewed by Vietnamese and Turkish bilingual research assistants, respectively, and the first author conducted interviews with Australian women and with Vietnamese and Turkish women who were fluent in English.

The questionnaire was developed specifically for the study. There were detailed questions on women's birth experiences (McLachlan & Forster 2006); socio-demographic data were collected; and questions were asked regarding women's breastfeeding intentions, attitude towards colostrum, current method of feeding, timing of first feed and breastfeeding problems during the first days after birth. Women were also asked about their partners' attitude towards infant feeding. The definitions used in this chapter include 'breast milk only', that is, breast milk is the only nutritional intake, either at the breast or expressed; 'any breast milk' that is, a combination of breast milk and formula or 'formula', that is, formula only.

The questionnaire was first developed in English and then translated into Turkish and Vietnamese by professionally trained and qualified translators who were accredited by the National Accreditation Authority for Translators and Interpreters. Questionnaires were then translated back into English by a different qualified translator who had no knowledge of the original version, known as 'blind back translation' (McDermott & Palchanes 1994; Small, Yelland, Lumley, & Liamputtong Rice 1999a, Small, Yelland, Lumley, Liamputtong Rice, Cotronei et al. 1999b). Using this method, the original questionnaire could be compared to the back translated version. The back translation was reviewed by the first author and discussed with three qualified Turkish and Vietnamese interpreters. Discussion centred on the accuracy, meaning, clarity and appropriateness of the questions. Only one question pertaining to breastfeeding posed any issues in translation. There was some discussion related to the translation to Vietnamese regarding 'problems attaching the baby to the breast', which was translated incorrectly to 'my child always wants to suckle'. This was translated and back translated a second time and was discussed with three qualified interpreters with a final back translation 'The baby has difficulty grabbing hold of the nipple with its mouth'. Original translations were accurate on the whole with few modifications made to the final translation.

The Victorian Perinatal Data Collection Unit (PDCU) provided data on all Turkish, Vietnamese and Australian women who gave birth in Victoria during the study period to assess the representativeness of the study sample. Ethical approval for the study was obtained from the Royal Women's Hospital and La Trobe University Human Research Ethics Committees.

The data were first described using descriptive statistics, then comparisons between the groups were conducted using the chi square statistic to test the independence between categorical variables. T-tests were used to compare means of continuous variables. Logistic regression was used to explore the association between country of birth and breastfeeding outcomes and to adjust for the effect of demographic and obstetric variables. The univariate association between each of the independent variables and the breastfeeding outcomes at the time of interview (i.e. feeding 'breast milk only' and 'any breast milk') was tested and only those that had a p value of <0.2 were included in the regression model with each outcome variable. Factors explored at the univariate level were number of years since migration to Australia (Vietnamese and Turkish women only), ability to understand spoken English, secondary education, higher education, parity, age, episiotomy, smoking, induction of labour, pharmacological pain relief and country of birth. Statistical analysis was undertaken using SPSS for Windows (SPSS Statistical Packages for the Social Sciences 1998) and STATA (Stata Corporation 2003).

21.3 Findings

21.3.1 Participants: Background Characteristics

During the recruitment period (January 1998–May 1999), 289 Turkish, 274 Vietnamese and 4281 Australian women gave birth as public patients at the RWH, and of these 110 Turkish and 102 Vietnamese women met the study inclusion criteria and were invited to participate. Ten Turkish, two Vietnamese and no Australian women declined participation in the study.

The Turkish and Vietnamese women in the study were of approximately the same average age as other women born in these countries who gave birth in Victoria during the recruitment period (Turkish women: 27.7 vs. 27.8 years; Vietnamese women: 29.9 vs. 29.3 years). The proportion of married women was also similar (Turkish women: 99 percent vs. 95 percent; Vietnamese women: 82 percent vs. 81 percent) (Victorian Perinatal Data Collection Unit 2000). Australian women in our sample were on average younger (27.9 vs. 29.1 years) and significantly less likely to be married (45 percent vs. 74 percent) compared with the population of Australian women who gave birth in Victoria during the study period (Victorian Perinatal Data Collection Unit 2000).

Table 21.1 shows that compared with the Australian group, Turkish women were more likely to be Muslim, multiparous, married, less educated, on a lower family income, and less likely to smoke. Vietnamese women were more likely to be Buddhist, married, older and on a lower family income compared with Australian women. Greater variation was observed regarding Vietnamese women's educational background not only with a larger proportion having completed secondary school than Australian women but also a larger proportion having only limited education. Vietnamese women were less likely to smoke prior to becoming pregnant. Vietnamese women migrated to Australia more often as a refugee or for family reunion compared with Turkish women who migrated for marriage or a better quality of life. The two migrant groups also differed in religious background, with the majority of Turkish women being Muslim, and Vietnamese women Buddhist. Turkish women were more likely than Vietnamese women to speak English. All the women in the study had a normal birth at term. The groups were similar in obstetric outcomes including augmentation and length of labour. However, Vietnamese women were less likely to be induced (12 percent) compared with Australian (27 percent) and Turkish women (25 percent), and were more likely to have an episiotomy (29 percent) compared with Australian and Turkish women (16 percent and 18 percent respectively). Vietnamese women also had less pharmacological and non-pharmacological pain relief (McLachlan & Waldenstrom 2005).

Table 21.1 Background characteristics of study participants

Characteristics	Australian-born women (*n*=100)[a] *n* (percent)[b]	Turkish-born women (*n*=100)[a] *n* (percent)[b]	Vietnamese-born women (*n*=100)[a] *n* (percent)[b]
Marital status			
Married	45	99	82
De facto	47	0	11
Single/divorced/separated	8	1	7
Age, mean (sd)	27.9 (6.17)	27.7 (5.11)	29.9 (6.09)
Education			
Secondary school to final year	38	32	54
Secondary school but not completed	62	36	26
Primary school only	0	31	18
Did not attend school	0	1	2
Further studies			
Degree/diploma	9	9	14
Apprenticeship/traineeship	23	6	25
None	68	85	61
Total family income per year (AUD)[c]	(*n*=90)	(*n*=63)	(*n*=43)
$20,000 or less	25 (27.8)	27 (42.9)	18 (41.9)
$20,000–$30,000	22 (24.4)	16 (25.4)	8 (19.6)
$30,000–$40,000	13 (14.4)	7(11.1)	7 (16.3)
More than $40,000	30 (33.3)	13 (21.6)	10 (23.3)
Language of interview English	100	38	27
Ability to understand spoken English		(n=92)	(n=92)
Very well		25 (27.2)	9 (9.8)
Fairly well		14 (15.2)	18 (19.6)
Not very well		47 (51.0)	48 (52.2)
Does not speak English		6 (6.5)	17 (18.5)
Religion			(*n*=98)
Christian	53	0	22 (22.4)
Muslim	2	98	1 (1)
Buddhist	0	0	60 (61.2)
No religion	43	2	14 (14.3)
Other	2	0	1 (1)
Reason for migration			
Refugee		3	35
Family reunion		9	40
Marriage		59	23
Economic/quality of life		29	2
Years in Australia, mean (sd)		12.5 (9.4)	9.0 (5.3)
Smoked prior to pregnancy	51	30	2
Primiparas	41	30	41

[a]n = 100 in each group unless otherwise stated
[b]Percentages only reported when *n* not equal to 100
[c]AUD—Australian dollars

21.3.2 Breastfeeding Initiation

Seventy-five percent of the Vietnamese women initiated breastfeeding, compared with 84 percent of Australian women and 98 percent of Turkish women (see Table 21.2). In the following sections, we compare breastfeeding outcomes and attitudes between Vietnamese-born and Australian-born women then Turkish-born and Australian-born women.

21.3.3 Comparing Vietnamese and Australian Women

Significantly fewer Vietnamese women (60 percent) were exclusively breastfeeding during the first days after birth compared with Australian women 81 percent (see Table 21.2). There was no statistical difference in the number of women who fed any breast milk at the univariate level (Vietnamese 75 percent, Australian 84 percent). However, the difference became statistically significant after adjusting for confounders that had been significant at the univariate level, that is, secondary education and ability to understand spoken English (Table 21.2). Forty percent of Vietnamese women fed their baby formula in hospital compared with 19 percent of Australian women.

Compared with Australian women, the Vietnamese women were less likely to have planned to breastfeed (90 percent vs 79 percent) and did not value the health benefits of colostrum to the same extent (Table 21.3). There were no differences between Vietnamese and Australian women in their perception of their partner's infant feeding preference. Of those Australian and Vietnamese women who were breastfeeding, there were no differences in the proportion of women who reported having a 'great' or 'good deal' of trouble breastfeeding (14 percent and 8 percent respectively). However, of those women reporting having difficulty feeding, the reasons given for the breastfeeding problems varied, with Australian women being more likely to cite difficulties with attachment (83 percent) compared with the Vietnamese women (31 percent). Vietnamese women more often described sore nipples as their main problem (63 percent) compared with Australian women (17 percent) (see Table 21.3).

21.3.4 Comparing Turkish and Australian Women

Almost all Turkish women breastfed their baby (98 percent) compared with 84 percent of Australian women, and they were more likely to exclusively breastfed in the first days of life (92 percent Vs 81 percent) (see Table 21.2). Women born in Turkey were more likely to perceive that their partners wanted them to breastfeed (83 percent) compared with Australian women (64 percent) (see Table 21.4). The majority of Turkish women considered colostrum to be healthier for the baby than breast milk (60 percent), which was similar to the views of the Australian women (55 percent).

Table 21.2 Method of feeding in hospital

Outcomes	Australian-born women (n=100)	Turkish-born women (n=100)	Vietnamese-born women (n=100)	Unadjusted odds ratio (95 percent CI)	p^a	Adjusted odds ratio (95 percent CI)	p^a
Breast milk only							
Turkish c/w Australian	81	92	–	2.70 (1.05, 7.14)	0.04	2.90 (1.2, 7.03)	0.02
Vietnamese c/w Australian	81	–	60	0.35 (0.18, 0.70)	0.002	0.29 (0.15, 0.56)	<0.001
Secondary education completed	38	32	54	1.74 (0.97, 3.09)	0.06	2.71 (1.43, 5.14)	0.002
No/poor English	0	53	65	0.51 (0.29, 0.88)	0.02	ns	
Any breast milk[b]							
Turkish c/w Australian	84	98	–	9.33 (2.08,85.25)	0.001[c]	10.12 (2.25,45.5)	0.003
Vietnamese c/w Australian	84	–	75	0.57 (0.27,1.21)	0.16	0.47 (0.23, 0.98)	0.04
Secondary education completed	38	32	54	1.20 (0.98, 4.10)	0.06	2.93 (1.38, 6.22)	0.005
Formula only							
Turkish c/w Australian	16	2	–	0.11 (0.01,0.48)	0.001[c]	n/a	
Vietnamese c/w Australian	16	–	25	1.75 (0.82,3.74)	0.16	n/a	

Adjusted for country of birth, secondary education, ability to understand spoken English
ns: not significant in final model
n/a: not presented as is opposite to 'any' breast milk calculations
c/w: compared with
[a]Australian women reference group
[b]Combination of breast milk and formula
[c]Exact confidence limits reported

Table 21.3 Breastfeeding attitudes, intentions and problems: Vietnamese-born women compared with Australian-born women

Breastfeeding attitudes, intentions and problems	Australian-born women *n* (percent)[c]	Vietnamese-born women *n* (percent)[b]	Odds ratio (95 percent CI)	p^a
Planned to breastfeed	(*n*=100)	(*n*=100)		
	90	79	0.42 (0.17, 1.00)	0.05
Breastfeeding preferred by partner	(*n*=95)	(*n*=85)		
(women's perceptions)	61 (64.2)	62 (73.0)	1.50 (0.76, 2.98)	0.27
If breastfeeding, attitude towards colostrum compared with milk produced later	(*n*=84)	(*n*=75)		
More healthy for baby	46 (54.8)	19 (25.7)	0.28 (0.13, 0.58)	<0.001
Equally healthy	20 (23.8)	48 (64.9)	5.69 (2.71, 12.06)	<0.001
Less healthy	0	1 (1.3)	c	
Not sure	18 (21.4)	7 (9.3)	0.38 (0.13, 1.04)	0.06
Breastfed within 1 h of birth	(n=93)	(n=68)		
	65 (69.9)	38 (55.9)	0.55 (0.27, 1.10)	0.10
Problems breastfeeding	(*n*=84)	(*n*=75)		
Great/good deal	12 (14.3)	6 (8.0)	0.52 (0.15, 1.61)	0.32
Moderate	17 (20.2)	10 (13.3)	0.61 (0.24, 1.53)	0.34
Very little/none	55 (65.5)	59 (78.7)	1.94 (0.90, 4.22)	0.09
Type of breastfeeding problems	(*n*=29)	(*n*=16)		
Attachment	24 (82.8)	5 (31.3)	0.09 (0.02, 0.48)	0.002
No/insufficient milk	1 (3.4)	3 (18.8)	c	
Baby unsettled	4 (13.8)	1 (6.3)	c	
Sore nipples	5 (17.2)	10 (62.5)	8.00 (1.65, 42.48)	0.006
Other	2 (6.9)	2 (12.5)	c	

[a]Australian women reference group
[b]Percentages only reported when *n* not equal to 100
[c]Numbers too small to undertake statistical test

Of the Turkish women who were breastfeeding, they were more likely to say they were having a 'good' or 'great deal' of trouble breastfeeding (33 percent) than women from Australia (14 percent). The reasons given for the breastfeeding problems also varied, with Australian women being more likely to cite difficulties with attachment (83 percent) compared with Turkish women (51 percent). Turkish women having breastfeeding problems more often described sore nipples as their main problem (77 percent) compared with Australian women (17 percent) (see Table 21.4).

21.3.5 Multivariate Analysis

Regression analysis was used to explore whether country of birth differences in breastfeeding in hospital remained significant after adjusting for other potentially

Table 21.4 Breastfeeding attitudes, intentions and problems: Turkish-born women compared with Australian-born women

Breastfeeding attitudes, intentions and problems	Australian-born women *n* (percent)[b]	Turkish-born women *n* (percent)[b]	Odds ratio (95 percent CI)	p[a]
Planned to breastfeed	(*n*=100) 90	(*n*=100) 93	1.48 (0.49, 4.52)	0.61
Breastfeeding preferred by partner (women's perceptions)	(*n*=95) 61 (64.2)	(*n*=99) 82 (82.8)	2.69 (1.31, 5.56)	0.005
If breastfeeding, attitude towards colostrum compared with milk produced later	(*n*=84)	(*n*=98)		
More healthy for baby	46 (54.8)	59 (60.2)	1.25 (0.66, 2.35)	0.55
Equally healthy	20 (23.8)	4 (4.0)	0.14 (0.03,44)	<0.001
Less healthy	0	3 (3.1)	c	
Not sure	18 (21.4)	32 (32.7)	1.78 (0.86, 3.68)	0.12
Breastfed within 1 h of birth	(*n*=93) 65 (69.9)	(*n*=98) 63 (64.3)	0.78 (0.40, 1.48)	0.50
Problems breastfeeding	(*n*=84)	(*n*=98)		
Great/good deal	12 (14.3)	32 (32.7)	2.91 (1.31, 6.55)	0.007
Moderate	17 (20.2)	19 (19.4)	0.95 (0.43, 2.09)	0.96
Very little/none	55 (65.5)	47 (48.0)	0.49 (0.25, 0.92)	0.03
Type of breastfeeding problems	(*n*=29)	(*n*=51)		
Attachment	24 (82.8)	26 (51.0)	0.22 (0.06, 0.72)	0.009
No/insufficient milk	1 (3.4)	9 (17.6)	c	
Baby unsettled	4 (13.8)	2 (3.9)	c	
Sore nipples	5 (17.2)	39 (76.5)	15.6 (4.39,61.55)	<0.001
Other	2 (6.9)	2 (3.9)	c	

[a]Australian women reference group
[b]Percentages only reported when *n* not equal to 100
[c]Numbers too small to undertake statistical test

confounding factors. Factors that were found to be not significantly associated with either any or exclusive breastfeeding at the univariate level were number of years since migration to Australia (Vietnamese and Turkish women only), higher education, parity, age, smoking status, induction of labour, pharmacological pain relief in labour and episiotomy. Secondary education was negatively associated with *any* and *exclusive* breastfeeding, and poor/no ability to understand spoken English was negatively associated with *exclusive* breastfeeding. These were entered in regression models with country of birth and each of the two breastfeeding outcomes (see Table 21.2).

Turkish women remained significantly more likely to give *any* breast milk (adjusted OR 10.12; 95 percent CI 2.25, 45.5) and to exclusively breastfeed (adjusted OR 2.90; 95 percent CI 1.2, 7.03) in hospital than Australian women.

Vietnamese women remained significantly less likely than Australian women to exclusively breastfeed their babies in hospital (adjusted OR 0.29; 95 percent CI 0.15,

0.56). After accounting for confounders, Vietnamese women were also significantly less likely to give any breast milk than Australian women (adjusted OR 0.47; 95 percent CI 0.23, 0.98).

For all women, completing secondary school was associated with an increased likelihood of giving *any* breast milk (adjusted OR 2.93; 95 percent CI 1.38, 6.22) and *exclusively* breastfeeding (adjusted OR 2.71; 95 percent CI 1.43, 5.14).

21.4 Discussion

Overall, Vietnamese women had the lowest breastfeeding initiation, which was consistent with their breastfeeding intentions. They did not value the health benefits of colostrum to the same extent as Australian women. Turkish women were more likely to commence breastfeeding and they were more likely to perceive that breastfeeding was preferred by their partners when compared with Australian women. Turkish women also reported more breastfeeding problems.

The variation in the proportion of women breastfeeding between cultural groups found in this study is consistent with many other studies. Australian women breastfed at a similar rate (84 percent) to that reported in the most recent Australian national data using the 2004–5 National Health Survey, which estimated that the proportion of children breastfed at discharge from hospital was 88 percent (Amir & Donath 2008).

21.4.1 Vietnamese Women

The results of this study add to the previously reported finding that immigrant Vietnamese women are less likely to initiate exclusive breastfeeding following migration to a new country (Mathews & Manderson 1980; Henderson & Brown 1987; Fishman et al. 1988; Rossiter 1992b; Tuttle & Dewey 1994; Yelland et al. 1998; Rossiter & Yam 2000; Yelland et al. 2003; Nguyen et al. 2004; Groleau, Soulière, & Kirmayer 2006; Mistry, Freedman, Sweeney, & Hollenbeck 2008). Reasons previously cited for low breastfeeding rates among immigrant women are convenience (Yoshida & Davies 1982; Fishman et al. 1988; Rossiter & Yam 2000); perceptions of impaired quality of milk (Fishman et al. 1988; Rossiter 1992b; Groleau et al. 2006); difficulties communicating with caregivers (Rossiter & Yam 2000); economic reasons such as the need to return to work (Rossiter 1992a; Rossiter & Yam 2000); a decrease in social support (Rossiter 1992a; Rossiter & Yam 2000); perceptions that more affluent families do not breastfeed their own babies (Rossiter 1992a); availability of infant formula (Mistry et al. 2008); and a desire to conform to the perceived cultural norm of the new country (Rossiter 1992b). A number of studies have reported that Vietnamese women will breastfeed for a shorter period of time if they have been unable to undertake traditional postpartum practices such as an eating an appropriate diet and receiving adequate rest, which is needed to restore maternal health after childbirth and to maximise the quality of breast milk (Fishman et al. 1988; Rossiter & Yam 2000; Groleau et al. 2006). In this study, reasons for breastfeeding outcomes were not explored in-depth and it is therefore, not possible to draw conclusions. See Chapter 20 for the case of rural Vietnamese women in Vietnam.

The beliefs of people from many Asian countries that colostrum is not as healthy for the baby does not seem to have been changed by the strong evidence of its benefits (Morse et al. 1990). Traditionally in Vietnam, the newborn is fed rice water or other liquid while the colostrum is expressed and discarded and the baby is then put to the breast around day three (Henderson & Brown 1987; Liamputtong Rice 1998, 2000). Perhaps the negative view of colostrum is one reason why breastfeeding Vietnamese women were more likely than Turkish or Australian women to give supplementary formula whilst in hospital. It is also possible that the lower rates of breastfeeding were only temporary because of cultural beliefs regarding colostrum, although other studies suggest that this is not likely to be the case, and that breastfeeding rates for Vietnamese women remain low after the first few days (Mathews & Manderson 1980; Fishman et al. 1988; Rossiter 1992b; Tuttle & Dewey 1994; Rossiter & Yam 2000; Nguyen et al. 2004; Groleau et al. 2006).

21.4.2 Turkish Women

Our finding that 98 percent of Turkish women breastfed in hospital is consistent with the finding by Yelland and colleagues (1998) that 97 percent of Turkish women who had migrated to Australia, initiated breastfeeding. Almost all Turkish women in this study were Muslim; in the Quran, mothers are encouraged to breastfeed for 2 years (Ali 1975). Despite reports of women from some migrant groups initiating breastfeeding less often following migration to a new country, this does not seem to be the case with Turkish women in this study. Studies of breastfeeding women in Turkey, however, have reported that women are ceasing breastfeeding earlier due to little support for breastfeeding in the workplace, a lack of maternity leave (Camurdan et al. 2008; Yilmaz et al. 2002) and formula supplementation in hospital (Alikasifoglu et al. 2001). We do not have data on the duration of breastfeeding so we do not know if these factors influenced the Turkish women in our study.

Women were asked whether or not they thought their partner wanted them to breastfeed. Women born in Turkey were more likely to state that their partner wanted them to breastfeed (83 percent) than Australian (64 percent) and Vietnamese women (73 percent). This is consistent with studies which have shown that social support from a partner, or the influence of family, friends or health professionals affect infant feeding methods and rates of breastfeeding (Nolan & Goel 1995; Taveras et al. 2003; Lande et al. 2003). However, it is possible that women's partners were also influenced about infant feeding methods in the same way as the women themselves and therefore shared the same views.

Of those women who commenced breastfeeding, Turkish women were significantly more likely to say that they had trouble breastfeeding. This may be related to

Turkish women acknowledging any difficulties they had and attempting to resolve them. There is a cultural expectation that Turkish women can and do breastfeed. (Alikasifoglu et al. 2001; Camurdan et al. 2008; Karacam 2008; Yesildal et al. 2008; see also Chapter 18 in this volume). It is also possible that Turkish women felt more able to express their difficulties. Another possibility is related to the level of breastfeeding support whilst in hospital. We suggest that midwives may offer less help to Turkish women either due to language difficulties or possibly because of a perception that Turkish women usually breastfeed successfully. Australian women may have received more help because they asked for it or because they were more likely to be offered help.

Australian women's breastfeeding problems were usually related to difficulties with attachment compared with Turkish women who more often reported sore nipples. Australian women may have been more aware that problems with attachment may lead to sore nipples. 'Attachment problems' is a relatively newly derived term for unsuccessful breastfeeding and it is a term used by midwives.

21.4.3 Care in Hospital

The majority of breastfeeding women in this study breastfed within one hour of the birth. This finding may be related to the fact that the hospital in which the study was conducted had been accredited as a Baby Friendly Hospital (BFHI), a joint World Health Organization (WHO) and United Nations Children's Fund (UNICEF) global initiative, which encourages the first breastfeed within half an hour of the birth (UNICEF) (see also Chapter 4 in this volume). However, despite the BFHI status of the hospital, there were marked differences between the groups in infant feeding during the first days after the birth, with 40 percent of Vietnamese women giving their baby formula. The hospital environment is a key area where care providers may be able to help make a difference to breastfeeding initiation, particularly for women of non-English-speaking background who are less likely to attend childbirth education classes (Hoang 2008).

A question that arises from our findings is how to deal with traditional cultural practices that do not encourage optimal health outcomes. In this study, the lower rate of breastfeeding may have health implications for Vietnamese mothers and babies. How health professionals tackle this issue is complex. Some cultural awareness and knowledge of the evidence of findings in studies such as this one may be essential to allow early interventions to occur. However, Vietnamese, Turkish and Australian women are not homogenous cultural groups and should not be stereotyped as such. They will be influenced by a range of social, personal and cultural circumstances that are not generalisable, and care providers need be sensitive and accepting of these differences.

Some studies have suggested targeting breastfeeding education programs for migrant women in Western countries (Chan-Yip & Kramer 1983; Young & Kaufman 1988; Rossiter 1994; Golin et al. 2003; Mistry et al. 2008). In a culture-specific education program to promote breastfeeding among Vietnamese women in Sydney,

Australia, Rossiter (1994) reported significant effects on knowledge, attitudes and initiation of breastfeeding, although the study had some design problems including using a convenience sample, questionnaires not being translated back into English and the researcher and interpreters being used as support people for breastfeeding problems experienced by women in the study. The study by Yelland and colleagues (2003) found higher rates of breastfeeding among Vietnamese women who had attended an antenatal model of care designed specifically for Vietnamese women. The model employs midwives, medical practitioners, a community development worker and interpreters and operates with a philosophy of continuity and an individualised approach to care. This may be a model which could be further explored.

21.5 Conclusion

We found significant differences in breastfeeding initiation between Turkish, Vietnamese and Australian women in this study. The hospital environment is one place where care providers have the opportunity to influence breastfeeding behaviour. Despite the hospital where the study was conducted being accredited as baby-friendly, 40 percent of Vietnamese women fed their baby formula in hospital. Future research should include well-designed randomised controlled trials to test interventions specifically aimed at increasing breastfeeding initiation among Vietnamese women.

In this study, a variety of strategies were used in an attempt to ensure validity and reliability. These included translation, followed by 'blind' back translation by qualified translators, consultation with bilingual interpreters and translators, piloting and re-piloting of questionnaires, and careful selection, training and support of bilingual interviewers. However, working with translated research instruments is complex; and despite extensive and careful translation and back translation, we cannot completely rule out the possibility that words such as those used as response alternatives may have slightly different meanings in the three languages and cultures (Liamputtong 2010). Although we used a rigorous translation process, it is possible that differences in the perception of words such as 'attachment', for example, related to subtle translation differences.

Our results suggest that the Turkish and Vietnamese women in this study were more representative of the general Victorian populations from these countries than the Australian sample. One explanation of these findings was the selection of only public patients into the study. During the recruitment period, 35 percent of Australian women who gave birth in Victoria were admitted for the birth as private patients compared with only 4 percent of Turkish and 8 percent of Vietnamese women (Victorian Perinatal Data Collection Unit 2000). It is likely that if private patients were included in the study, the disparity found between Australian women and Vietnamese women would have been greater, given the higher rate of breastfeeding among women from higher socio-economic groups (Amir & Donath 2008).

Acknowledgments We thank the women who participated in the study and the bicultural interviewers and translators: Aygul Dogangun, Tran Pham, Alev Gurlek, Dondu Guneydin and Tuong Tran. We also thank the funding bodies: The Royal Women's Hospital Division of Research and Education, the Australian College of Midwives Incorporated, La Trobe University Faculty of Health Sciences, and the Royal Women's Hospital Foundation. We are grateful to Professor Ulla Waldenström who initially conceived the study, and the Victorian Perinatal Data Collection Unit for provision of data.

The chapter incorporates material originally published in BMC International Breastfeeding Journal (McLachlan HL and Forster DA. Initial breastfeeding attitudes and practices of women born in Turkey, Vietnam and Australia after giving birth in Australia. *BMC International Breastfeed Journal.* 2006 Apr 7, 1, 7).

References

Ali, A. (1975). *The holy Quran*, 1st ed. Leicester: The Islamic Foundation.

Alikasifoglu, M., Erginoz, E., Gur, E., Baltas, Z., Beker, B., & Arvas, A. (2001). Factors influencing the duration of exclusive breastfeeding in a group of Turkish women. *Journal of Human Lactation, 17*(3), 220–226.

Almroth, S., Arts, M., Quang, N., Hoa, P., & Williams, C. (2008). Exclusive breastfeeding in Vietnam: An attainable goal. *Acta Pædiatrica, 97*(8), 1066–1069.

Amir, L. H., & Donath, S. M. (2008). Socioeconomic status and rates of breastfeeding in Australia: Evidence from three recent national health surveys. *Medical Journal of Australia, 189*(5), 254–256.

Camurdan, A. D., Ilhan, M. N., Beyazova, U., Sahin, F., Vatandas, N., & Eminoglu, S. (2008). How to achieve long-term breast-feeding: Factors associated with early discontinuation. *Public Health Nutrition, 11*(11), 1173–1179.

Chan-Yip, A., & Kramer, M. (1983). Promotion of breastfeeding in a Chinese community in Montreal. *Canadian Medical Association Journal, 129*, 955–958.

Committee for Population Family and Children (2003). *Vietnam Demographic and Health Survey 2002*. Hanoi: Committee for Population Family and Children.

Consultative Council on Obstetric and Paediatric Mortality and Morbidity (2008). *Births in Victoria 2005 and 2006*. Melbourne: Victorian Department of Human Services.

Duong, D., Lee, A., & Binns, C. (2005). Determinants of breastfeeding within the first 6 months post-partum in rural Vietnam. *Journal of Paediatrics and Child Health, 41*, 338–343.

Duong, D. V., Binns, C. W., & Lee, A. H. (2004). Breast-feeding initiation and exclusive breastfeeding in rural Vietnam. *Public Health Nutrition, 7*(06), 795–799.

Dyson, L., McCormick, F., & Renfrew, M. J. (2005). Interventions for promoting the initiation of breastfeeding. *Cochrane Database of Systematic Reviews* (2), CD001688.

Fishman, C., Evans, R., & Jenks, E. (1988). Warm bodies, cool milk: Conflicts in post partum food choice for Indo-Chinese women in California. *Social Science and Medicine, 26*(11), 1125–1132.

Gatrad, A. (1994). Attitudes and beliefs of Muslim mothers towards pregnancy and infancy. *Archives of Disease in Childhood, 71*, 170–174.

Gibson-Davis, C. M., & Brooks-Gunn, J. (2006). Couples' immigration status and ethnicity as determinants of breastfeeding. *American Journal of Public Health, 96*(4), 641–646.

Golin, R., Marzarib, F., & Zanardo, V. (2003). Incidence and correlates of breast-feeding practices in the non-European Community migrant women. *Nutrition Research, 23*(8), 983–990.

Groleau, D., Soulière, M., & Kirmayer, L. J. (2006). Breastfeeding and the cultural configuration of social space among Vietnamese immigrant woman. *Health & Place, 12*(4), 516–526.

Henderson, S., & Brown, J. (1987). Infant feeding practices of Vietnamese immigrants to the Northwest United States. *Scholarly Inquiry for Nursing Practice, 1*(2), 153–169.

Hizel, S., Ceyhun, G., Tanzer, F., & Sanli, C. (2006). Traditional beliefs as forgotten influencing factors on breast-feeding performance in Turkey. *Saudi Medical Journal, 27*(4), 511–518.

Hoang, H. (2008). Language and cultural barriers of Asian migrants in accessing maternal care in Australia. *The International Journal of Language Society and Culture, 26*, 55–61.

Jones, D. A., West, R. R., & Newcombe, R. G. (1986). Maternal characteristics associated with the duration of breast-feeding. *Midwifery*, 2, 141–146.

Karacam, Z. (2008). Factors affecting exclusive breastfeeding of healthy babies aged zero to four months: a community-based study of Turkish women. *Journal of Clinical Nursing, 17*(3), 341–349.

Kocturck, T., & Zetterstrom, R. (1986). Breastfeeding among Turkish mothers living in suburbs of Istanbul and Stockholm – a comparison. *Acta Pædiatrica, 75*(2), 216–221.

Lande, B., Andersen, L., Baerug, A., Trygg, K., Lund-Larsen, K., Veierod, M., et al. (2003). Infant feeding practices and associated factors in the first six months of life: The Norwegian Infant Nutrition Survey. *Acta Paediatrica*, 92, 152–161.

Liamputtong, P. (2007). On childrearing and infant care: A cross-cultural perspective. In P. Liamputtong (Ed.), *Childrearing and infant care issues: A cross-cultural perspective* (pp. 3–29). New York: Nova Science.

Liamputtong Rice, P. (1998). Culture and infant feeding practices among Southeast Asian mothers living in Melbourne. *Birth Issues Journal, 7*(1), 15–22.

Liamputtong Rice, P. (2000). *Hmong women and reproduction*. Westport: Bergin & Garvey.

Liamputtong, P. (2010). Performing cross-cultural research. Cambridge University Press. New York. 2010.

Liubai, L., Doan Thi Phuong, l., Nguyen-Thi, H., & Hiroshi, U. (2002). Prevalence of breastfeeding and its correlates in Ho Chi Minh City, Vietnam. *Pediatrics International, 44*(1), 47–54.

Manderson, L., & Mathews, M. (1981). Vietnamese attitudes towards maternal and infant health. *Medical Journal of Australia, 24*, 69–72.

Mathews, M., & Manderson, L. (1980). Infant feeding practices and lactation diets amongst Vietnamese immigrants. *Australian Paediatric Journal, 16*, 263–266.

McDermott, M., & Palchanes, K. (1994). A literature review of the critical elements of translation theory. *Journal of Nursing Scholarship, 26*(2), 113–117.

McLachlan, H., & Forster, D. (2006). Initial breastfeeding attitudes and practices of women born in Turkey, Vietnam and Australia after giving birth in Australia. *International Breastfeeding Journal*. 2006 doi: 10.1186/1746-4358-1-7.

McLachlan, H., & Waldenstrom, U. (2005). Experience of childbirth and labour pain of women born in Turkey, Vietnam and Australia on giving birth in Australia. *Birth, 32*(4), 272–282.

Mistry, Y., Freedman, M., Sweeney, K., & Hollenbeck, C. (2008). Infant-feeding practices of low-income Vietnamese American women. *Journal of Human Lactation, 24*(4), 406–414.

Morrow, M. (1996). Breastfeeding in Vietnam: Poverty, tradition, and economic transition. *Journal of Human Lactation, 12*(2), 97–103.

Morse, J., Jehle, C., & Gamble, D. (1990). Initiating breastfeeding: a world survey of the timing of postpartum breastfeeding. *International Journal of Nursing Studies, 27*(3), 303–313.

Neyzi, O., Olgun, P., Kutluay, T., Uzel, N., Saner, G., Gokcay, G., et al. (1991). An educational intervention on promotion of breastfeeding. *Paediatric and Perinatal Epidemiology, 5*, 286–298.

Nguyen, N., Allen, J., Peat, J., Schofield, W., Nossar, V., Eisenbruch, M., et al. (2004). Growth and feeding practices of Vietnamese infants in Australia. *European Journal of Clinical Nutrition, 58*, 356–362.

Nolan, L., & Goel, V. (1995). Sociodemographic factors related to breastfeeding in Ontario: Results from the Ontario Health Survey. *Canadian Journal of Public Health, 86*(5), 309–312.

Piper, S., & Parks, P.L. (1996). Predicting the duration of lactation: evidence from a national survey. *Birth, 23*(1), 7–12.

Rossiter, J. (1992a). Attitudes of Vietnamese women to baby feeding practices before and after immigration to Sydney, Australia. *Midwifery, 8*, 103–112.
Rossiter, J. (1992b). Maternal-infant health beliefs and the perception and experience of immigrant Vietnamese women in Sydney. *Contemporary Nurse, 1*(2), 75–81.
Rossiter, J. (1994). The effect of a culture specific education program to promote breastfeeding among Vietnamese women in Sydney. *International Journal of Nursing Studies, 31*(4), 369–379.
Rossiter, J., Ledwidge, H., & Coulon, L. (1993). IndoChinese women's breastfeeding practices following immigration to Sydney: A pilot study. *The Australian Journal of Advanced Nursing, 10*(3), 3–9.
Rossiter, J., & Yam, B. (2000). Breastfeeding: How could it be enhanced? The perceptions of Vietnamese women in Sydney, Australia. *Journal of Midwifery and Women's Health, 45*(3), 271–276.
Small, R., Yelland, J., Lumley, J., & Liamputtong Rice, P. (1999a). Cross-cultural research: Trying to do it better 1. Issues in study design. *Australian and New Zealand Journal of Public Health, 23*(4), 385–389.
Small, R., Yelland, J., Lumley, J., Liamputtong Rice, P., Cotronei, V., & Warren, R. (1999b). Cross-cultural research: Trying to do it better 2. Enhancing data quality. *Australian and New Zealand Journal of Public Health, 23*(4), 390–395.
SPSS Statistical Packages for the Social Sciences (1998). Statistical Packages for the Social Sciences (Version 9). Chicago.
Stata Corporation (2003). STATA statistical data analysis (Version 8). College Station: Stata Corporation.
Taveras, E., Capra, A., Braveman, P., Jensvold, N., Escobar, G., & Lieu, T. (2003). Clinician support and psychosocial risk factors associated with breastfeeding discontinuation. *Pediatrics, 112*(1), 108–115.
Tuttle, C., & Dewey, K. (1994). Determinants of infant feeding choices among Southeast Asian immigrants in Northern California. *Journal of the American Dietetic Association, 94*(3), 282–286.
UNICEF. Baby Friendly Hospital Initiative. Retrieved 14 August 2009, from http://www.unicef.org/nutrition/index_24806.html
UNICEF. Monitoring the situation of children and women. Retrieved 5 August 2009, from http://www.childinfo.org/breastfeeding_countrydata.php.
Victorian Perinatal Data Collection Unit (2000). *Unpublished report on Turkish, Vietnamese and Australian born women who gave birth in Victoria in 1998*. Melbourne: Victorian Department of Human Services, Victoria.
Wiles, L. (1984). The effect of prenatal breastfeeding education on breastfeeding success and maternal perception of the infant. *Journal of Gynaecological and Neonatal Nursing*, (July/August), 253–257.
World Health Organization. Global Data Bank on Breastfeeding. Retrieved 10 August, 2009, from http://apps.who.int/research/iycf/bfcf/
World Health Organization. (2001). *The optimal duration of exclusive breastfeeding. Results of a WHO systematic review*. Geneva: World Health Organization.
Yelland, J., Small, R., Lumley, J., & Liamputtong Rice, P. (1997). *Choice or constraint? Infant feeding amongst Vietnamese, Turkish and Filipino women.* Paper presented at the Nursing Mothers' Association of Australia International Conference Proceedings, Sydney.
Yelland, J., Small, R., Lumley, J., Liamputtong Rice, P., Contronei, V., & Warren, R. (1998). Support, sensitivity, satisfaction: Filipino, Turkish and Vietnamese women's experiences of postnatal hospital stay. *Midwifery, 14*, 144–154.
Yelland, J., Small, R., Krastev, A., & Brown, S. (2003). *Evaluating practice and the organisation of care at Southern Health and Sandringham Hospital: Report 2. Interviews with Vietnamese women*. Melbourne: Centre for the Study of Mothers' and Children's Health.

Yesildal, N., Aytar, G., Kocabay, K., Senih Mayda, A., Cetin Dagli, S., & Bahcebasi, T. (2008). Breastfeeding practices in Duzce, Turkey. *Journal of Human Lactation, 24*(4), 393–400.

Yilmaz, G., Gurakan, B., Akgun, S., & Ozbek, N. (2002). Factors influencing breastfeeding for working mothers. *The Turkish Journal of Paediatrics, 44*, 30–34.

Yoshida, M., & Davies, M. (1982). Parenting in a new culture: Experiences of East Indian, Portuguese, and Caribbean mothers. *Multiculturalism, 5*(3), 3–5.

Young, S., & Kaufman, M. (1988). Promoting breastfeeding at a migrant health centre. *American Journal of Public Health, 78*, 523–525.

Index

Note: The letters 'f' and 't' following the locators refer to figures and tables respectively.

P. Liamputtong (ed.), *Infant Feeding Practices*, DOI 10.1007/978-1-4419-6873-9,
© Springer Science+Business Media, LLC 2011

C

E

F

G

J

FSC
www.fsc.org
MIX
Papier | Fördert
gute Waldnutzung
FSC® C083411

Kolibri 360 GmbH
Ferdinand-Jühlke-Straße 7
99095 Erfurt, Deutschland
produktsicherheit@kolibri360.de